Precision Medicine in Neurodevelopmental Disorders: Personalized Characterization of Autism from Molecules to Behavior

Precision Medicine in Neurodevelopmental Disorders: Personalized Characterization of Autism from Molecules to Behavior

Editor

Elizabeth B. Torres

MDPI • Basel • Beijing • Wuhan • Barcelona • Belgrade • Manchester • Tokyo • Cluj • Tianjin

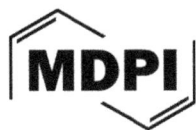

Editor
Elizabeth B. Torres
Rutgers The State University of New Jersey (New Brunswick Campus)
USA

Editorial Office
MDPI
St. Alban-Anlage 66
4052 Basel, Switzerland

This is a reprint of articles from the Special Issue published online in the open access journal *Journal of Personalized Medicine* (ISSN 2075-4426) (available at: https://www.mdpi.com/journal/jpm/special_issues/Molecules_Behavior).

For citation purposes, cite each article independently as indicated on the article page online and as indicated below:

LastName, A.A.; LastName, B.B.; LastName, C.C. Article Title. *Journal Name* **Year**, *Volume Number*, Page Range.

ISBN 978-3-0365-5127-2 (Hbk)
ISBN 978-3-0365-5128-9 (PDF)

© 2022 by the authors. Articles in this book are Open Access and distributed under the Creative Commons Attribution (CC BY) license, which allows users to download, copy and build upon published articles, as long as the author and publisher are properly credited, which ensures maximum dissemination and a wider impact of our publications.
The book as a whole is distributed by MDPI under the terms and conditions of the Creative Commons license CC BY-NC-ND.

Contents

About the Editor vii

Preface to "Precision Medicine in Neurodevelopmental Disorders: Personalized Characterization of Autism from Molecules to Behavior" ix

Elizabeth B. Torres
Special Issue "Precision Medicine in Neurodevelopmental Disorders: Personalized Characterization of Autism from Molecules to Behavior"
Reprinted from: *J. Pers. Med.* **2022**, *12*, 918, doi:10.3390/jpm12060918 1

Elizabeth B. Torres
Precision Autism: Genomic Stratification of Disorders Making Up the Broad Spectrum May Demystify Its "Epidemic Rates"
Reprinted from: *J. Pers. Med.* **2021**, *11*, 1119, doi:10.3390/jpm11111119 5

Jihye Ryu, Tami Bar-Shalita, Yelena Granovsky, Irit Weissman-Fogel and Elizabeth B. Torres
Personalized Biometrics of Physical Pain Agree with Psychophysics by Participants with Sensory over Responsivity
Reprinted from: *J. Pers. Med.* **2021**, *11*, 93, doi:10.3390/jpm11020093 31

Alina Demiy, Agata Kalemba, Maria Lorent, Anna Pecuch, Ewelina Wolańska, Marlena Telenga and Ewa Z. Gieysztor
A Child's Perception of Their Developmental Difficulties in Relation to Their Adult Assessment. Analysis of the INPP Questionnaire
Reprinted from: *J. Pers. Med.* **2020**, *10*, 156, doi:10.3390/jpm10040156 47

Elizabeth B. Torres
Reframing Psychiatry for Precision Medicine
Reprinted from: *J. Pers. Med.* **2020**, *10*, 144, doi:10.3390/jpm10040144 59

Peter Washington, Emilie Leblanc, Kaitlyn Dunlap, Yordan Penev, Aaron Kline, Kelley Paskov, Min Woo Sun, Brianna Chrisman, Nathaniel Stockham, Maya Varma, Catalin Voss, Nick Haber and Dennis P. Wall
Precision Telemedicine through Crowdsourced Machine Learning: Testing Variability of Crowd Workers for Video-Based Autism Feature Recognition
Reprinted from: *J. Pers. Med.* **2020**, *10*, 86, doi:10.3390/jpm10030086 85

Jihye Ryu and Elizabeth Torres
The Autonomic Nervous System Differentiates between Levels of Motor Intent and End Effector
Reprinted from: *J. Pers. Med.* **2020**, *10*, 76, doi:10.3390/jpm10030076 99

Nadire Cavus, Abdulmalik A. Lawan, Zurki Ibrahim, Abdullahi Dahiru, Sadiya Tahir, Usama Ishaq Abdulrazak and Adamu Hussaini
A Systematic Literature Review on the Application of Machine-Learning Models in Behavioral Assessment of Autism Spectrum Disorder
Reprinted from: *J. Pers. Med.* **2021**, *11*, 299, doi:10.3390/jpm11040299 125

Cristina Panisi, Franca Rosa Guerini, Provvidenza Maria Abruzzo, Federico Balzola, Pier Mario Biava, Alessandra Bolotta, Marco Brunero, Ernesto Burgio, Alberto Chiara, Mario Clerici, Luigi Croce, Carla Ferreri, Niccolò Giovannini, Alessandro Ghezzo, Enzo Grossi, Roberto Keller, Andrea Manzotti, Marina Marini, Lucia Migliore, Lucio Moderato, Davide Moscone, Michele Mussap, Antonia Parmeggiani, Valentina Pasin, Monica Perotti, Cristina Piras, Marina Saresella, Andrea Stoccoro, Tiziana Toso, Rosa Anna Vacca, David Vagni, Salvatore Vendemmia, Laura Villa, Pierluigi Politi and Vassilios Fanos
Autism Spectrum Disorder from the Womb to Adulthood: Suggestions for a Paradigm Shift
Reprinted from: *J. Pers. Med.* **2021**, *11*, 70, doi:10.3390/jpm11020070 . . . . **141**

About the Editor

Elizabeth B. Torres

Elizabeth B. Torres, PhD is a tenured Full Professor at Rutgers, the State University of New Jersey. She holds joint appointments at the Psychology Department, the Center for Biomedicine Imaging and Modeling (CBIM) of the Computer Science Department and the Rutgers University Center for Cognitive Science (RUCCS). She is also Graduate Faculty at the Rutgers Biomedical Engineering Department and at the Neuroscience and Cell Biology program. Torres has pioneered several analytical platforms to integrate data from disparate levels of inquiry in autism aimed at advancing diagnostics and treatments of autism subtypes. As an educator, she has graduated multiple students and sent them to high profile universities, medical schools, and industry jobs. As a translational-science researcher, she directs the Sensory Motor Integration Laboratory of Rutgers University, located at the Busch campus. As a public servant, she is the Executive and Scientific Director of the New Jersey Autism Center of Excellence from 2018–2023, a unique innovative center initiative of the New Jersey Governor's office that integrates scientists, educators, and service providers with the autistic community, to address the critical needs identified by the families and self-advocates of the autism spectrum. Her research spans over 100 peer-reviewed publications, multiple peer-reviewed books, and multiple patents in use by industry. Her work as a scientist and as a public servant has been praised by the autistic community not only for reflecting their needs and wants, but more importantly for respecting their agency and promoting their dignity. In 2021, Torres received a joint legislative resolution from the New Jersey Senate and the assembly in honor of her meritorious records of service, leadership, and commitment to transform autism research, education, and treatments.

Preface to "Precision Medicine in Neurodevelopmental Disorders: Personalized Characterization of Autism from Molecules to Behavior"

The precision medicine (PM) platform has emerged as a powerful model for the development of personalized targeted treatments in cancer research. It may be advantageous to adapt this model to psychiatric and psychological disorders that are now defined within the realm of mental illness and without reference to their underlying neurology.

Among such disorders are autism, currently defined through observation and description of behaviors, with an emphasis on social inappropriateness. One of the barriers to translating the PM model to autism has been the subjective nature of its current definition of behaviors. The current criteria (problems with social communication and repetitive ritualistic behaviors), defined by observation, have led to a highly heterogeneous phenomenology. There is now a consensus that there may be different autism subtypes. However, in view of such heterogeneity, it has proven difficult to advance basic scientific research to develop personalized targeted treatments tailored to each person within a subphenotypic group.

The present book brings together diverse perspectives from different subfields of autism research, treatments, and services across the world. The authors' contributions help redefine the layers of behaviors of the PM model by leveraging the wearable sensors, neuroscience, and genomic revolutions while considering the neurological underpinnings of currently defined autistic behaviors. The work examines such issues as they evolve from the womb through infancy and beyond, throughout a person's lifespan, and across different layers of the PM knowledge network. By redefining autism as a problem at the crosstalk of nervous and immune systems' development and by pairing new telemedicine approaches with objective criteria derived from biosensors' physical data, we see how autism can be stratified into different subtypes according to the genomics, which determine the structure and function of the nervous and immune systems. This approach leverages ontogenetic and phylogenetic orders of maturation that neurobiology already defines, spanning from molecules to complex social interactions, to bring a paradigm shift to autism diagnostics, research, and treatment.

We are most grateful to the autistic individuals and their families who participated in the presented work. We thank the governmental funding bodies and private foundations who generously funded the presented work.

Elizabeth B. Torres
Editor

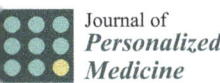

Editorial

Special Issue "Precision Medicine in Neurodevelopmental Disorders: Personalized Characterization of Autism from Molecules to Behavior"

Elizabeth B. Torres [1,2,3]

1. Department of Psychology, Rutgers the State University of New Jersey, Piscataway, NJ 08854, USA; ebtorres@psych.rutgers.edu
2. Center for Biomedicine Imaging and Modeling, Computer Science Department, Rutgers University, Piscataway, NJ 08854, USA
3. Center for Cognitive Science, Rutgers University, Piscataway, NJ 08854, USA

The Precision Medicine (PM) platform [1] has emerged as an important transformative model to help advance personalized medicine and transform translational research and clinical practices. In PM, multiple layers of the knowledge network are interconnected (Figure 1) to integrate the patient's clinical information derived from a multitude of tests, with different levels of objectivity and subjectivity, into targeted treatments that rely on specific signatures of the patient's health, in relation to population signatures.

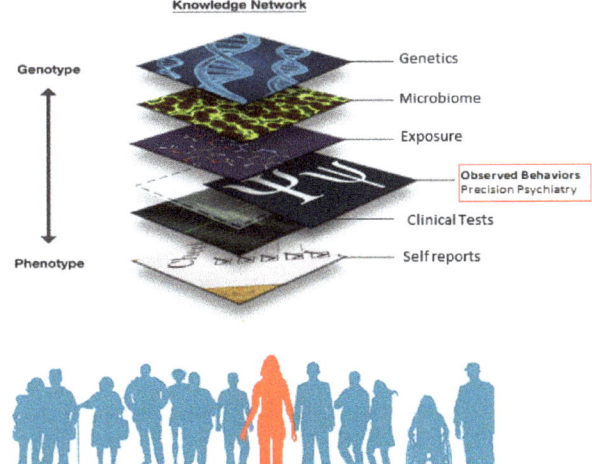

Figure 1. The Precision Medicine platform applied to the fields of Psychiatry and Psychology, can integrate information from several layers of the knowledge network, to help develop targeted behavioral and genomic personalized treatments to improve mental health. The layer of observed behaviors can now be digitized thanks to the wearable sensors revolution and integrated with clinical criteria and self-reports, to provide interpretable digital biomarkers for Precision Psychiatry (Figure courtesy of Dr. C.P. Whyatt and the Rutgers University Sensory Motor Integration lab).

The present Special Issue, entitled "Precision Medicine in Neurodevelopmental Disorders: Personalized Characterization of Autism from Molecules to Behavior", brings together researchers from multiple disciplines to address research at various layers of the

Citation: Torres, E.B. Special Issue "Precision Medicine in Neurodevelopmental Disorders: Personalized Characterization of Autism from Molecules to Behavior". *J. Pers. Med.* **2022**, *12*, 918. https://doi.org/10.3390/jpm12060918

Received: 18 May 2022
Accepted: 23 May 2022
Published: 1 June 2022

Publisher's Note: MDPI stays neutral with regard to jurisdictional claims in published maps and institutional affiliations.

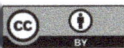

Copyright: © 2022 by the author. Licensee MDPI, Basel, Switzerland. This article is an open access article distributed under the terms and conditions of the Creative Commons Attribution (CC BY) license (https://creativecommons.org/licenses/by/4.0/).

knowledge network and offer contemporary solutions to the implementation of some of the current research in autism and other neurodevelopmental disorders.

Cristina Panisi, et al. [2] discussed "Autism Spectrum Disorder from the Womb to Adulthood: Suggestions for a Paradigm Shift", offering new avenues of inquiry and integration of research across different stages of neurodevelopment. In their manuscript, the authors highlight the need to move towards a more fluid, dynamic conception of autism, one that integrates genetics, environment, and epigenetics in a holistic manner, taking into consideration individual systemic variations, rather than doing so linearly and in a piecemeal fashion. They discuss the embryo–fetal period and the first two years of life (so-called 'First 1000 Days'), as a critical window to detect differences at its earliest point and intervene accordingly. The work invites possible interventions while considering immune activation, gut dysbiosis, and mitochondrial impairment/oxidative stress affecting neurodevelopment during pregnancy and undermining the health of autistic individuals throughout life. The review argues for intervention at the molecular levels during early embryonic stages of neural development, as a path forward that is now realizable thanks to recent advances in omics. A comprehensive and exhaustive pathogenic research approach to autism is advanced in this paper, as an actionable medical resource that can go beyond theoretical ideas, into practical implementation. This work offers a bird's view of this lifelong condition while integrating these multiple layers of knowledge, while the papers below address relevant issues at each one of the individual layers of the knowledge network.

At the important level of patient's self-reports and observational behavioral inventories, encompassing the perception of autistic individuals by others, we find the manuscript by Demiy, et al. [3], entitled "A Child's Perception of Their Developmental Difficulties in Relation to Their Adult Assessment: Analysis of the INPP Questionnaire". In this paper, the authors compare the perception of teachers, parents, and clinicians to those of the child, using clinical questionnaires from the Institute for Neuro-Psychological Psychology (INPP). The questions focus primarily on psychomotor problems related to balance, motor coordination and concentration, as well as school skills. The work reports that children self-perceived these issues significantly stronger than their parents did, and educators and therapists differed from the parents' opinion, particularly in matters related to attention and concentration. The results highlight the important amount of information that escapes the naked eye of the observer. They underscore the need to consider the internal states of the autistic person, as expressed by the autistic individuals. The study concludes that "Children perceive their difficulties much more seriously than adults." and suggests that "Talking and the support of adults can make it easier for a child to overcome developmental difficulties."

Insights into automated behavioral assessments at the intersection of clinical reports and the layer of behaviors are offered by Cavus, et al. [4], in their paper, entitled "A Systematic Literature Review on the Application of Machine-Learning Models in Behavioral Assessment of Autism Spectrum Disorder". The authors address the critical need for computationally driven assessments in an exponentially growing ASD phenomenon that requires, but lacks, trained diagnosticians with high scoring reliability. Despite good evaluation metrics achieved by the ML models, there remains scarce evidence on their readiness for clinical implementation. The review highlights numerous challenges associated with data-centric techniques and their misalignment with the conceptual basis upon which professionals diagnose ASD. Their systematic review proposes vital considerations for real-life implementation of ML-based ASD screening and diagnostic systems that other authors in the Special Issue take on.

The work by Washington, et al. [5], entitled "Precision Telemedicine through Crowdsourced Machine Learning: Testing Variability of Crowd Workers for Video-Based Autism Feature Recognition", provides a clear example of implementation of ML methods and innovative approaches to diagnosing ASD. The results from their work demonstrate that while the crowd can produce accurate diagnoses, there are intrinsic differences in crowd-worker ability to rate behavioral features. The authors propose a novel strategy for the recruitment of crowdsourced workers, to ensure high-quality diagnostic evaluations of autism, and potentially many other pediatric behavioral health conditions. This work represents a viable step in the direction of crowd-based approaches for more scalable and affordable precision medicine.

Moving along to the layer of behavioral analyses, Ryu, et al. [6] offer new methods to assess pain in their paper, entitled "Personalized Biometrics of Physical Pain Agree with Psychophysics by Participants with Sensory over Responsivity". This work underscores the importance of combining digital data from biosensors with clinical inventories, to produce clinically interpretable digital biomarkers of pain. Using EEG activity and new analytical methods, the researchers from a multitude of fields collaboratively joined efforts with clinicians to study sensory issues commonly found in autism. The group characterizes pain by standardizing the moment-by-moment fluctuations in biophysical signals derived from EEG brain activity. These signals from the central nervous systems (CNS) reflect the person's experience of temperature-based stimulation at the periphery. A type of gross data that is often disregarded as noise by traditional analytic methods, here, precisely characterizes the lingering sensation of discomfort raising to the level of pain, individually, for each participant. The work shows fundamental differences between the SOR group in relation to controls and provides an objective account of pain that is congruent with the subjective self-reported data. This integrative approach offers the potential to build a standardized scale useful to profile pain levels in a personalized manner across the general population.

Within the layer of behavioral assessments, another paper by Ryu and Torres [7], entitled "The Autonomic Nervous System Differentiates between Levels of Motor Intent and End Effector", examines differences in volitional control that are capturable in personalized form, through the person's fluctuations in heart-rate variability. The work alludes to the potential to bridging motor control and cognitive science by tracking peripheral activity as reafferent input that is convolved with micro-motor (kinesthetic) reafference, harnessed from continuous streams of interleaved intentional and spontaneous movements. Using new analytics that do not discard the so-called "gross data" as noise, the authors find that when the action is intended, the heart signal from the Autonomic Nervous Systems (ANS) leads the body kinematics signals. In stark contrast, when the action segment spontaneously occurs without instructions, the heart signal lags the bodily kinematics signals. They conclude that the ANS can differentiate levels of intent, a result that has translational value, and actionable scalability, given the ubiquitous presence of commercially available, off-the-shelf wearable biosensors embedded in smart watches and phones. These biosensors reliably register heart-rate variability in natural situations, as the person, e.g., wears a smart watch and checks the outputs in an app. In this sense, using such signals combined with the analytics reported in the methods, it becomes feasible to study and infer moment-by-moment cognitive states from motor and autonomic data streams.

Finally, a path forward integrating these disparate layers of knowledge is offered by Torres in their paper, entitled "Reframing Psychiatry for Precision Medicine" [8], with a direct application to autism in a paper, entitled "Precision Autism: Genomic Stratification of Disorders Making Up the Broad Spectrum May Demystify Its Epidemic Rates" [9]. These two papers lay out a possible way to help cope with the heterogeneous nature of developmental disorders on a spectrum by leveraging the genomics revolution and automatically stratifying the disorder into subgroups with common genetic pools, according to genes' expressions on fundamental tissues underlying all social behaviors that define the disorders in the first place. Combining digitized behaviors (naturally and unobtrusively attainable during clinical tests), with observational data informed by clinical criteria, and integrating genomic information, will help treat such disorders in autism by leveraging advances from different fields. This approach could significantly help improve a person's quality of life and redirect resources differently towards fields that offer real solutions for everyday independent living. Further advancing research questions in autism informed by the person's self-reports on internal states is also possible under a new statistical platform that harnesses individual variations present in the continuous stream of data that we collect at each of these layers of the knowledge network in Figure 1. From variations in genes' expression to variations in genes' network interactions, to variations in fluctuations of biophysical rhythms registered from the CNS, the PNS and the ANS, we can help integrate these disparate layers of information under a common computational framework that does not throw away data and relies on a systemic approach, integrating information from the human body and brain, as they dynamically change over time.

This Special Issue provides an example of interdisciplinary collaboration occurring today at multiple levels of inquiry across complex, nonlinear dynamics, and the stochastic variations that continuous streams of data offer to contemporary medicine. A new unifying model that helps us integrate such information and track it over time has already made its presence visible in our labs, clinics, and homes. Indeed, we are at an inflection point in medicine [1], poised for a clinical revolution that has leveraged neuroscience, genomics, and the wearable biosensor revolution of the last decade. Personalized Medicine has already arrived.

Funding: This research was funded by the New Jersey Governor's Council for Autism grant number CAUT18ACE. The APC was funded by CAUT18ACE.

Conflicts of Interest: The authors declare no conflict of interest.

References

1. Hawgood, S.; Hook-Barnard, I.G.; O'Brien, T.C.; Yamamoto, K.R. Precision medicine: Beyond the inflection point. *Sci. Transl. Med.* **2015**, *7*, 300ps17. [CrossRef]
2. Panisi, C.; Guerini, F.R.; Abruzzo, P.M.; Balzola, F.; Biava, P.M.; Bolotta, A.; Brunero, M.; Burgio, E.; Chiara, A.; Clerici, M.; et al. Autism Spectrum Disorder from the Womb to Adulthood: Suggestions for a Paradigm Shift. *J. Pers. Med.* **2021**, *11*, 70. [CrossRef] [PubMed]
3. Demiy, A.; Kalemba, A.; Lorent, M.; Pecuch, A.; Wolańska, E.; Telenga, M.; Gieysztor, E.Z. A Child's Perception of Their Developmental Difficulties in Relation to Their Adult Assessment. Analysis of the INPP Questionnaire. *J. Pers. Med.* **2020**, *10*, 156. [CrossRef] [PubMed]
4. Cavus, N.; Lawan, A.; Ibrahim, Z.; Dahiru, A.; Tahir, S.; Abdulrazak, U.; Hussaini, A. A Systematic Literature Review on the Application of Machine-Learning Models in Behavioral Assessment of Autism Spectrum Disorder. *J. Pers. Med.* **2021**, *11*, 299. [CrossRef] [PubMed]
5. Washington, P.; Leblanc, E.; Dunlap, K.; Penev, Y.; Kline, A.; Paskov, K.; Sun, M.; Chrisman, B.; Stockham, N.; Varma, M.; et al. Precision Telemedicine through Crowdsourced Machine Learning: Testing Variability of Crowd Workers for Video-Based Autism Feature Recognition. *J. Pers. Med.* **2020**, *10*, 86. [CrossRef] [PubMed]
6. Ryu, J.; Bar-Shalita, T.; Granovsky, Y.; Weissman-Fogel, I.; Torres, E. Personalized Biometrics of Physical Pain Agree with Psychophysics by Participants with Sensory over Responsivity. *J. Pers. Med.* **2021**, *11*, 93. [CrossRef] [PubMed]
7. Ryu, J.; Torres, E. The Autonomic Nervous System Differentiates between Levels of Motor Intent and End Effector. *J. Pers. Med.* **2020**, *10*, 76. [CrossRef] [PubMed]
8. Torres, E. Reframing Psychiatry for Precision Medicine. *J. Pers. Med.* **2020**, *10*, 144. [CrossRef] [PubMed]
9. Torres, E.B. Precision Autism: Genomic Stratification of Disorders Making Up the Broad Spectrum May Demystify Its "Epidemic Rates". *J. Pers. Med.* **2021**, *11*, 1119. [CrossRef] [PubMed]

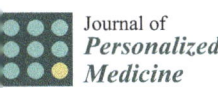

Article

Precision Autism: Genomic Stratification of Disorders Making Up the Broad Spectrum May Demystify Its "Epidemic Rates"

Elizabeth B. Torres [1,2,3]

1. Psychology Department, Rutgers the State University of New Jersey, Piscataway, NJ 08854, USA; ebtorres@psych.rutgers.edu; Tel.: +1-848-445-8909
2. Center for Biomedicine Imaging and Modeling, Computer Science Department, Rutgers University, Piscataway, NJ 08854, USA
3. Center for Cognitive Science, Rutgers University, Piscataway, NJ 08854, USA

Abstract: In the last decade, Autism has broadened and often shifted its diagnostics criteria, allowing several neuropsychiatric and neurological disorders of known etiology. This has resulted in a highly heterogeneous spectrum with apparent exponential rates in prevalence. I ask if it is possible to leverage existing genetic information about those disorders making up Autism today and use it to stratify this spectrum. To that end, I combine genes linked to Autism in the SFARI database and genomic information from the DisGeNET portal on 25 diseases, inclusive of non-neurological ones. I use the GTEx data on genes' expression on 54 human tissues and ask if there are overlapping genes across those associated to these diseases and those from SFARI-Autism. I find a compact set of genes across all brain-disorders which express highly in tissues fundamental for somatic-sensory-motor function, self-regulation, memory, and cognition. Then, I offer a new stratification that provides a distance-based orderly clustering into possible Autism subtypes, amenable to design personalized targeted therapies within the framework of Precision Medicine. I conclude that viewing Autism through this physiological (Precision) lens, rather than viewing it exclusively from a psychological behavioral construct, may make it a more manageable condition and dispel the Autism epidemic myth.

Keywords: Autism; genes; tissues; stratification; neurodevelopment; neurological disorders; neuropsychiatric disorders

1. Introduction

According to the CDC, in the span of 16 years, the US moved from 6.7/1000 to 18.5/1000 autistics in the population of school age children [1]. Reportedly, this increase continues to move along an exponential rate, while maintaining a near 5:1 males-to-females ratio [2,3]. This ratio prevents researchers from spontaneously reaching statistical power in any random draw of the population, when attempting to characterize the autistic female phenotype. Yet, motor features derived from endogenous neural signals in motor patterns, do identify the female phenotype [4–7]. This is the case even when digitizing the current clinical criteria that would otherwise miss females because of exclusive reliance on external observation [8,9]. Likewise, subtle cultural biases built into the social-appropriateness criteria of the current instruments skew identification of underserved populations [1]. Consequentially, current interventions are far from being inclusive, or advocating for neurodiversity in the clinical data driving best-practices and evidence-based criteria for treatment recommendation [10,11].

Despite sparse sampling in certain sectors of society, the shifts in diagnostic criteria have significantly broadened the detection rates to include now children with sensory issues and to allow comorbidity with ADHD under the Diagnostic Statistical Manual (DSM-5) [11]. This inclusion of ADHD in ASD contrasts with the former DSM-IV criteria, which would not allow comorbidities of ASD and ADHD, nor would it recognize sensory issues in Autism.

The challenges that broadening the diagnostics criteria bring to the science and practices of Autism are manifold [12], albeit some clinicians are discouraged from trying to stratify the spectrum into subtypes [13,14]. Under current standards, motor, kinesthetic sensing, and vestibular issues are not part of the core symptoms of the original diagnosis in the DSM. These criteria also remain absent from psychological instruments like the ADOS test, currently used to diagnose different age groups [10,15,16]. However, kinesthetic sensing and motor/vestibular issues define several of the many disorders that today received the Autism diagnosis [17]. Among them are Cerebral Palsy [18,19], Dystonia [20,21], Tourette's Syndrome [22] and obsessive-compulsive disorders (OCD) thought to be related to ADHD [23]. Besides these neurological disorders in ASD [24], others of known genetic origins enter in the broad criteria for Autism. Among them, various types of Ataxias [25] and Fragile X [26,27] make up for a large percentage of individuals with Autism today. Despite profound physiological, systemic alterations and somatic-sensory-motor differences, these individuals will very likely go on to receive blanket-style behavioral modification-treatments-for-all, during early interventions. Furthermore, these behavioral modification interventions in the US, will continue later at the school, through the individualized education plan. Such treatments neither recognize, nor address individual phenotypic physiological features of these disorders of known genetic origins that, nevertheless, do enter in the Autism spectrum today.

Phenotypically, these disorders that currently also go on to receive the Autism diagnosis, are precisely defined by somatic, sensory-motor issues [28,29] that manifest throughout the lifespan [30]. Their definition in their fields of origin, is nevertheless at odds with the current clinical "gold standard" criteria. In the DSM-5 [11] we read *"Hyper- or hypoactivity to sensory input or unusual interests in sensory aspects of the environment (e.g., apparent indifference to pain/temperature, adverse response to specific sounds or textures, excessive smelling or touching of objects, visual fascination with lights or movement)."* And in the DSM-5 criteria, motor issues are excluded owing to the confounds of symptoms induced by psychotropic medication, *"Medication-induced movement disorders are included in Section II because of their frequent importance in (1) the management by medication of mental disorders or other medical conditions and (2) the differential diagnosis of mental disorders (e.g., anxiety disorder versus neuroleptic-induced akathisia; malignant catatonia versus neuroleptic malignant syndrome). Although these movement disorders are labeled 'medication induced', it is often difficult to establish the causal relationship between medication exposure and the development of the movement disorder, especially because some of these movement disorders also occur in the absence of medication exposure. The conditions and problems listed in this chapter are not mental disorders."* This neglecting of motor issues is enforced despite scientific evidence that even without medication, there are profound motor issues in Autism [5] that intensify with aging [30].

Further sidelining sensory-motor issues in Autism, within the ADOS booklet [10], under the guidelines for selecting a module, we read *"Note that the ADOS-2 was developed for and standardized using populations of children and adults without significant sensory and motor impairments. Standardized use of any ADOS-2 module presumes that the individual can walk independently and is free of visual or hearing impairments that could potentially interfere with use of the materials or participation in specific tasks"*.

Despite these caveats explicitly stated on their manuals, children with profound and highly visible motor, kinesthetic sensing and vestibular issues [17] go on to receive the Autism diagnosis that places them on a behavioral modification therapeutic pipeline that does not consider the brain-body physiology [31]. Clearly, there is a contradiction between the somatic-sensory-motor medical-physiological criteria and the social-appropriateness behavioral-psychological criteria explicitly denying the former. Which one is it? And why are these important medical-physiological factors deemed secondary or co-morbid, when they are at the core of the basic building blocks necessary to develop and maintain social behaviors?

To better understand this tension between psychological criteria (dominating Autism research, diagnostics, therapies, and services) and medical-physiological issues reported by peer-reviewed science [32], I here examine the genes linked to these neurological and neuropsychiatric disorders making up a large portion of the autistic population today and manifesting profound somatic and sensory-motor differences.

I investigate the pool of genes linked to a purely behavioral diagnosis of Autism attained through instruments that precisely sideline the somatic sensory-motor physiology (i.e., the ADOS/DSM-5). Specifically, the ADOS-2 research criteria inform the studies that support the confidence scores of the Autism-linked genes hosted by the Simons Foundation Research Initiative (SFARI). I leverage this research-based data repository of Autism-linked genes and use it as reference to compare its gene pool to the genes from other sources identifying neurological and neuropsychiatric disorders making up the Autism spectrum today. Given that those other disorders of known genetic origin are visibly affected by somatic-sensory-motor differences, but also receive the Autism diagnosis, I here ask if the gene pool of those disorders could help us stratify the broad spectrum of Autism into subtypes.

Stratifying the broad spectrum of autism based on available genetic information, would help us advance at least two areas of intervention. At the non-drug intervention level, if we were to learn that a subtype of autism shares phenotypic characteristics with another disorder of the nervous system, we could repurpose treatments and accommodations working well in that other disorder and import them, adapting them to the autism subtype. In autism, we have a blanket treatment for all that is not working for many. This heterogeneous disorder with such homogeneous behavioral intervention has proven a poor model to aid neurodevelopment and is in fact stunting it. At the drug intervention level, we face a similar problem as we do with non-drug interventions. The broad heterogeneity that the current diagnostic criteria produce impedes tailoring interventions appropriately to the responsive features of the person's nervous system. Subtyping autism into different categories, each one with similar genomic make up, could help us repurpose drug research in a more targeted manner (as explained in Figure 1). For example, if we were to target genes responsive to certain compounds and those compounds were to alleviate symptoms of a physiological ailment, then knowing that those responsive genes are present in both a subtype of autism and another disorder (e.g., ataxia) for which such compounds may have started research, we could leverage that research, bring it to autism, and advance drug discovery for a particular cluster sharing genes responsive to the compound. It is the same humankind, the human brain and body share fundamental similarities across the human population, whether one has an autism label or not. Why not repurpose the scientific advances led by physiology and medicine in other fields, instead of being informed and guided exclusively by rather subjective psychological criteria [32]?

I find that we can indeed automatically and categorically stratify Autism through the gene pool of neurological and neuropsychiatric disorders that make up its broad spectrum today. I discuss our results in the context of the Precision Medicine (PM) model (Figure 1A) aimed at the development of personalized targeted treatments that integrate several layers of the knowledge network [33]. Under this PM platform I can better situate the person on the landscape of existing disorders for which there are more effective treatments than those currently offered in Autism. Based on this genomic stratification of Autism, I here propose a paradigm shift whereby the pipeline of diagnosis-to-treatment is based on the known physiology of these disorders (Figure 1B), addressing specific capabilities, predispositions and needs of each neurological phenotype. This new line of scientific inquiry not only leverages existing genomic information but more importantly, it responds to the quest of the autistic community to improve the prognosis and the future lives of those who receive this diagnosis.

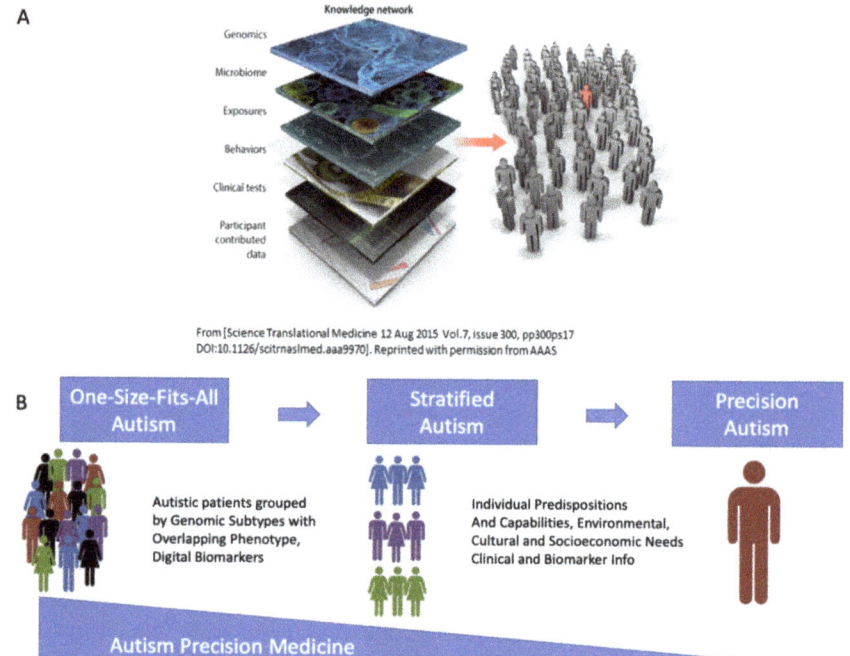

Figure 1. Leveraging existing genomic data to stratify the broad Autism Spectrum. (**A**) Reprinted with permission from AAAS Science Translational Medicine 12 August 2015 Vol. 7, Issue 300, pp300ps17 [33], Copyright AAAS 2015. The Precision Medicine model aims at the design of personalized targeted treatments that integrate all layers of the knowledge network to support the person's needs under the genetic and epigenetic individual makeup. (**B**) Proposed model to stratify the broad spectrum of Autism based on existing genomic information causally defining the origins of neurological and neuropsychiatric disorders making up Autism today. This Precision Autism model can identify, relative to other disorders of known origin, the person's best predispositions and capabilities, the environmental, cultural, and socio-economic needs, and design a personalized treatment that targets the medical-physiological issues rather than modifying behavior to conform to a grand average norm -a norm arbitrarily defined by current clinical criteria.

2. Materials and Methods

I examine the genetic data base from the Simons Foundation Research Initiative (SFARI), which has been scored according to the evidence provided in the scientific literature linking the behavioral Autism diagnosis with a pool of genes. I then extract from that set those genes that overlap with the pool of genes linked to other disorders that are fundamentally defined by somatic-sensory-motor issues. Among them I use the genes associated with cerebral palsy (CP), Dystonia, Attention Deficit Hyperactivity Disorder (ADHD), obsessive compulsive disorder (OCD), Tourette's, the Ataxias (autosomal dominant, recessive and X-linked) and Fragile X (FX). I also use the genes associated with Parkinson's disease (PD) [34,35], as symptoms of Parkinsonism abound in autistic adults after 40 years of age [30,36].

While the SFARI genes circularly depend on the ADOS and the DSM behavioral Autism criteria (i.e., they were obtained precisely based on those clinical inventories describing presumed socially inappropriate behaviors), the latter genes come from the disease-association network (the DisGeNET portal) which did not rely on an Autism diagnosis. These individuals are likely to receive an Autism diagnosis at present, because of the shifts and broadening of the criteria [23,24,37–41]. However, they have their own clinical definition and known genetic origins [19,42].

In Autism research, when the person has both diagnoses (ASD and a neurological or neuropsychiatric one) the former is coined idiopathic Autism, whereas the latter are called Autism of known etiology. Yet in a random draw of the population, we have identified clusters differentiating subtypes by relying on gait [6,17], voluntary reaches [4,28,43,44] and involuntary head motions [5,7,30,45,46].

I blindly took these genes associated to other disorders of the nervous system (clinically and physiologically defined) and interrogated them in terms of their expression on brain and bodily tissues. I asked how much overlapping one would find (if any) with the SFARI Autism-linked genes (coined hereafter SFARI-Autism) defined by observation and descriptions of behaviors.

Upon this compilation of genes from several sources in the DisGeNET portal and the literature, I used the Genotype-Tissue Expression (GTEx) project involving human RNA-seq, expressed in Transcripts Count Per Million (TCM) to examine the genes' expression across the 54 tissues sampled in their database [47] (Figure 2A). Using this atlas of genetic regulatory effects across human tissues, I compare across diseases, for those genes overlapping with the SFARI Autism-linked genes, the common tissues where the expression of these genes is maximal. To zoom into these overlapping genes expressed on tissues from the GTEx project (Figure 2A), I included the 11 distinct brain regions along with other 7 tissues representative of three fundamental muscle types: cardiac, smooth, and skeletal (Figure 2B), supporting the generation and maintenance of all physiological processes underlying all human functions and behaviors. Specifically, brain tissues included: the amygdala, the anterior cingulate cortex, the basal ganglia (caudate, putamen, nucleus accumbens), the brain cortex and the brain frontal cortex, the cerebellum and the cerebellar hemisphere, the hippocampus, the hypothalamus, and the substantia nigra.

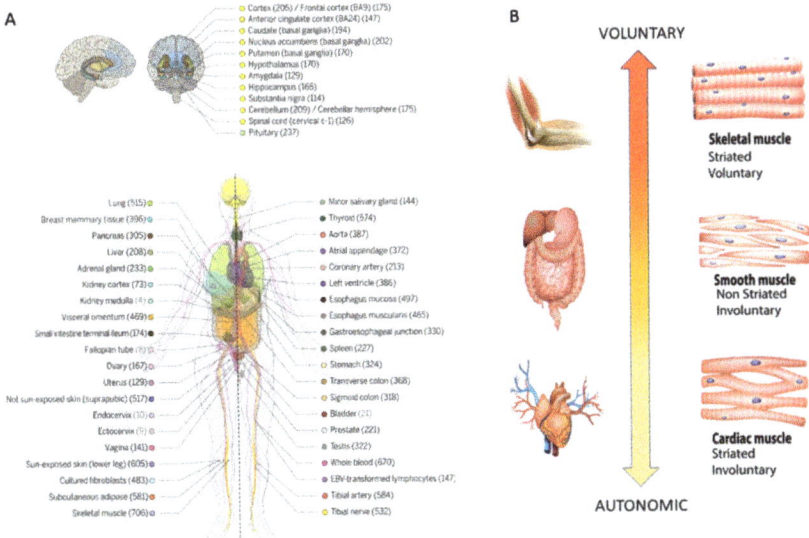

Figure 2. Genomic and Physiological criteria used in this study. (**A**) GTEx v8 study atlas of 54 tissues including 11 distinct brain regions and two cell lines. Genotyped sample donors' numbers in parenthesis and color coding to indicate the tissue in the adjacent circles (Reprinted with permission from AAAS Science 2020, 369, pp 1318–1330, Copyright AAAS 2020 [47]). (**B**) Three fundamental types of muscles supporting autonomic, involuntary and voluntary actions in humans can help us categorize behavioral functional levels according to related tissues affected [25].

Representative tissues of the different muscle types are: (cardiac) the heart left ventricle and the heart atrial appendage, (smooth) the esophagus muscularis and the bladder, (skeletal) skeletal muscle. Given their foundational role in all behavioral functions, I also examined these genes' expression on the tibial nerve and the spinal cord (Figure 2A).

The SFARI Autism categories that I used to determine the level of confidence that the gene is linked to Autism, were those reported as of 03-04-2020. Quoting from their site:

- CATEGORY 1

Genes in this category are all found on the SPARK gene list. Each of these genes has been clearly implicated in Autism Spectrum Disorders, ASD—typically by the presence of at least three de novo likely-gene-disrupting mutations being reported in the literature—and such mutations identified in the sequencing of the SPARK cohort are typically returned to the participants. Some of these genes meet the most rigorous threshold of genome-wide significance; all at least meet a threshold false discovery rate of <0.1.

- CATEGORY 2

Genes with two reported de novo likely-gene-disrupting mutations.

A gene uniquely implicated by a genome-wide association study, either reaching genome-wide significance or, if not, consistently replicated and accompanied by evidence that the risk variant has a functional effect.

- CATEGORY 3

Genes with a single reported de novo likely-gene-disrupting mutation.

Evidence from a significant but unreplicated association study, or a series of rare inherited mutations for which there is not a rigorous statistical comparison with controls.

- SYNDROMIC (former category 4)

The syndromic category includes mutations that are associated with a substantial degree of increased risk and consistently linked to additional characteristics not required for an ASD diagnosis. If there is independent evidence implicating a gene in idiopathic ASD, it will be listed as "#S" (e.g., 2S, 3S). If there is no such independent evidence, the gene will be listed simply as "S".

The GTEx dataset is as the 06-05-2017 v8 release [47]. For every gene in the disorders and diseases of interest, I first confirmed the presence of the gene in the GTEx dataset and then incorporated it into the analyses. This was necessary to provide the tissue expression from GTEx.

The genes from the DisGeNET portal were found by interrogation of their dataset under disease type and saving the outcome to excel files containing all pertinent information.

I follow our previously proposed roadmap to adapt the Precision Medicine platform [33] to Autism research and treatments [48] linking other disorders to the broad Autism phenotype (Figure 1). I first isolate the genes common to Autism and each disorder under consideration, sort them according to their median gene expression over the above mentioned 18 tissues of interest and then, for each tissue of interest, I highlight the top genes with expression above ($\log(e^{60})$) TMP (using the natural logarithm, Euler's base 2.7183), to further help visualize common top genes across these diseases. I note that this is an arbitrary threshold used only to help visualize the top genes, since other thresholds could be used to visualize more genes in common expressing on tissues of interest. I report in the Supplementary Materials the full set of genes common to these disorders and the SFARI-Autism set. Then, for each of the 54 tissues, I obtain the gene in the unique intersection set with the maximal expression and plot this information for the brain tissues of interest along with the SFARI-Autism score assigned to that gene.

In addition to genes linked to neurological disorders, I examined genes linked to neuropsychiatric conditions such as depression, schizophrenia, ADHD, and post-traumatic stress syndrome (PTSD), the latter owing to the tendencies in ASD to develop trauma and depression reportedly induced by current behavioral therapies [49], and to the known overlap between Autism and schizophrenia [50]. Furthermore, since the DSM 5 now accepts ASD and ADHD as coexisting diagnoses, I included ADHD-linked genes and asked about their overlap with Autism. I also tallied the shared genes pairwise across all the neurological and neuropsychiatric disorders under consideration, to learn about shared genes across these diseases.

Finally, other non-neurological and non-neuropsychiatric diseases were considered, to ascertain their overlap with the Autism-linked genes and with the genes linked to the neurological and neuropsychiatric disorders. I tallied their genes in common and interrogated the genes' expression reported in the GTEx tissues. These included several forms of cancer (colon 49 genes, breast 488 genes, pancreas 114 genes), diabetes 5545 genes, autoimmune disorders (lupus systemic 1743 genes, psoriasis 1221 genes, irritable bowel syndrome 1483 genes), and congenital heart disease 252 genes, totaling 10,895 genes in addition to 10,028 genes associated to neural disorders (a random draw across 25 diseases of 20,923 genes and their expression on 54 tissues). Here I hypothesized that the overlap between the genes linked to Autism and those linked to neurological and neuropsychiatric conditions would be much higher than the overlap between the Autism-linked genes and the genes linked to other non-neurological diseases.

Methods to Obtain Pairwise Comparisons of Genes' Expression in Autism and Various Disorders

I obtained for each set of reported DisGeNET genes liked to each disorder, their expression across the 54 tissues from the GTEx project. This yielded a matrix of N genes × 54 tissues, where each entry in the matrix is the gene's expression in that tissue. Taking the median across all rows for each column (i.e., the number of genes in the disorder) gives a 1 × 54 vector array of median genes' expression per tissue, which I normalize by the total number of genes in that disorder (scaling it to range between 0 and 1 unitless quantity). This is depicted in stem form in Figure 3A for each of 3 different representative disorders (ASD, ADHD and Lupus Systemic.) I then take the histogram of the values (represented by red dots in Figure 3A) and obtain the Earth Mover's Distance (EMD) [51–53] between histograms, to code the distance in some probability space where I can represent these histograms according to an empirically fit continuous family of probability distributions. I obtain the EMD quantity pairwise between disorders, normalize it by the maximum value across the entire set, and represent it in matrix form for neuropsychiatric, neurological disorders and non-neurological diseases. I ask if clusters self-emerge from this representation of the median genes' expression across the 54 tissues.

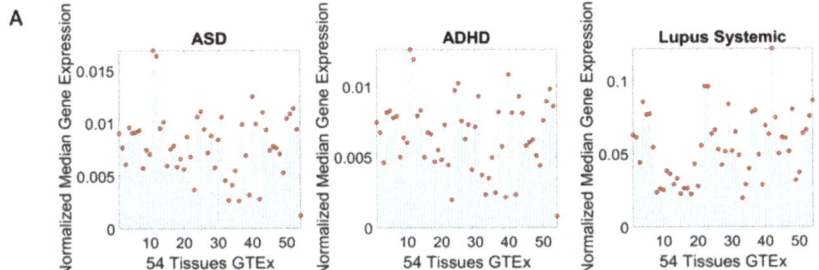

Figure 3. *Cont.*

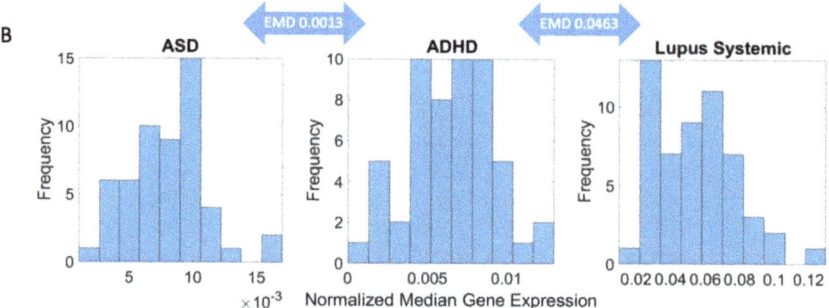

Figure 3. Pipeline of analysis to obtain pairwise similarity measurements between disorders. (**A**) The matrix of N genes × 54 tissues whereby is *ij* entry is the gene expression from the row *i* in the tissue *j*, is transformed into a 1 × 54 vector of median gene expression values (across the matrix rows) represented here in stem form, from the normalized values accounting for the number of genes in each disorder. Each red dot represents the median gene expression at the jth tissue. Three representative disorders are shown. (**B**) Histogram of the genes' normalized expression correspond to the stem plots of panel (**A**). I take the earth mover's distance (EMD) pairwise between two disorders (represented in the arrow) and build a matrix of EMD values representing the distance (similarity) between two disorders in the precise sense of genetic information contributing to genes' expression on tissues.

3. Results

3.1. Neuropsychiatric Disorders and Autism Share Common Genes Expressed in Brain Tissues for Motor, Emotional and Self-Regulatory Control

Quantification of genes common to Autism and neuropsychiatric disorders is depicted in Table 1. Figure 4A shows the pairwise shared genes color-coded (in log N color scale, where N is the number of genes in common with the SFARI-Autism set.) The inset in Figure 4A shows the distribution of genes common to the Autism linked SFARI database and each of the neuropsychiatric disorders under consideration, schizophrenia, ADHD, depression, and bipolar depression and including the neurological disorders. Notice that ADHD and Schizophrenia share the highest number of genes followed by depression and bipolar depression. Interestingly, I included PTSD owing to the tendency of trauma reported in Autism [49,54,55] and found 55 genes of those linked to PTSD in the SFARI-Autism set. I also included lupus systemic, owing to the known relations between autism and autoimmune disorders [56,57].

Table 1. Overlap between Autism-linked genes in SFARI and known neuropsychiatric disorders, ranked by the % of genes obtained relative to the number of genes in the SFARI set under consideration here.

Neuropsychiatric Condition	Number of Genes in DISGENET	Number of Genes Shared with SFARI ASD-Linked Genes	% (Relative to DisGeNET, Relative to 906 SFARI Genes)
Schizophrenia	2697	336	(24.58, 37.08)
ADHD	795	188	(23.64, 20.75)
Depression	1407	158	(11.22, 17.43)
PTSD	395	55	(13.92, 6.07)
Bipolar Depression	116	33	(28.34, 3.6)

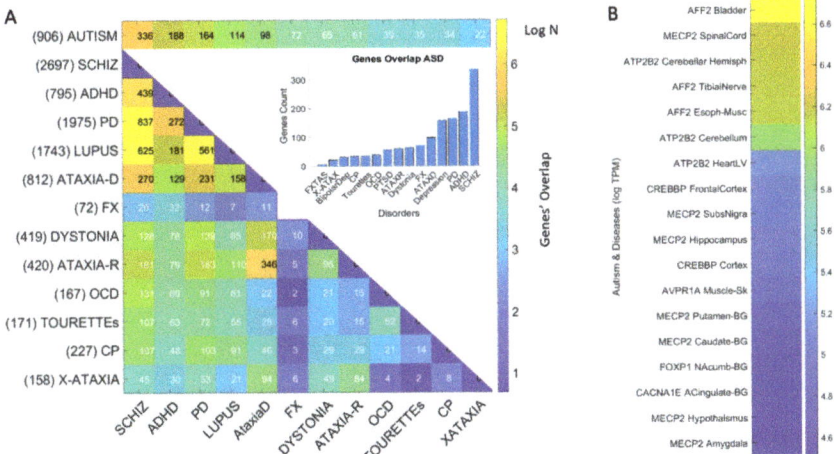

Figure 4. Number of genes common to Autism and selected neuropsychiatric, neurological, and autoimmune disorders. (**A**) Inset shows bar plot tallying the number of genes in each disorder that are also present in the SFARI dataset linking genes to Autism according to a confidence score (see the Section 2) Colormap depicting the number of genes in Autism and each disorder on the top row. Pairwise shared genes between disorder in row *i* and column *j* is the number on each entry of the matrix. Color is in log N, where N is the number of genes common to Autism and the disorder, or common to a disorder and another disorder (pairwise intersect.) (**B**) Color bar reflecting the 18 tissues with maximal gene expression and the corresponding gene at the intersection of SFARI-Autism and all shared genes in (**A**).

3.2. Neurological Disorders and Autism Share Common Genes Expressed in Brain Tissues for Motor, Emotional and Regulatory Control

Likewise, quantification of genes linked to well-known neurological disorders and present in the SFARI-Autism dataset yielded up to 164 overlapping genes. These are depicted in Tables 1 and 2 for neuropsychiatric and neurological disorders respectively. I ranked them in each category by % relative to the 906 genes in the SFARI set under consideration, and by the number of genes associated to each disorder in DisGeNET. The shared genes are also shown in Figure 4A, color coded according to the number of genes in the intersection of SFARI-Autism and each disorder, and between disorders, taking the pairwise intersection. Table 1 shows that among the neuropsychiatric conditions, schizophrenia is the one with the highest percentage of genes shared with the SFARI-Autism set. Table 2 shows that among the neurological conditions, Parkinson's disease has the highest percent shared with the SFARI-Autism set. This result came as a surprise, but it helps explain why as autistics age, the onset of Parkinson-like symptoms is reported by 40 years of age in 20% of the autistic adult population. This contrasts with 0.09% after 65 years of age in the general population [36]. Furthermore, this shared genetic pool between SFARI-Autism and the DisGeNET genes associated to Parkinson's disease helps explain the marked stochastic shift away from typical ranges of noise levels found in autistics at 40 years of age, when examining their involuntary head micro-motions at rest [30].

Surprisingly also was the finding concerning schizophrenia in Figure 4A, whereby 837 genes are shared between Parkinson's disease and the schizophrenia set, while 439 are shared between ADHD and schizophrenia. Furthermore, 625 genes are shared between lupus systemic and schizophrenia. This figure depicts the shared gene pool across these selected disorders that also show their genes overlapping with Autism-linked genes (on the top row.) The numbers next to the disorder are the number of genes reported in DisGeNET. The numbers in the color map entries are those shared pairwise between the disorders in row *i* and column *j* of the matrix. Figure 4B shows the tissues with the maximal gene expression using a color bar (in log median TCM) sorted in descending order. These are the genes common to all the disorders under consideration that overlap with SFARI-Autism genes.

Table 2. Overlap between Autism-linked genes in SFARI and known neurological disorders of genetic origins ranked based on % relative to the set of 906 SFARI genes under consideration here.

Neurological Disorder	Number of Genes Reported in DISGENET	Number of Genes Shared with SFARI ASD-Linked Genes	% (Relative to DisGeNET, Relative to 906 SFARI Genes)
Parkinson's	1975	164	(8.3, 18.10)
Ataxia Autosomal Dominant	812	98	(12.06, 10.81)
FX	72	72	(100.0, 7.94)
Dystonia	419	65	(15.51, 7.17)
Ataxia Autosomal Recessive	420	61	(14.52, 6.73)
OCD	167	39	(23.35, 4.30)
Tourette's	171	35	(20.46, 3.86)
CP	227	34	(14.97, 3.75)
X-Ataxia	158	22	(13.92, 2.42)
FXTAS	63	22	(34.9, 2.42)
Progressive Cerebellar Ataxia	134	13	(9.70, 1.43)

3.3. Examination of the Maximal Gene Expression on the Tissues for Genes Common to Autism and These Disorders Revealed a Compact Gene Pool

I found that 12 genes are common to autism, and these disorders are maximally ex-pressed on the 54 tissues. They are depicted in Table 3 along with the tissues where they maximally express, while Figure 4B shows the genes maximally expressed on the 18 tissues of interest (brain, spinal cord, tibial nerve, and those key to cardiac, smooth, and skeletal muscles.) I discuss later some of the literature on these known genes. I also provide Supplementary Text Files containing for each disorder, the pairwise genes in common between Autism and each disorder or disease under consideration.

Table 3. Compact set of genes common to Autism and the neurological and neuropsychiatric disorders maximally and selectively expressed across the 54 tissues.

Genes Common to ASD and Neuro-Disorders	Tissue with Max Expression
ACTB	Liver
AFF2	Adipose Subcutaneous, Adipose Visceral Omentum, AdrenalGland, Artery Aorta, Artery Coronary, Artery Tibial, Bladder, Breast Mammary Tissue, Cervix Ectocervix, Cervix Endocervix, Colon Sigmoid, Colon Transverse, Esophagus Gastro esophageal Junction, Esophagus Muscularis, Fallopian Tube, Heart AtrialAppendage, Kidney Cortex, Kidney Medulla, Lung, Minor Salivary Gland, Nerve Tibial, Pituitary, Prostate, Small Int ileum, Spleen, Stomach, Thyroid, Uterus, Vagina
AKAP9	Whole Blood
ALDH5A1	Esophagus Mucosa

Table 3. *Cont.*

Genes Common to ASD and Neuro-Disorders	Tissue with Max Expression
ATP2B2	Heart Left, Ventricle, Ovary, Cerebellar Hemi, Cerebellum
AVPR1A	Skeletal Muscle
CACNA1E	Ant Cingulate Cortex
CHD7	Pancreas, Skin not Sun Exposed Suprapubic, Skin Sun Exposed Lower Leg
CREBBP	Cortex, Frontal Cortex, Fibroblasts, Cell-Lymphocytes
FOXP1	Nucleus Accumbens of the Basal Ganglia (BG)
MECP2	Amygdala, Caudate-BG, Hippocampus, Hypothalamus, Putamen-BG, Spinal Cord-Cervical, Substantia Nigra
SMAD4	Testis

3.4. Genomic Stratification of Neurological and Neuropsychiatric Diseases Making Up Autism Today

The EMD taken pairwise between Autism and each disorder, and pairwise across all neuropsychiatric, neurological disorders and non-neurological diseases revealed an orderly stratification of disorders, whereby a common gene pool and expression on the tissues can clearly separate neuropsychiatric and neurological from non-neurological diseases. This is shown in Figure 5A, where we can also appreciate that in the non-neurological diseases, the autoimmune ones share a common gene pool and tissue expression. Notably, colon cancer is also close in a probability distance sense, to neurological disorders of known genetic origin, namely, Fragile X, FXTAS, the ataxias, dystonia, and Parkinson's disease.

Zooming into the entries with lowest EMD value, corresponding to the neuropsychiatric and neurological disorders, we see in Figure 5B, that other patterns self-emerge further refining the clusters. There, we can appreciate that ASD is close to ADHD and Schizophrenia, as well as close to Depression, PTSD and Cerebral Palsy. Furthermore, OCD and Tourette's cluster close together, also showing a common gene pool and genes' expression across the tissues. In the group of the neurological disorders of known etiology, we can visualize self-grouping of FX and the ataxias (dominant and recessive), while X-ataxia, dystonia, Progressive cerebellar ataxia, and Parkinson self-cluster and separate from FXTAS.

To further test this visualization, I ran a common clustering procedure using MATLAB linkage function applying Euclidean distance and plotting the output as a dendogram. This shows the orderly binary tree structure of these genes-tissues grouping in Figure 5C. We can see that there are three main subtrees of the binary tree, i.e., two subtrees comprised of neurological disorders, and one with neuropsychiatric disorders of the types diagnosed by the DSM. Further refinement reveals FXTAS as a leaf of its own, close to progressive cerebellar ataxia, dystonia, and X-ataxia, all under the same subtree. The other subtree contains Parkinson's disease, ataxia dominant and recessive and Fragile X.

At the neuropsychiatric end, we see that Tourette's and OCD group in a branch and bipolar depression is a leaf of its own, while schizophrenia and SFARI-Autism fall the closest together in one branch of the same subtree. That subtree also groups PTSD, Depression and ADHD under one branch and shows CP as a leaf of its own. These gene pools and their expression on the 54 GTEx tissues define an orderly stratification aided by genes common to autism spectrum disorders, according to DisGeNET and SFARI genomic reports.

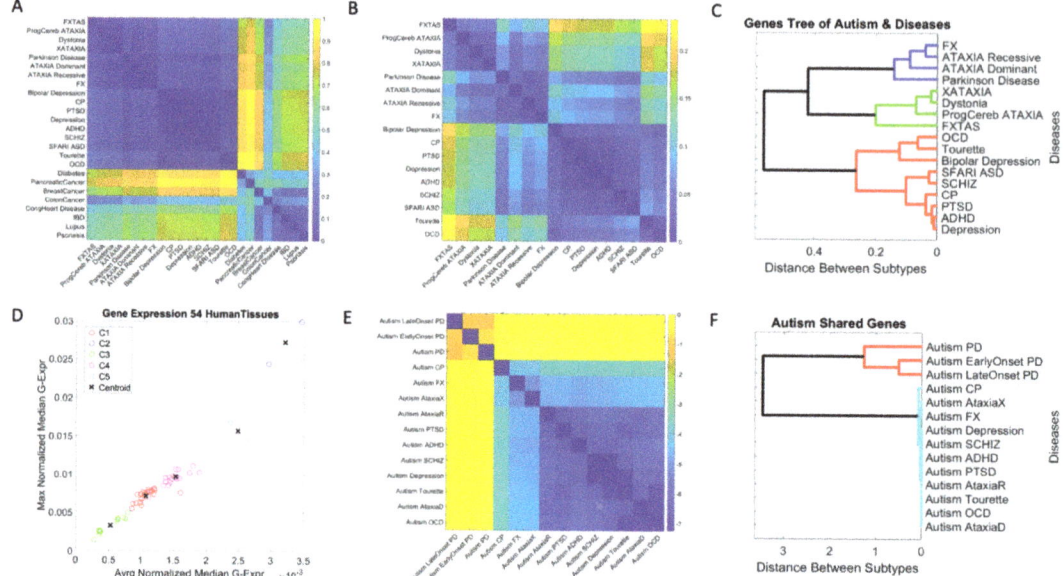

Figure 5. Genomic stratification of Autism and diseases obtained by leveraging the gene pool that overlaps with other known neurological and neuropsychiatric diseases and their expression on the 54 tissues defined by GTEx. (**A**) EMD-based separation between neuropsychiatric, neurological disorders and non-neurological diseases, also identifying common gene pool in autoimmune diseases. Color scale is the normalized EMD value taken pairwise between the vector of median gene expression across 54 tissues of GTEx. (**B**) Zooming into the neuropsychiatric and neurological diseases whose gene pool overlaps with Autism, I see different self-emerging subclusters further refining the stratification. (**C**) Dendogram showing the binary tree orderly organization that groups and categorizes diseases according to genes' overlap and tissue expression with respect to ASD. (**D**) Output of K-Means algorithm with 5 tissue-cluster criteria taken on shared genes between SFARI-Autism and each disorder/disease in (**B**,**C**). Cluster 1 (red) includes the amygdala, hippocampus, putamen, and substantia nigra. Cluster 2 (blue) in a category of its own, includes the cerebellar hemisphere and the cerebellum. Cluster 3 (green) does not contain brain tissues but contains tissues important for cardiac (heart atrial appendage, heart left ventricle), smooth (esophagus mucosa, bladder) and skeletal muscles (muscle skeletal.) Cluster 4 (magenta) contains the anterior cingulate cortex, the basal ganglia's caudate and nucleus accumbens, the brain cortex, the hypothalamus. Cluster 5 (cyan) contains the frontal cortex and the pituitary gland. (**E**) Similarity matrix built by taking the normalized Earth Mover's distance metric pairwise between the genes in the intersection of Autism and each of the 14 disorders under consideration. Higher distances (yellow) indicate more effort to transform the distribution of median values of genes' expression (taken across the 54 tissues) from one set of SFARI-Autism shared genes and a given disorder, with another set of SFARI-Autism shared genes and another disorder. (**F**) Hierarchical clustering of these shared genes identifies two main groups of shared genes with SFARI-Autism, one formed by those SFARI-Autism genes found in the genes linked to PD, early onset PD and late onset PD, and the other formed by the genes shared (pairwise) with each of the other neuropsychiatric and neurological disorders under consideration.

Clustering by tissues maximally expressing the shared genes across disorders (Figure 5D), we can see 5 groups of tissues whereby, the cerebellum and cerebellar hemisphere are by far the tissues with the highest gene expression, followed by the prefrontal cortex and pituitary gland. The following group is comprised of the anterior cingulate cortex, the basal ganglia's caudate and nucleus accumbens, the brain cortex, the hypothalamus, followed by the cluster containing the amygdala, hippocampus, putamen, and substantia nigra. The lowest expression is in the cluster containing no brain tissues, but tissues important for survival and overall functioning of cardiac (heart atrial appendage, heart left ventricle), smooth (esophagus mucosa, bladder) and skeletal muscles (muscle skeletal).

Furthermore, I examined the pairwise intersection sets of genes shared between SFARI-Autism and each of these disorders in the neurological and neuropsychiatric sets. These are found in Figure 5E, as they grouped according to the EMD metric (expressed here in log scale.) The hierarchical clustering revealed two main subtrees in this case, one comprising PD and early and late onset PD in the intersection with SFARI-Autism. The other branch revealed an orderly grouping of neurological disorders surrounding the neuropsychiatric disorders (depression, schizophrenia, ADHD, and PTSD.)

Figures 6 and 7 reveal the genes expression for values above ($\log(e^{60})$ TCM) with the SFARI confidence score on the horizontal axis and the expression value log TCM on the vertical axis. Figure 6 shows the brain tissues and genes above this level of expression along with the confidence score in the SFARI data repository. Tissues that are fundamental for the development and maintenance of motor learning, motor coordination and motor adaptation include the substantia nigra (maximal expressed gene AFF2-AUT1 signifying this gene is scored in SFARI as score 1 confidence), basal ganglia with caudate, putamen and nucleus accumbens also with AFF2-AUT1 as top expressing gene. Other tissues involved in motor control are the cerebellar hemisphere (ATP2B2-AUT2) and the cerebellum (CREBBP-AUT1). Tissues known to be involved in executive function are the brain frontal cortex (MECP2-AUT1) and the brain cortex (CACNA1E-AUT2). Tissues known for their involvement in emotions (amygdala (AFF2-AUT1)) and memory (hippocampus (BRSK2-AUT1)) and the anterior cingulate cortex (BRSK2-AUT1) are also depicted in Figure 6, along with the schematics of the brain from Figure 1 with the locations of these areas.

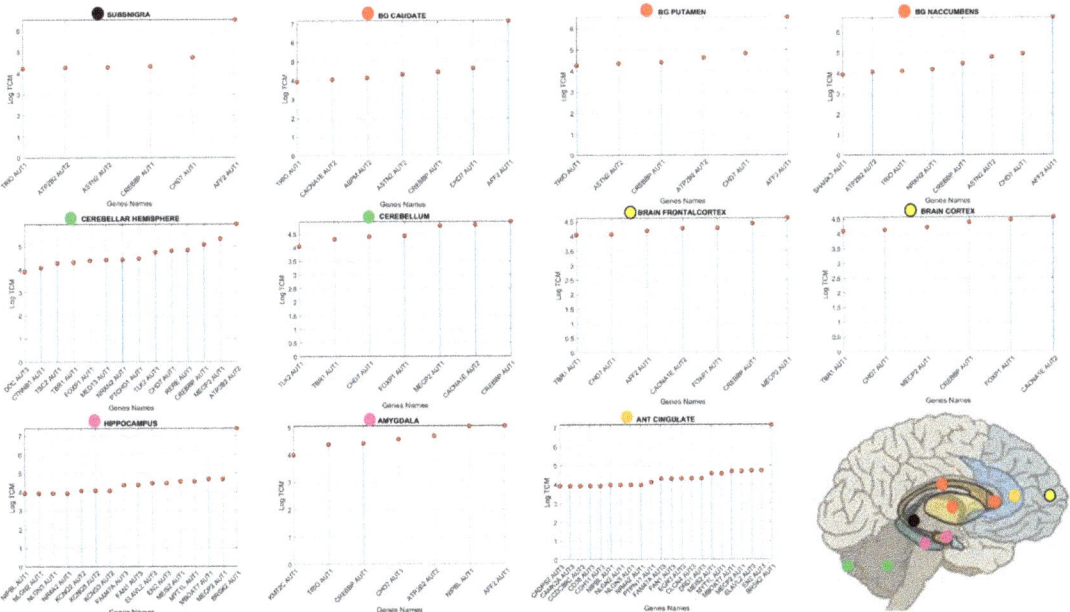

Figure 6. Common genes to Autism and all other neurological and neuropsychiatric disorders maximally express on brain tissues involved in the initiation, generation, control, coordination, and adaptation of movements, as well as in tissues necessary for the creation, retrieval and maintenance of memories and executive function. Genes' expression is threshold above $\log(e^{60})$ to show the top expressing genes from DisGenNet overlapping with those in the SFARI set (Full list of shared genes are in the Supplementary Materials Files.) The AUT# reflects the confidence score assigned to the gene at the SFARI repository. Horizontal axis shows the genes above threshold and vertical axis gives the expression level (log transcripts count per million, TCM.) Each colored dot is shown at the brain tissue in Figure 2A schematic form.

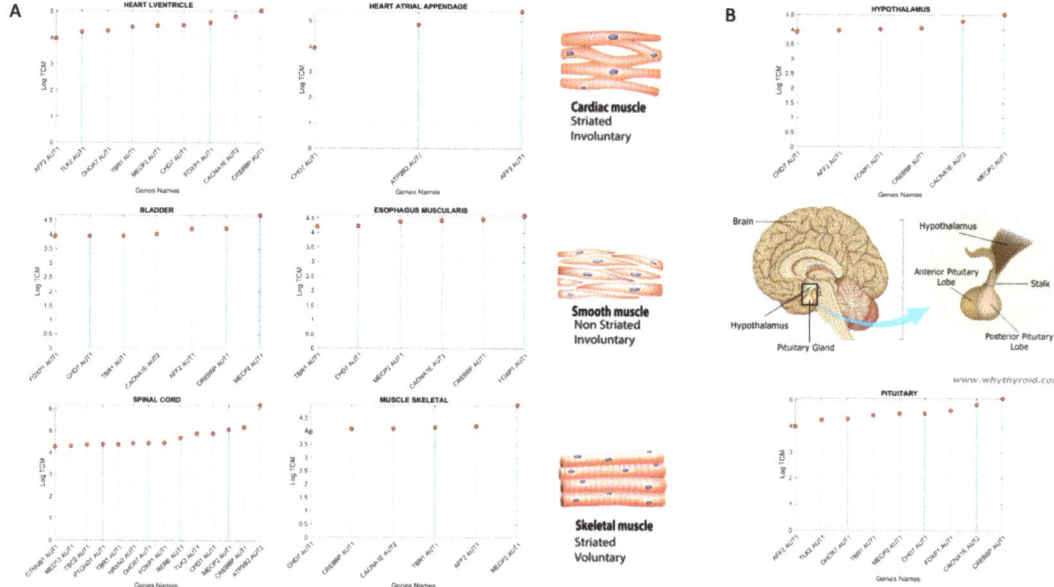

Figure 7. Genes present in Autism and all other neurological and neuropsychiatric disorders maximally expressed (above $\log(e^{60})$) on tissues involved in all vital functions associated with cardiac, smooth, and skeletal muscles and the spinal cord (**A**), and with self-systemic regulation (**B**). Top genes and corresponding SFARI confidence score are also plotted on the horizontal axis. Vertical axis reflects the expression in log TCM units. Schematics reflect the locations of the hypothalamus and pituitary gland in the brain (from www.whythyroide.com) (accessed on 28 October 2021).

In Figure 7, I also reveal those genes' expression and SFARI scores for the cardiac (heart left ventricle and the heart atrial appendage), skeletal (muscle skeletal), and smooth muscle (esophagus muscularis and bladder) tissues and for the nerve tibial. The latter is critical to develop kinesthetic reafference and proper gait, known to be disrupted in several of these disorders (autism, PD, FX [17]). Common to all these disorders are well known genes in the Autism literature with SFARI score confidence 1 (e.g., *MECP2*, *AFF2*, *FOXP1*, *CREBBP*, *CACNA1E*, *CHD7*, *TRIO* and *SHANK3*, among others.) I will later discuss the known roles of some of these genes in the development of synapses and circuits necessary to form and dynamically maintain neural networks.

I further plot in Supplementary Figures S1–S3 genes common to Autism and some of the disorders, for the top 20 genes with maximal expression (in log TCM units) across the brain and spinal cord tissues, as well as tissues involving skeletal muscle, cardiac, and smooth muscle types. These figures in the Supplementary Materials show the matrix with genes across the rows (top 20 expressed genes) and 18/54 tissues across the columns. Each entry is color coding the expression of these genes in log TCM units. From these plots, I note that e.g., MECP2 is present at the highest expression on the spinal cord in Autism and Schizophrenia, Autism and Depression, Autism and ADHD, Autism and OCD, Autism and Cerebral Palsy, Autism and Dystonia, Autism and Autosomal Dominant Ataxia, Autism and Autosomal Recessive Ataxia, Autism and Fragile X, Autism and X-ataxia, Autism and PTSD but not in Tourette's & Autism, where MECP2 is not among the top 20 genes expressed on these tissues. Instead, CHD2 is expressed on the spinal cord, and highly expressed on the cerebellum and cerebellar hemisphere. Indeed, Tourette's is closer to OCD (Figure 5C) than to the cluster formed by ASD, ADHD and Schizophrenia (though located on the same subtree as these neuropsychiatric disorders, but in a separate branch containing bipolar depression too.)

4. Discussion

This work provides support to the idea of reframing Autism under the model of Precision Medicine [25,48], while also addressing the notion of an "Autism epidemic" recently portrayed as an exponential rise in prevalence [58] and its costly consequences [58]. Re-examining Autism as the conglomerate of disorders and diseases, many of known origins, comprising this heterogeneous spectrum, I conclude that such "epidemic" or "tsunami" is bound to be an artifact of the current behavioral diagnosis-to-treatment pipeline. This pipeline allows such comorbidities and often shifts criteria, discouraging stratification. I invite the thought that stratifying the spectrum according to underlying genetic, causal information would provide far more viable strategies to cope with the overall increase in neurodevelopmental disorders in general, than continuing the use of Autism as a blanket label grouping all these disorders. Furthermore, I argue that several of the disorders in question already have therapies designed to address issues in their corresponding phenotype. As such, the general Autism label, when funneled through genetic subtypes, could leverage the accommodations, and offer support pertinent to each of the neurological and neuropsychiatric groups conforming its broad spectrum today. Here we report that they have a considerable genetic overlap with the genes linked to SFARI-Autism.

Autism serves as an umbrella term encompassing many disorders and diseases, some of which have precise etiology (e.g., Down Syndrome [59], Fragile X Syndrome [60], etc.) I therefore combined multiple open access data sets with the label of Autism and with the label of a disorder or disease that often receives the Autism diagnosis. I included neuropsychiatric disorders, and neurological and non-neurological diseases associated with some sets of genes. Then, I applied common computational techniques to attempt to automatically and orderly stratify a cohort of 25 diseases and 20,923 genes expressed on 54 brain and bodily tissues, vital for the survival and functioning of the individual

I show that given a random draw of genes linked to disorders with high penetrance in Autism, and even some which are not officially associated with autism, one could find self-emerging clusters at their intersection. Using (probabilistic) distance metric assessing the similarity between genes associated to autism and those associated to the other disorders, and examining their expression in brain-body tissues, several important patterns self-revealed. Among them, DisGeNET Parkinson's disease emerged as the neurological condition with maximal number of shared genes associated to the SFARI-Autism set under consideration. Schizophrenia appeared as the neuropsychiatric disorder with maximal number of genes shared with Parkinson's disease. Both SFARI-Autism and Schizophrenia shared the maximum number of genes with the SFARI set, strongly suggesting that movement disorders are at the core of both autism and schizophrenia.

I found self-emerging clusters that clearly (and automatically) differentiated neuropsychiatric and neurological disorders from non-neurological diseases and within the brain-related disorders, I established an orderly distance to Autism in the sense of overlapping genes and their expression on tissues critical for motor control (initiation-termination, learning, coordination, sequencing, and adaptation), cognition, memory, and self-regulation. I also found that the autoimmune disorder lupus systemic shares 114 genes with those linked to Autism in SFARI (12.6% relative to the 906 genes in SFARI), a result congruent with recent links between Autism and autoimmune disorders [56,57,61].

The overall conclusions from these results are several folds: (1) Autism is a movement disorder and should be accordingly redefined and treated as such, rather than treated as a misbehavior; (2) The broad spectrum of Autism, as we know it today, i.e., inclusive of disorders and diseases of known etiology, share a common set of genes with genetic disorders and consequentially can be stratified into Autism subtypes. (3) Given this automatic clustering, it is safe to conclude that Autism prevalence rates are an artifact of current surveillance methods relying exclusively on the clinical (behavioral) diagnosis that welcomes other disorders. Incidentally, it has been shown that such methods of diagnoses use fundamentally flawed statistics in the criteria, thus inflating false positives [9]. Furthermore, digitizing them with wearable biosensors, captures the fundamental differences in females, saves time, thus being less taxing on the children and offering a new level of finer granularity of physiological function, well beyond the limits of the naked eye. As such, digitized dyadic interactions during the ADOS opens a new avenue for precision (physiological) phenotyping that, when combined with genomics results here, stands to reformulate autism research under the tenets of Precision Medicine [8,25].

The genetically-based subtypes reported here might be more manageable and less costly to treat and service, than forecasted by current epidemiological accounts relying only on the psychological construct of "appropriate" social behaviors [58]. Since there are therapies for other disorders that share genes associated with Autism, it may be possible to repurpose such therapies and adapt them to corresponding Autism subtypes.

4.1. The Genetically Informed Autism Subtypes

Given a mixture of genes and their median expression on the 54 tissues defined by GTEx, across multiple neuropsychiatric and neurological disorders, I found that Autism-linked genes in SFARI overlap with genes defining those disorders in DisGeNET, which would also likely receive the Autism label. Such overlapping showed an orderly stratification using a binary tree structure that rendered schizophrenia as the closest to SFARI-Autism (sharing 363/906 genes reported in SFARI) and FXTAS as the farthest (nonetheless sharing 22/906 genes reported in SFARI.) I note that DisGeNET ASD (autism spectrum disorders; CUI: C1510586) is a superset of SFARI, 1071 vs. 906 genes and SFARI genes are ranked according to the literature. I also note that since our last download, the number of genes in SFARI may have increased.

In good concordance with clinical criteria, two main subtypes automatically self-emerged according to the distance metric that I used (Figure 5C) comprising neuropsychiatric and neurological disorders, all sharing a compact set of genes described below. The neuropsychiatric branch includes the Autism linked genes in DisGeNET (overlapping with a subset of those in SFARI) and disorders in the Diagnostic Statistical Manual, 5th edition, DSM-5 and the International Classification of Diseases, 10th edition, ICD-10. In order of distance to SFARI-Autism, on one end we have schizophrenia (the closest sharing the same sub-branch), CP, PTSD, ADHD (allowed to be co-diagnosed with Autism in the DSM5) and depression. Then, the other branch has bipolar depression, Tourette's, and OCD. Among the neurological disorders conforming the second cluster, I have in order of distance from the SFARI-Autism set, FXTAS, progressive cerebellar ataxia, dystonia, and X-ataxia. The last cluster has Parkinson's disease, ataxia dominant, ataxia recessive and Fragile X, with Parkinson's disease sharing the largest percent of SFARI-Autism genes. This natural breakdown of the (Autism) spectrum according to the shared genetic pool and genes' expression on tissues fundamental to form the building blocks of any human behavior, is far more manageable (using physiological and medical knowledge today) than considering the full spectrum in a monolithic form, as suggested by psychological surveillance methods [1,58] and the behaviorists' recommendations [13].

4.2. The Genes Common to Autism and Each Subtype

Each neuropsychiatric or neurological subtype identified by the genes-tissue analysis shared genes with the SFARI-Autism set. The full list in Supplementary Materials for each disorder/disease, offers clues with regards to the tissues whereby these intersecting genes maximally express. Furthermore, Figure 5D revealed several clusters of tissues common to all these pairwise-shared genes between the disorders and SFARI-Autism. Among these clusters, the cerebellar hemisphere and the cerebellum emerged as a separate group, common to all these disorders, with the maximum average median gene expression. This cluster of tissues was followed by a cluster that included the frontal cortex and the pituitary gland, also far apart from the other three clusters in Figure 5D.

Autism and schizophrenia, Autism and ADHD, Autism and Depression, Autism and OCD, Autism and FX, Autism and ataxia-X, Autism and PTSD, Autism and CP, Autism and dystonia, Autism and Ataxia autosomal dominant and Autism and Ataxia autosomal recessive, all share METHYL-CpG-binding protein 2, MECP2, with cytogenetic location at Xq28 (according to the Online Mendelian Inheritance in Man, OMIM site). It is reported as implicated in severe neonatal encephalopathy, mental disability and Rett syndrome, as well as to have high Autism susceptibility. MECP2, binds methylated CpGs. It is a chromatin-associated protein that can both activate and repress transcription; it is required for maturation of neurons and is developmentally regulated [62].

Furthermore, Autism and schizophrenia and Autism and ADHD (the two top neuropsychiatric disorders sharing the highest percentages of genes with the genes linked to SFARI-Autism) shared the CREP-Binding Protein (CREBBP), among the top 10 genes expressed maximally across the 54 tissues and common to the Autism and Schizophrenia gene pool. It is located in 16p12.3, a chromosomal region linked to Autism.

Autism and Tourette's syndrome did not share MECP2, but shared CHD2 as the top gene maximally expressed across all 18 tissues of the brain, spinal cord and tissues associated with cardiac, smooth, and skeletal muscles. Maximal expression at the cerebellar hemisphere and the cerebellum suggests involvement in motor control, coordination, and adaptation, while high expression in other tissues for memory, cognition, and self-systemic regulation suggest that this gene is rather important. Indeed, prior work in Autism [63] and other neurodevelopmental disorders [64] had conferred importance to this gene for neural development.

Among highly expressed genes in Autism and other disorders, I also found AFF2 [65] and BRSK2 [66], both with score 1 in SFARI and reportedly critical for neurodevelopment. Indeed, the X-linked gene AFF2 has been found in patients with fragile X E (FRAXE) intellectual disability, while the gene encoding the serine/threonine-protein kinase BRSK2 was recently detected in individuals with developmental and intellectual disability.

To further understand the possible links that have been suggested between Autism and PD (particularly during adulthood), I also examined the genes from DisGeNET linked to early (50 genes) and late (238 genes) onset of PD, along with those linked to PD in general (1975 genes.) This revealed that DisGeNET PD shares 164 genes with SFARI-Autism, whereas early onset PD shares 8 and late onset PD shares 32 genes with those in SFARI-Autism. Among the genes maximally expressed in the tissues of the brain and the cardiac, smooth, and skeletal muscles in PD, *AFF2* and *TSC2* were found. In early onset PD, RAB39B and SLC6A3 were found. Mutations in RAB39B cause X-linked intellectual disability and early-onset Parkinson disease with alpha-synuclein pathology, also linked to X-linked mental disability associated with Autism, epilepsy, and macrocephaly [67–70]. SLC6A3 provides instructions for making the dopamine transporter protein (DAT) embedded in dopaminergic neurons. Variations (polymorphisms) of the *SLC6A3* gene have been linked to PD, ADHD [71] and ASD [72]. Dopamine is a known neurotransmitter important for multiple cognitive and motor functions, as well as for the functioning of the reward systems of the brain. In late onset PD, TET2, ADA and PTGS2 (COX2) were found. Located in 4q24, TET methylcytosine dioxygenase 2 is listed in OMIM as a TET protein playing a key role in the regulation of DNA-methylation status serving both as a stable epigenetic mark and participating in active demethylation [73]. TET2 has been described as early and essential stage in somatic cell reprogramming preceding the induction of transcription at endogenous pluripotency loci. It is said to contribute to an epigenetic program that directs subsequent transcriptional induction at pluripotency loci during somatic cell reprogramming [74]. Adenosine deaminase (or adenosine aminohydrolase) ADA is located at 20q13.12 and is associated with severe immunodeficiency [75].

These genes and their expression in relevant tissues are shown in the Supplementary Materials Figure S4. It will be interesting to track the evolution of these shared genes on induced pluripotent stem cell models, as cells develop into neuronal classes. Research along those lines is warranted [60]. Prostaglandin-endoperoxide synthase 2 PTGS2 or cyclooxygenase 2 COX2, is in 1q31.1. High-level induction of COX2 in mesenchymal-derived inflammatory cells suggests a role for COX2 in inflammatory conditions [76] and CNS-inflammatory pain hypersensitivity [77].

4.3. The Genes Common to Autism and All Subtypes

MECP2 and CREBBP were found to be shared pairwise with Autism and the above-mentioned disorders, but also present at the intersection set, taken across disorders. MECP2 expressed maximally in tissues related to emotion (amygdala) and memory (hippocampus) and tissues important for motor control (basal ganglia's caudate and putamen regions, the substantia nigra, the cerebellum and cerebellar hemisphere, and the spinal cord) and for self-regulation (hypothalamus.) CREBBP was found to be maximally expressed at the cortex and frontal cortex, both of which are important for high-level cognitive and executive functions. Another important forkhead transcription factor FOXP1 was found to be maximally expressed in the basal ganglia's nucleus accumbens, a structure important for developing striatal function and differentiation in medium spiny neurons from precursors to maturity [78–80]. CACNA1E was found maximally expressed across disorders in the anterior cingulate cortex, a region associated with impulse control, emotion and decision making, and previously known in connection to epilepsy, Autism, schizophrenia, and major depressive disorder [81–83].

Cluster analyses revealed that across all disorders under consideration, the cerebellum and cerebellar hemisphere had the maximal gene expression. Yet, different genes shared with the SFARI-Autism set contributed across disorders. MECP2 was maximally expressed in both the cerebellum and the cerebellar hemisphere in CP, Dystonia, OCD, Depression, PTSD and Lupus. In ADHD, MECP2 was maximally expressed in the cerebellum but the cerebellar hemisphere maximally expressed CREBBP. As mentioned, in PD, TSC2 was maximally expressed in both cerebellar tissues, while early onset had RAB39B and late onset had TET2 maximally expressed in both cerebellar tissues. Tourette's had CHD2. Bipolar depression had SHANK2. Infantile Schizophrenia had ATP1A, and Schizophrenia had ATP2B2. These are shown in Supplementary Figures S4–S6 along with other brain tissues and tissues important for cardiac, smooth, and skeletal muscles. The mixture of neuropsychiatric, neurological, and autoimmune disorders all had the cerebellar tissues with maximal gene expression of the genes shared with the SFARI-Autism set. These genes are thus bound to play an important role in motor control, coordination, initiation-termination, sequencing and adaptation, all critical components of basic building blocks to develop proper motor dynamics in social interactions. It is not surprising then that Autism has so many motor issues, as it sits squarely at the intersection of these neurological, neuropsychiatric, and autoimmune disorders. Why are motor issues not seriously considered in Autism research and clinical practices? Continuing to sideline the motor and motor sensing axes misses a superb opportunity to finally turn the science of Autism into a rigorous quantitative practice, beyond opinions or political agendas currently dominating the field and obfuscating important neurodevelopmental issues.

4.4. Implications of This Genomic Categorization for Treatment Selection in Autism

Approaching Autism as genotypically defined orderly subtypes may also be more humanely relevant to the affected individuals. Today, they receive recommendations for a "one-size-fits-all" behavioral-modification or conversion-therapy to reshape "socially inappropriate behaviors" without informing such treatments by brain-body physiological and medical issues. This approach disregards possible adverse effects linked to their genomic characteristics [84]. Indeed, despite advances in genetics, it has been reported that the current paradigm neglects the physiological phenotypes in favor of psychological constructs [32]. The literature reports that this model for Autism treatment selection promotes stigma, causes harm in the form of trauma, increases the person's stress and ultimately results in PTSD [85]. Along those lines, there is a pool of genes linked to PTSD and depression overlapping with a subset of the SFARI-Autism data set, and very close to the Autism branch of the binary tree in Figure 5C. These genes may interact in ways that could increase the predisposition of the Autistic system to develop PTSD and depression, explaining the rise as well in suicidal ideation [49,86–88].

The outcome of this work highlights the relevance of considering, when choosing treatments, the medical and physiological issues linked to the phenotypic characteristics that these genes forecast. This proposed approach contrasts with choosing treatments that exclusively focus on the social appropriateness criteria. The latter model has been said to lead to high societal cost [58,89], to offer no future to the affected individuals and their families and has recently been shown to be polluted with conflict of interests and nonscientific practices [90,91].

In the present study, I reasoned that stratifying Autism based on the genetic makeup of the diseases that today go on to receive the Autism clinical diagnosis, could help us in various ways. One was to find the diseases genetically closer to Autism itself (as defined by the SFARI genes.) Another was to leverage existing clinical information in other fields, amenable to create support and accommodations for the individuals affected by those disorders undergoing physiologically relevant treatments in other fields. Such accommodations could then be tailored to the autistic person, according to the phenotype that these genetic pools express for each of these other diseases of known etiology. Furthermore, since Autism today includes all these other disorders in its broad spectrum, utilizing the information that has already been verified (e.g., in the SFARI repository) would bring us a step closer to the Personalized Medicine approach, coined here Precision Autism (Figure 1B).

It has been recently proposed that the behavioral definition of Autism, which recommends against stratifying the spectrum [13], feeds the Autism Industrial Complex (AIC) [89] and opens a behavioral diagnosis-to-treatment pipeline contributing to their claimed societal burden [58]. It is almost perverse to create a problem and sustain the problem by sidelining existing solutions, or alternative scientific routes, when the same model practiced over 40 years has not worked. It is as though to remain relevant and well-funded, that group steering autism research through the behavioral diagnostic-to-treatment pipeline, persists in neglecting the physiological issues.

The stratification of Autism revealed by the gene pool under consideration underscores the need to seriously consider the somatic-sensory-motor issues in the spectrum. This spectrum of disorders today includes diseases of known origins (e.g., Timothy Syndrome, SYNGAP1, SHANK3 deletion syndrome, Fragile X, Cerebral Palsy and Dystonia, among others) with life-threatening conditions that could seriously harm the affected child under the type of stress that a behavioral modification technique has been said to bring to their nervous systems [54,84,92].

This work revealed a compact set of top genes shared by SFARI-Autism and all diseases demonstrating that they too share tissues critical for (i) somatic-sensory-motor functioning, (ii) memory and cognition and (iii) systemic self-regulation. This compact set of genes for each of these functions in (i)–(iii) underly all critical physiological ingredients for social communication and smooth, well-coordinated actions. These basic functions are essential to all human autonomic, involuntary, and voluntary behaviors. As such, they should not be sidelined when recommending and selecting treatments for Autism. I provided a distance from each disorder to SFARI-Autism based on the genes' expression on these 54 tissues defined by GETx, in the hopes of offering new ways to converge to truly personalized interventions that agree with the individual's physiological phenotype and with the endophenotype of a genetically informed group.

I concluded from these analyses that the highly publicized exponential rate in prevalence reported by the US CDC surveillance network is a myth. This myth has been built by broadening and shifting the criteria over time and by allowing diseases of known etiology be part of the Autism spectrum. The increase in neurodevelopmental disabilities is real, as evidenced by the compact set of genes identified to be common to SFARI-Autism and all other diseases under consideration. All these genes play a fundamental role on the development of synapses via proteins that are necessary for channels functioning and neurotransmitters balance, neuronal differentiation, the formation of circuits and networks, etc., during neurodevelopment [93]. Yet, these disorders exist independent of Autism. Calling them Autism, under the current definition of inappropriate social behaviors may be doing more harm than benefit. The current model stigmatizes the affected individuals [58], their families and negatively impacts the entire ecosystem inclusive of research, services and education, by promoting an erroneous perception of Autism as a behavioral issue [85]. By neglecting the physiology of the disorders that make up Autism today, the current approach skews the therapy recommendations for Autism in ways that may in fact harm their nascent nervous systems, induce trauma, and lower quality of life.

Given these results, I invite rethinking the epidemiology of autism spectrum disorders, to go beyond the behavioral diagnosis when surveying the spectrum to estimate prevalence. I also offer a new avenue to adapt the platform of Precision Medicine to Autism and disclose the implications of these results for the design of truly personalized therapies aimed at helping the affected individuals become an integral part of society.

4.5. The Importance of Reframing Autism under the Precision Medicine Paradigm

This notion of personalized medicine for Autism that I have proposed [25,48], contrasts with the current behavioral diagnosis-to-treatment pipeline that discourages stratification of Autism and advocates for a general (one-size-fits-all) model of behavioral modification. Indeed, the last study from the U.S. National Academy of Science (NAS) considering how to educate autistic children, recommended that Autism shall not be stratified [13]. Since then, practice and services do not distinguish e.g., between a child with Cerebral Palsy and a child with ADHD. Both receive the Autism diagnosis, and both will receive a form of behavioral modification to reshape social behaviors in compliance with a set of social norms that bear no scientific empirical evidence for their recommendations. As mentioned, such imposed norms were never informed, in any way, by the nervous systems physiology [9]. The accreditation programs enabling such behavioral diagnoses and interventions in fact lack training on basic neuroscience (https://accreditation.abainternational.org/apply/accreditation-standards.aspx (accessed on 28 October 2021). https://www.wpspublish.com/ados-2-autism-diagnostic-observation-schedule-second-edition (accessed on 28 October 2021)). In the US, these treatments will be administered at the school and the home, under a type of insurance coverage that other therapies do not have.

Our results show that contrary to the recommendations of the 2001 NAS study, such stratification is not only possible today, but more importantly, it is much needed to help guide and inform the design of new targeted therapies for Autism. Such new therapies could be truly personalized to address phenotypic features of the CNS, including tissues linked to self-regulating systemic structures, memory, cognition, and motor control. They would consider the physiology of numerous networks in the human brain-body complex, serving as the building blocks of all behaviors.

The methods used in this work are rather simple and parsimonious. They also rely on open access data sets. These sets are reliable and provide the grounds for reproducibility of this and related works [25,48]. I encourage the community to stratify Autism into the appropriate phenotypes with capabilities, predispositions and needs causally linked to the genetic origins of each subtype. Continuing the blanket approach also misses three important revolutions of the 21st Century: the genomic, the neuroscience and the wearables sensors revolution. The latter brings a level of precision to analyze continuous streams of behaviors beyond the limits of the naked eye, capable of automatically separating genetic-based disorders from natural, simple behaviors like walking and yet uncovering individual stochastic signatures of the person's biorhythms with causal dynamics [17].

If we follow the medical and physiological scientific path, we will be able to advance Autism research, treatments, and services. But if we continue to follow the circular behaviorist approach, we will not make headways in identifying personalized targeted treatments. Worse yet, this antiquated approach, dating back to Skinner's ideas of the 1950s, developed for research involving pigeons and rats, will continue to cause trauma to the individual in the spectrum. How come such methods for use with animals were translated to human children, without providing any validated scientific evidence that they would work in humas? Such methods violate the natural autonomy of nascent nervous systems and go against the development of social agency [31,94]. The current generation of adults that underwent such horror has informed us of this outcome. They have created the neurodiverse movement to alert researchers of the dangers of applying behaviorism to human babies in early intervention programs and throughout school age.

An alternative route to the current research paradigm in Autism is possible, by leveraging the work from other fields of science and engineering, and by stratifying the broad spectrum that otherwise purportedly keeps exponentially growing [1,58]. Contrary to archaic recommendations from behaviorists [13], here I show that Autism can and should be stratified to take the first steps toward a paradigm shift toward *Precision Autism*.

Supplementary Materials: The following are available online at https://www.mdpi.com/article/10.3390/jpm11111119/s1, Figure S1: Colormaps of top 20 genes expressed in 54 tissues at the intersection of SFARI-Autism and other disorders-I, Figure S2: Colormaps of top 20 genes expressed in 54 tissues at the intersection of SFARI-Autism and other disorders-II, Figure S3: Colormaps of top 20 genes expressed in 54 tissues at the intersection of SFARI-Autism and another disorders-III, Figures S4–S6 colormaps of genes shared between SFARI-Autism and other disorders, maximally expressed in brain tissues and tissues linked to cardiac, smooth and skeletal muscles across disorders. Text files list the genes at the intersection of SFARI-Autism and other disorders.

Funding: This research was funded by New Jersey Governor's Council for the Medical Research and Treatments of Autism, grant number CAUT15APL038.

Institutional Review Board Statement: Not applicable.

Informed Consent Statement: Not Applicable.

Data Availability Statement: Data supporting the results can be found at https://www.sfari.org/resource/sfari-gene/ (accessed on 28 October 2021), https://gtexportal.org/home/ (accessed on 28 October 2021) and https://www.disgenet.org/ (accessed on 28 October 2021).

Acknowledgments: I support open access data repositories SFARI, GTEx and DisGeNET and OMIM used in this study.

Conflicts of Interest: The authors declare no conflict of interest.

References

1. Maenner, M.J.; Shaw, K.A.; Baio, J.; Washington, A.; Patrick, M.; DiRienzo, M.; Christensen, D.L.; Wiggins, L.D.; Pettygrove, S.; Andrews, J.G.; et al. Prevalence of Autism Spectrum Disorder Among Children Aged 8 Years—Autism and Developmental Disabilities Monitoring Network, 11 Sites, United States, 2016. *MMWR Surveill. Summ.* **2020**, *69*, 1–12. [CrossRef] [PubMed]
2. Mandy, W.; Chilvers, R.; Chowdhury, U.; Salter, G.; Seigal, A.; Skuse, D. Sex differences in autism spectrum disorder: Evidence from a large sample of children and adolescents. *J. Autism Dev. Disord.* **2012**, *42*, 1304–1313. [CrossRef] [PubMed]
3. Russell, G.; Stapley, S.; Newlove-Delgado, T.; Salmon, A.; White, R.; Warren, F.; Pearson, A.; Ford, T. Time trends in autism diagnosis over 20 years: A UK population-based cohort study. *J. Child Psychol. Psychiatry* **2021**, *69*, 1–12. [CrossRef]
4. Torres, E.B.; Isenhower, R.W.; Yanovich, P.; Rehrig, G.; Stigler, K.; Nurnberger, J.; Jose, J.V. Strategies to develop putative biomarkers to characterize the female phenotype with autism spectrum disorders. *J. Neurophysiol.* **2013**, *110*, 1646–1662. [CrossRef]
5. Torres, E.B.; Denisova, K. Motor noise is rich signal in autism research and pharmacological treatments. *Sci. Rep.* **2016**, *6*, 37422. [CrossRef]
6. Torres, E.B.; Nguyen, J.; Mistry, S.; Whyatt, C.; Kalampratsidou, V.; Kolevzon, A. Characterization of the Statistical Signatures of Micro-Movements Underlying Natural Gait Patterns in Children with Phelan McDermid Syndrome: Towards Precision-Phenotyping of Behavior in ASD. *Front. Integr. Neurosci.* **2016**, *10*, 22. [CrossRef]
7. Torres, E.B.; Mistry, S.; Caballero, C.; Whyatt, C.P. Stochastic Signatures of Involuntary Head Micro-movements Can Be Used to Classify Females of ABIDE into Different Subtypes of Neurodevelopmental Disorders. *Front. Integr. Neurosci.* **2017**, *11*, 10. [CrossRef] [PubMed]
8. Bokadia, H.; Rai, R.; Torres, E.B. Digitized Autism Observation Diagnostic Schedule: Social Interactions beyond the Limits of the Naked Eye. *J. Pers. Med.* **2020**, *10*, 159. [CrossRef] [PubMed]
9. Torres, E.B.; Rai, R.; Mistry, S.; Gupta, B. Hidden Aspects of the Research ADOS Are Bound to Affect Autism Science. *Neural Comput.* **2020**, *32*, 515–561. [CrossRef] [PubMed]

10. Lord, C.; Risi, S.; Lambrecht, L.; Cook, E.H., Jr.; Leventhal, B.L.; DiLavore, P.C.; Pickles, A.; Rutter, M. The autism diagnostic observation schedule-generic: A standard measure of social and communication deficits associated with the spectrum of autism. *J. Autism Dev. Disord.* **2000**, *30*, 205–223. [CrossRef]
11. American Psychiatric Association. *Diagnostic and Statistical Manual of Mental Disorders*, 5th ed.; American Psychiatric Association: Arlington, VA, USA, 2013. [CrossRef]
12. Mottron, L. A radical change in our autism research strategy is needed: Back to prototypes. *Autism Res.* **2021**, *14*, 2213–2220. [CrossRef]
13. Council, N.R. *Educating Children with Autism*; National Academy of Science: Washington, DC, USA, 2001.
14. Constantino, J.N. Response to "A Radical Change in Our Autism Research Strategy is Needed: Back to Prototypes" by Mottron et al. *Autism Res.* **2021**, *14*, 2221–2223. [CrossRef]
15. Gotham, K.; Pickles, A.; Lord, C. Standardizing ADOS scores for a measure of severity in autism spectrum disorders. *J. Autism Dev. Disord.* **2009**, *39*, 693–705. [CrossRef] [PubMed]
16. Esler, A.N.; Bal, V.H.; Guthrie, W.; Wetherby, A.; Ellis Weismer, S.; Lord, C. The Autism Diagnostic Observation Schedule, Toddler Module: Standardized Severity Scores. *J. Autism Dev. Disord.* **2015**, *45*, 2704–2720. [CrossRef] [PubMed]
17. Bermperidis, T.; Rai, R.; Ryu, J.; Torres, E.B. Optimal Time Lags from Causal Prediction Model Help Stratify and Forecast Nervous System Pathology. *Sci. Rep.* **2021**, *11*, 20904. [CrossRef]
18. Sanger, T.D.; Kukke, S.N. Abnormalities of tactile sensory function in children with dystonic and diplegic cerebral palsy. *J. Child. Neurol.* **2007**, *22*, 289–293. [CrossRef] [PubMed]
19. Pham, R.; Mol, B.W.; Gecz, J.; MacLennan, A.H.; MacLennan, S.C.; Corbett, M.A.; van Eyk, C.L.; Webber, D.L.; Palmer, L.J.; Berry, J.G. Definition and diagnosis of cerebral palsy in genetic studies: A systematic review. *Dev. Med. Child. Neurol.* **2020**, *62*, 1024–1030. [CrossRef]
20. Lin, J.P.; Nardocci, N. Recognizing the Common Origins of Dystonia and the Development of Human Movement: A Manifesto of Unmet Needs in Isolated Childhood Dystonias. *Front. Neurol.* **2016**, *7*, 226. [CrossRef] [PubMed]
21. Xiao, R.; Zhong, H.; Li, X.; Ma, Y.; Zhang, R.; Wang, L.; Zang, Z.; Fan, X. Abnormal Cerebellar Development Is Involved in Dystonia-Like Behaviors and Motor Dysfunction of Autistic BTBR Mice. *Front. Cell Dev. Biol.* **2020**, *8*, 231. [CrossRef] [PubMed]
22. Geurts, H.M.; Grasman, R.P.; Verte, S.; Oosterlaan, J.; Roeyers, H.; van Kammen, S.M.; Sergeant, J.A. Intra-individual variability in ADHD, autism spectrum disorders and Tourette's syndrome. *Neuropsychologia* **2008**, *46*, 3030–3041. [CrossRef] [PubMed]
23. Zablotsky, B.; Bramlett, M.D.; Blumberg, S.J. The Co-Occurrence of Autism Spectrum Disorder in Children With ADHD. *J. Atten. Disord.* **2020**, *24*, 94–103. [CrossRef]
24. Bell, L.; Wittkowski, A.; Hare, D.J. Movement Disorders and Syndromic Autism: A Systematic Review. *J. Autism Dev. Disord.* **2019**, *49*, 54–67. [CrossRef] [PubMed]
25. Torres, E.B. Reframing Psychiatry for Precision Medicine. *J. Pers. Med.* **2020**, *10*, 144. [CrossRef] [PubMed]
26. Hagerman, R.; Hoem, G.; Hagerman, P. Fragile X and autism: Intertwined at the molecular level leading to targeted treatments. *Mol. Autism* **2010**, *1*, 12. [CrossRef] [PubMed]
27. Wang, L.W.; Berry-Kravis, E.; Hagerman, R.J. Fragile X: Leading the way for targeted treatments in autism. *Neurotherapeutics* **2010**, *7*, 264–274. [CrossRef]
28. Torres, E.B.; Brincker, M.; Isenhower, R.W.; Yanovich, P.; Stigler, K.A.; Nurnberger, J.I.; Metaxas, D.N.; Jose, J.V. Autism: The micro-movement perspective. *Front. Integr. Neurosci.* **2013**, *7*, 32. [CrossRef] [PubMed]
29. Torres, E.B. Atypical signatures of motor variability found in an individual with ASD. *Neurocase* **2011**, *19*, 150–165. [CrossRef] [PubMed]
30. Torres, E.B.; Caballero, C.; Mistry, S. Aging with Autism Departs Greatly from Typical Aging. *Sensors* **2020**, *20*, 572. [CrossRef]
31. Torres, E.B.; Whyatt, C. *Autism: The Movement Sensing Perspective*; CRC Press/Taylor & Francis Group: Boca Raton, FL, USA, 2018; p. xviii. 386p.
32. Whyatt, C.P.; Torres, E.B. Autism Research: An Objective Quantitative Review of Progress and Focus Between 1994 and 2015. *Front. Psychol.* **2018**, *9*, 1526. [CrossRef] [PubMed]
33. Hawgood, S.; Hook-Barnard, I.G.; O'Brien, T.C.; Yamamoto, K.R. Precision medicine: Beyond the inflection point. *Sci. Transl. Med.* **2015**, *7*, 300ps317. [CrossRef] [PubMed]
34. Scott, W.K.; Nance, M.A.; Watts, R.L.; Hubble, J.P.; Koller, W.C.; Lyons, K.; Pahwa, R.; Stern, M.B.; Colcher, A.; Hiner, B.C.; et al. Complete genomic screen in Parkinson disease: Evidence for multiple genes. *JAMA* **2001**, *286*, 2239–2244. [CrossRef] [PubMed]
35. Klein, C.; Westenberger, A. Genetics of Parkinson's disease. *Cold Spring Harb. Perspect. Med.* **2012**, *2*, a008888. [CrossRef] [PubMed]
36. Starkstein, S.; Gellar, S.; Parlier, M.; Payne, L.; Piven, J. High rates of parkinsonism in adults with autism. *J. Neurodev. Disord.* **2015**, *7*, 29. [CrossRef] [PubMed]
37. Pahlman, M.; Gillberg, C.; Wentz, E.; Himmelmann, K. Autism spectrum disorder and attention-deficit/hyperactivity disorder in children with cerebral palsy: Results from screening in a population-based group. *Eur. Child. Adolesc. Psychiatry* **2020**, *29*, 1569–1579. [CrossRef] [PubMed]
38. Riccio, M.P.; Siracusano, R.; d'Alessandro, I.; Marino, M.; Bravaccio, C. Dystonic Movement Disorder as Symptom of Catatonia in Autism Spectrum Disorder. *Case Rep. Psychiatry* **2020**, *2020*, 8832075. [CrossRef]

39. Dell'Osso, L.; Carpita, B.; Cremone, I.M.; Gesi, C.; D'Ermo, A.; De Iorio, G.; Massimetti, G.; Aguglia, E.; Bucci, P.; Carpiniello, B.; et al. Autism spectrum in patients with schizophrenia: Correlations with real-life functioning, resilience, and coping styles. *CNS Spectr.* **2021**, 1–11. [CrossRef]
40. Gecz, J.; Berry, J.G. Cerebral palsy with autism and ADHD: Time to pay attention. *Dev. Med. Child. Neurol.* **2021**, *63*, 247–248. [CrossRef]
41. Ghaziuddin, M.; Ghaziuddin, N. Bipolar Disorder and Psychosis in Autism. *Psychiatr. Clin.* **2021**, *44*, 1–9. [CrossRef]
42. Pan, P.Y.; Bolte, S.; Kaur, P.; Jamil, S.; Jonsson, U. Neurological disorders in autism: A systematic review and meta-analysis. *Autism* **2021**, *25*, 812–830. [CrossRef]
43. Torres, E.B.; Yanovich, P.; Metaxas, D.N. Give spontaneity and self-discovery a chance in ASD: Spontaneous peripheral limb variability as a proxy to evoke centrally driven intentional acts. *Front. Integr. Neurosci.* **2013**, *7*, 46. [CrossRef]
44. Wu, D.; Jose, J.V.; Nurnberger, J.I.; Torres, E.B. A Biomarker Characterizing Neurodevelopment with applications in Autism. *Sci. Rep.* **2018**, *8*, 614. [CrossRef] [PubMed]
45. Caballero, C.; Mistry, S.; Vero, J.; Torres, E.B. Characterization of Noise Signatures of Involuntary Head Motion in the Autism Brain Imaging Data Exchange Repository. *Front. Integr. Neurosci.* **2018**, *12*, 7. [CrossRef] [PubMed]
46. Caballero, C.; Mistry, S.; Torres, E.B. Age-Dependent Statistical Changes of Involuntary Head Motion Signatures Across Autism and Controls of the ABIDE Repository. *Front. Integr. Neurosci.* **2020**, *14*, 23. [CrossRef]
47. Consortium, G.T. The GTEx Consortium atlas of genetic regulatory effects across human tissues. *Science* **2020**, *369*, 1318–1330. [CrossRef] [PubMed]
48. Torres, E.B.; Isenhower, R.W.; Nguyen, J.; Whyatt, C.; Nurnberger, J.I.; Jose, J.V.; Silverstein, S.M.; Papathomas, T.V.; Sage, J.; Cole, J. Toward Precision Psychiatry: Statistical Platform for the Personalized Characterization of Natural Behaviors. *Front. Neurol.* **2016**, *7*, 8. [CrossRef]
49. Haruvi-Lamdan, N.; Horesh, D.; Golan, O. PTSD and autism spectrum disorder: Co-morbidity, gaps in research, and potential shared mechanisms. *Psychol. Trauma* **2018**, *10*, 290–299. [CrossRef] [PubMed]
50. Pettersson, E.; Lichtenstein, P.; Larsson, H.; Song, J.; Attention Deficit/Hyperactivity Disorder Working Group of the iPSYCH-Broad-PGC Consortium; Autism Spectrum Disorder Working Group of the iPSYCH-Broad-PGC Consortium; Agrawal, A.; Borglum, A.D.; Bulik, C.M.; Daly, M.J.; et al. Genetic influences on eight psychiatric disorders based on family data of 4 408 646 full and half-siblings, and genetic data of 333 748 cases and controls. *Psychol. Med.* **2019**, *49*, 1166–1173. [CrossRef] [PubMed]
51. Monge, G. Memoire sur la Theorie des Deblais et des Remblais. In *Histoire de l' Academie Royale des Science; Avec les Memoires de Mathematique et de Physique*; De L'imprimerie Royale: Paris, France, 1781.
52. Rubner, Y.; Tomasi, C.; Guibas, L.J. Metric for Distributions with Applications to Image Databases. In Proceedings of the ICCV, Bombay, India, 4–7 January 1998.
53. Stolfi, J.; Guibas, L.J. The earth mover's distance as a metric for image retrieval. *Int. J. Comput. Vis.* **2000**, *40*, 99–121.
54. Hoover, D.W.; Kaufman, J. Adverse childhood experiences in children with autism spectrum disorder. *Curr. Opin. Psychiatry* **2018**, *31*, 128–132. [CrossRef]
55. Stack, A.; Lucyshyn, J. Autism Spectrum Disorder and the Experience of Traumatic Events: Review of the Current Literature to Inform Modifications to a Treatment Model for Children with Autism. *J. Autism Dev. Disord.* **2019**, *49*, 1613–1625. [CrossRef]
56. Yousef Yengej, F.A.; van Royen-Kerkhof, A.; Derksen, R.; Fritsch-Stork, R.D.E. The development of offspring from mothers with systemic lupus erythematosus. A systematic review. *Autoimmun. Rev.* **2017**, *16*, 701–711. [CrossRef]
57. Zhu, Z.; Tang, S.; Deng, X.; Wang, Y. Maternal Systemic Lupus Erythematosus, Rheumatoid Arthritis, and Risk for Autism Spectrum Disorders in Offspring: A Meta-analysis. *J. Autism Dev. Disord.* **2020**, *50*, 2852–2859. [CrossRef]
58. Blaxill, M.; Rogers, T.; Nevison, C. Autism Tsunami: The Impact of Rising Prevalence on the Societal Cost of Autism in the United States. *J. Autism Dev. Disord.* **2021**. [CrossRef]
59. Bradbury, K.R.; Anderberg, E.I.; Huang-Storms, L.; Vasile, I.; Greene, R.K.; Duvall, S.W. Co-occurring Down Syndrome and Autism Spectrum Disorder: Cognitive, Adaptive, and Behavioral Characteristics. *J. Autism Dev. Disord.* **2021**. [CrossRef]
60. Salcedo-Arellano, M.J.; Cabal-Herrera, A.M.; Punatar, R.H.; Clark, C.J.; Romney, C.A.; Hagerman, R.J. Overlapping Molecular Pathways Leading to Autism Spectrum Disorders, Fragile X Syndrome, and Targeted Treatments. *Neurotherapeutics* **2021**, *18*, 265–283. [CrossRef]
61. Tylee, D.S.; Sun, J.; Hess, J.L.; Tahir, M.A.; Sharma, E.; Malik, R.; Worrall, B.B.; Levine, A.J.; Martinson, J.J.; Nejentsev, S.; et al. Genetic correlations among psychiatric and immune-related phenotypes based on genome-wide association data. *Am. J. Med. Genet. B Neuropsychiatr. Genet.* **2018**, *177*, 641–657. [CrossRef] [PubMed]
62. Swanberg, S.E.; Nagarajan, R.P.; Peddada, S.; Yasui, D.H.; LaSalle, J.M. Reciprocal co-regulation of EGR2 and MECP2 is disrupted in Rett syndrome and autism. *Hum. Mol. Genet.* **2009**, *18*, 525–534. [CrossRef]
63. Platt, R.J.; Zhou, Y.; Slaymaker, I.M.; Shetty, A.S.; Weisbach, N.R.; Kim, J.A.; Sharma, J.; Desai, M.; Sood, S.; Kempton, H.R.; et al. Chd8 Mutation Leads to Autistic-like Behaviors and Impaired Striatal Circuits. *Cell Rep.* **2017**, *19*, 335–350. [CrossRef] [PubMed]
64. Talkowski, M.E.; Rosenfeld, J.A.; Blumenthal, I.; Pillalamarri, V.; Chiang, C.; Heilbut, A.; Ernst, C.; Hanscom, C.; Rossin, E.; Lindgren, A.M.; et al. Sequencing chromosomal abnormalities reveals neurodevelopmental loci that confer risk across diagnostic boundaries. *Cell* **2012**, *149*, 525–537. [CrossRef] [PubMed]
65. Mondal, K.; Ramachandran, D.; Patel, V.C.; Hagen, K.R.; Bose, P.; Cutler, D.J.; Zwick, M.E. Excess variants in AFF2 detected by massively parallel sequencing of males with autism spectrum disorder. *Hum. Mol. Genet.* **2012**, *21*, 4356–4364. [CrossRef]

66. Hiatt, S.M.; Thompson, M.L.; Prokop, J.W.; Lawlor, J.M.J.; Gray, D.E.; Bebin, E.M.; Rinne, T.; Kempers, M.; Pfundt, R.; van Bon, B.W.; et al. Deleterious Variation in BRSK2 Associates with a Neurodevelopmental Disorder. *Am. J. Hum. Genet.* **2019**, *104*, 701–708. [CrossRef]
67. Ciammola, A.; Carrera, P.; Di Fonzo, A.; Sassone, J.; Villa, R.; Poletti, B.; Ferrari, M.; Girotti, F.; Monfrini, E.; Buongarzone, G.; et al. X-linked Parkinsonism with Intellectual Disability caused by novel mutations and somatic mosaicism in RAB39B gene. *Parkinsonism Relat. Disord.* **2017**, *44*, 142–146. [CrossRef] [PubMed]
68. Giannandrea, M.; Bianchi, V.; Mignogna, M.L.; Sirri, A.; Carrabino, S.; D'Elia, E.; Vecellio, M.; Russo, S.; Cogliati, F.; Larizza, L.; et al. Mutations in the small GTPase gene RAB39B are responsible for X-linked mental retardation associated with autism, epilepsy, and macrocephaly. *Am. J. Hum. Genet.* **2010**, *86*, 185–195. [CrossRef] [PubMed]
69. Lesage, S.; Bras, J.; Cormier-Dequaire, F.; Condroyer, C.; Nicolas, A.; Darwent, L.; Guerreiro, R.; Majounie, E.; Federoff, M.; Heutink, P.; et al. Loss-of-function mutations in RAB39B are associated with typical early-onset Parkinson disease. *Neurol. Genet.* **2015**, *1*, e9. [CrossRef] [PubMed]
70. Wilson, G.R.; Sim, J.C.; McLean, C.; Giannandrea, M.; Galea, C.A.; Riseley, J.R.; Stephenson, S.E.; Fitzpatrick, E.; Haas, S.A.; Pope, K.; et al. Mutations in RAB39B cause X-linked intellectual disability and early-onset Parkinson disease with alpha-synuclein pathology. *Am. J. Hum. Genet.* **2014**, *95*, 729–735. [CrossRef] [PubMed]
71. Hansen, F.H.; Skjorringe, T.; Yasmeen, S.; Arends, N.V.; Sahai, M.A.; Erreger, K.; Andreassen, T.F.; Holy, M.; Hamilton, P.J.; Neergheen, V.; et al. Missense dopamine transporter mutations associate with adult parkinsonism and ADHD. *J. Clin. Investig.* **2014**, *124*, 3107–3120. [CrossRef] [PubMed]
72. Hamilton, P.J.; Campbell, N.G.; Sharma, S.; Erreger, K.; Herborg Hansen, F.; Saunders, C.; Belovich, A.N.; Consortium, N.A.A.S.; Sahai, M.A.; Cook, E.H.; et al. De novo mutation in the dopamine transporter gene associates dopamine dysfunction with autism spectrum disorder. *Mol. Psychiatry* **2013**, *18*, 1315–1323. [CrossRef] [PubMed]
73. Doege, C.A.; Inoue, K.; Yamashita, T.; Rhee, D.B.; Travis, S.; Fujita, R.; Guarnieri, P.; Bhagat, G.; Vanti, W.B.; Shih, A.; et al. Early-stage epigenetic modification during somatic cell reprogramming by Parp1 and Tet2. *Nature* **2012**, *488*, 652–655. [CrossRef] [PubMed]
74. Guallar, D.; Bi, X.; Pardavila, J.A.; Huang, X.; Saenz, C.; Shi, X.; Zhou, H.; Faiola, F.; Ding, J.; Haruehanroengra, P.; et al. RNA-dependent chromatin targeting of TET2 for endogenous retrovirus control in pluripotent stem cells. *Nat. Genet.* **2018**, *50*, 443–451. [CrossRef] [PubMed]
75. Shovlin, C.L.; Simmonds, H.A.; Fairbanks, L.D.; Deacock, S.J.; Hughes, J.M.; Lechler, R.I.; Webster, A.D.; Sun, X.M.; Webb, J.C.; Soutar, A.K. Adult onset immunodeficiency caused by inherited adenosine deaminase deficiency. *J. Immunol.* **1994**, *153*, 2331–2339. [PubMed]
76. Hla, T.; Neilson, K. Human cyclooxygenase-2 cDNA. *Proc. Natl. Acad. Sci. USA* **1992**, *89*, 7384–7388. [CrossRef] [PubMed]
77. Samad, T.A.; Moore, K.A.; Sapirstein, A.; Billet, S.; Allchorne, A.; Poole, S.; Bonventre, J.V.; Woolf, C.J. Interleukin-1beta-mediated induction of Cox-2 in the CNS contributes to inflammatory pain hypersensitivity. *Nature* **2001**, *410*, 471–475. [CrossRef] [PubMed]
78. Tamura, S.; Morikawa, Y.; Iwanishi, H.; Hisaoka, T.; Senba, E. Foxp1 gene expression in projection neurons of the mouse striatum. *Neuroscience* **2004**, *124*, 261–267. [CrossRef] [PubMed]
79. Hisaoka, T.; Nakamura, Y.; Senba, E.; Morikawa, Y. The forkhead transcription factors, Foxp1 and Foxp2, identify different subpopulations of projection neurons in the mouse cerebral cortex. *Neuroscience* **2010**, *166*, 551–563. [CrossRef]
80. Precious, S.V.; Kelly, C.M.; Reddington, A.E.; Vinh, N.N.; Stickland, R.C.; Pekarik, V.; Scherf, C.; Jeyasingham, R.; Glasbey, J.; Holeiter, M.; et al. FoxP1 marks medium spiny neurons from precursors to maturity and is required for their differentiation. *Exp. Neurol.* **2016**, *282*, 9–18. [CrossRef] [PubMed]
81. Peng, J.; Zhou, Y.; Wang, K. Multiplex gene and phenotype network to characterize shared genetic pathways of epilepsy and autism. *Sci. Rep.* **2021**, *11*, 952. [CrossRef] [PubMed]
82. Liao, X.; Li, Y. Genetic associations between voltage-gated calcium channels and autism spectrum disorder: A systematic review. *Mol. Brain* **2020**, *13*, 96. [CrossRef] [PubMed]
83. Yoshino, Y.; Roy, B.; Dwivedi, Y. Altered miRNA landscape of the anterior cingulate cortex is associated with potential loss of key neuronal functions in depressed brain. *Eur. Neuropsychopharmacol.* **2020**, *40*, 70–84. [CrossRef] [PubMed]
84. Bottema-Beutel, K.; Crowley, S.; Sandbank, M.; Woynaroski, T.G. Adverse event reporting in intervention research for young autistic children. *Autism* **2021**, *25*, 322–335. [CrossRef] [PubMed]
85. Thompson-Hodgetts, S.; Labonte, C.; Mazumder, R.; Phelan, S. Helpful or harmful? A scoping review of perceptions and outcomes of autism diagnostic disclosure to others. *Res. Autism Spectr. Disord.* **2020**, *77*, 101598. [CrossRef]
86. Chen, Y.Y.; Chen, Y.L.; Gau, S.S. Suicidality in Children with Elevated Autistic Traits. *Autism Res.* **2020**, *13*, 1811–1821. [CrossRef] [PubMed]
87. Costa, A.P.; Loor, C.; Steffgen, G. Suicidality in Adults with Autism Spectrum Disorder: The Role of Depressive Symptomatology, Alexithymia, and Antidepressants. *J. Autism Dev. Disord.* **2020**, *50*, 3585–3597. [CrossRef]
88. Hand, B.N.; Benevides, T.W.; Carretta, H.J. Suicidal Ideation and Self-inflicted Injury in Medicare Enrolled Autistic Adults with and Without Co-occurring Intellectual Disability. *J. Autism Dev. Disord.* **2020**, *50*, 3489–3495. [CrossRef]
89. Broderick, A.A.; Roscigno, R. Autism, Inc.: The Autism Industrial Complex. *J. Disabil. Stud. Educ.* **2021**, 1–25. [CrossRef]

90. Bottema-Beutel, K.; Crowley, S.; Sandbank, M.; Woynaroski, T.G. Research Review: Conflicts of Interest (COIs) in autism early intervention research—A meta-analysis of COI influences on intervention effects. *J. Child. Psychol. Psychiatry* **2021**, *62*, 5–15. [CrossRef] [PubMed]
91. Dawson, M.; Fletcher-Watson, S. Commentary: What conflicts of interest tell us about autism intervention research-a commentary on Bottema-Beutel et al. *J. Child Psychol. Psychiatry* **2021**, *62*, 16–18. [CrossRef] [PubMed]
92. Sandbank, M.; Bottema-Beutel, K.; Crowley, S.; Cassidy, M.; Dunham, K.; Feldman, J.I.; Crank, J.; Albarran, S.A.; Raj, S.; Mahbub, P.; et al. Project AIM: Autism intervention meta-analysis for studies of young children. *Psychol. Bull.* **2020**, *146*, 1–29. [CrossRef]
93. Carroll, L.; Braeutigam, S.; Dawes, J.M.; Krsnik, Z.; Kostovic, I.; Coutinho, E.; Dewing, J.M.; Horton, C.A.; Gomez-Nicola, D.; Menassa, D.A. Autism Spectrum Disorders: Multiple Routes to, and Multiple Consequences of, Abnormal Synaptic Function and Connectivity. *Neuroscientist* **2021**, *27*, 10–29. [CrossRef] [PubMed]
94. Torres, E.B. *Objective Biometric Methods for the Diagnosis and Treatment of Nervous System Disorders*; Academic Press: London, UK, 2018; 568p.

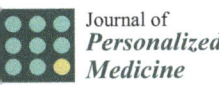

Article

Personalized Biometrics of Physical Pain Agree with Psychophysics by Participants with Sensory over Responsivity

Jihye Ryu [1], Tami Bar-Shalita [2], Yelena Granovsky [3], Irit Weissman-Fogel [4] and Elizabeth B. Torres [1,5,*]

1. Rutgers University Center for Cognitive Science, Psychology Department, Rutgers University, Piscataway, NJ 08854, USA; jihyeryu@mednet.ucla.edu
2. Department of Occupational Therapy, School of Health Professions, Faculty of Medicine, Sagol School of Neuroscience, Tel Aviv University, Tel Aviv 6997801, Israel; tbshalita@post.tau.ac.il
3. Laboratory of Clinical Neurophysiology, Department of Neurology, Faculty of Medicine, Rambam Health Care Campus, Technion, Haifa 3109601, Israel; y_granovsky@rambam.health.gov.il
4. Physical Therapy Department, Faculty of Social Welfare and Health Sciences, University of Haifa, Haifa 3498838, Israel; ifogel@univ.haifa.ac.il
5. Center for Biomedicine Imaging and Modeling, Computer Science Department, Rutgers University, Piscataway, NJ 08854, USA
* Correspondence: ebtorres@psych.rutgers.edu

Abstract: The study of pain requires a balance between subjective methods that rely on self-reports and complementary objective biometrics that ascertain physical signals associated with subjective accounts. There are at present no objective scales that enable the personalized assessment of pain, as most work involving electrophysiology rely on summary statistics from a priori theoretical population assumptions. Along these lines, recent work has provided evidence of differences in pain sensations between participants with Sensory Over Responsivity (SOR) and controls. While these analyses are useful to understand pain across groups, there remains a need to quantify individual differences more precisely in a personalized manner. Here we offer new methods to characterize pain using the moment-by-moment standardized fluctuations in EEG brain activity centrally reflecting the person's experiencing temperature-based stimulation at the periphery. This type of gross data is often disregarded as noise, yet here we show its utility to characterize the lingering sensation of discomfort raising to the level of pain, individually, for each participant. We show fundamental differences between the SOR group in relation to controls and provide an objective account of pain congruent with the subjective self-reported data. This offers the potential to build a standardized scale useful to profile pain levels in a personalized manner across the general population.

Keywords: EEG; pain biometrics; stochastic analyses; micro-movements spikes; sensory over responsivity; standardized scale; personalized pain

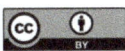

1. Introduction

The peripheral nervous systems include an interconnected network of afferent nerve fibers carrying information from the skin to the spinal cord and onto the brain [1]. This flow of activity can be modeled as it updates the brain moment by moment, reflecting the trajectories of our bodies in motion [2,3] or of the fluctuations in bodily signals at rest [4–7], within a given environment where sensory input is processed and integrated with ongoing movements making up intended [8,9] or spontaneous [10] behavioral states. The afferent fibers from the periphery carry information about touch, pressure and movements sensed by the mechanoreceptors [11], while thermoreceptors and nociceptors process information about temperature and pain, respectively [1,12]. Collectively, they give rise to the sense of touch, which is important to manipulate objects [13], to control our movements [14], to gain a sense of body ownership [15] and affection [16], and to develop and maintain our overall psychological and social wellbeing [17].

The experience of pain (i.e., its subjective perception) is comprised of sensory, affective-emotive, and cognitive processes of a noxious input. Pain experience can be measured in the lab applying quantitative sensory testing, namely inducing measurable pain stimuli of different modalities (e.g., heat, pressure), while subjects are required to rate their pain intensity/unpleasantness using various pain scales (e.g., visual analog scale, numerical rating scale). Thus, the individual's experience of pain though seemingly centrally processed, it is evoked at the periphery using different experimental assays. These may include (among others) the physical experience of sustained pressure [18,19] or sustained temperature [20–23], carried along peripheral afferent nerves to the central nervous systems, which is comprised of the spinal cord and the brain.

In recent years, we have learned about the central processing of movement-related reafference from a special participant (Ian Waterman, IW) who experienced a viral infection that killed the afferent fibers for light-touch, pressure, and movements. The infection spared the afferent fibers for pain and temperature [24–26]. IW has remastered motor control in the absence of proprioception and kinesthetic reafferent information, by sensory substituting with vision the senses of touch, pressure, and movement [27,28]. Perhaps using information about his central processing of peripheral activity during resting state [24], could help us develop new models of statistical inference and interpretations for use in other data sets. His case could help us interpret resting-state data from centrally processed sensory information in other patient populations with sensory processing dysfunctions mediated by disruptions in peripheral reafferent flow [29,30].

Ian Waterman's case is interesting as fluctuations in his electroencephalographic (EEG) activity at rest revealed the presence of the exponential distribution of peak amplitudes (Figure 1). This distribution represents a memoryless random process whereby past activity does not contribute to the probabilistic prediction of future events. In this case, events refer to moment-by-moment fluctuations in signals' amplitudes and timings. We posit that these fluctuations inform the nervous systems of dynamically adaptive states, as they transition from highly variable to steady-state. Based on our prior theoretical work on kinesthetic reafference [8], we have conjectured that this type of memoryless process may impede creating a proper memory buffer to sustain activity long enough to bring it to the brain's awareness, to consciously recognize it, or to use it effectively as reference to inform and predict impending states of the system [5,8,29].

Having found in IW these patterns at rest, reflecting the variability of the signals as a renewal process in "the here and now" in the absence of movement reafference sensations, may help us characterize other states related to pain sensation in neurotypical controls. More precisely, it may also help us characterize, stochastically, the departure from this memoryless state, in cases with atypical pain sensations. We know the stochastic signatures of not sensing touch, pressure, and movement, in a person that nevertheless senses temperature and pain. As such, we may use this prior information as reference to learn how the fluctuations in EEG activity may distribute during resting state for a person who does not have severed communication between the peripheral afferent fibers and the brain, but that nevertheless reports atypical sensation of pain. We would like to assess distributions of stochastic activities related to fluctuations in EEG peak-amplitudes on participants with sensory over-responsivity (SOR), a subtype of sensory modulation dysfunction (SMD) which in turn falls under the broader umbrella of sensory processing disorder [31].

The SOR subtype of SMD manifests clinically as a condition in which stimuli that are not typically painful are perceived as abnormally irritating, unpleasant, or even reportedly painful [32], sometimes interfering with activities of daily life [33]—as measured by several clinical scales. These clinical manifestations are also consistent in laboratory experiments, measured under controlled conditions [34]. Under these controlled settings, people with SOR express discomfort and hypersensitivity to experimental manipulations in pressure or temperature, whereby the lingering sensation of evoked peripheral activity leads to the conscious expression of pain and sustained pain aftersensation centrally experienced [34].

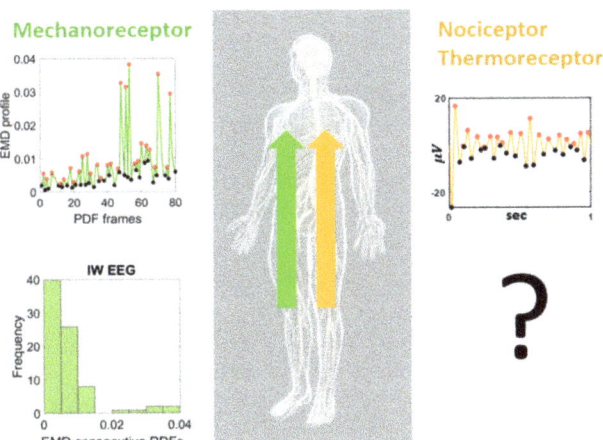

Figure 1. Proposed central characterization of lingering (pain) sensation. Special participant Ian Waterman (IW) lost his kinesthetic reafference but retained the sensations of pain and temperature. His electro-encephalographic (EEG) waveforms at rest, provide information about the shifts in probability density functions characterizing the distributions of fluctuations in peak activities in the lead electrodes with maximal clustering coefficient derived from the network of leads. Such shifts distribute exponentially, signaling a memoryless, random distribution of these activities, such that past events do not contribute to the prediction of future events. This type of distribution of his central EEG activities is congruent with the distribution of his movement-kinesthetic reafferent peripheral activities. What type of distributions could we find in individuals with intact kinesthetic reafference but sensory over-responsivity resulting in lingering sensations of temperature-induced pain?

Prior work has relied on population statistics and provided an account of full cohorts. A new detailed individualized characterization of minute fluctuations in EEG activities while experiencing pain could help us re-examine these issues to formulate a personalized account, useful to inform automatic groupings and stratifications of random draws of the population, with the overarching aim of defining a standardized scale of centrally processed pain. This would be beneficial to other disorders on a spectrum (e.g., autism, schizophrenia, and Parkinson's disease) whereby such sensory processing issues of pain abound too [35–38]. Across these various disorders of the nervous system, we need proper objective characterizations of pain sensation to complement and augment reports on the subjective sensations of pain captured by clinical inventories.

The type of analysis that we offer here, away from assumptions of theoretical population statistics, has been previously used on a characterization of stochastic variations in movement reafferent signals. This is a data-driven approach whereby we let the data reveal patterns and then, upon interpretation and inference, we propose possible lines of inquiry to pursue in future work. In our prior work, the results led to automatic clustering of the above-mentioned clinical disorders on a spectrum [39]. These in turn, have shown strong ties with other disorders of the nervous systems and various types of disruption in reafferent flow of movement information [40,41], thus allowing us to further pursue new lines of questions. Since pain and temperature share separable afferent channels from movement afference, and crosstalk can be quantified through central processing using controlled experimental assays, here we apply these new data-driven analytical methods to SOR participants who suffer from abnormally high pain sensation. We re-examine previously published EEG data [34] as well as explore pain-evoked EEG responses induced by sustained temperature in controls vs. SOR participants. We do so by analyzing the gross data commonly discarded as noise, by avoiding a priori assumptions of theoretical normal distributions of the fluctuations in EEG-waveforms' peak amplitudes. We discuss our

2. Materials and Methods

These details of the experiment have been explained in previous publications, but we report them here for completeness [34,42]. The Rutgers University Institutional Review Board approved this de-identified data sharing. The IRB committee of Rambam Health Care Campus approved this study in 2013. The IRB number is 3075, The Israeli ministry of health # HT4858.

2.1. Participants

The study included 21 healthy participants (5 males and 16 females) between the ages 18 and 40 years old recruited from a convenience sample in a laboratory database. Participants were naïve to the testing. Based on a medical survey, participants with no chronic pain history and no regular use of analgesic or psychiatric medication were included in the study. Participants with any psychological, psychosocial, metabolic, and neurological disorders were excluded from the study. This means that if the participant had a diagnosis of any of the above-mentioned disorders, they did not sign up, nor did they participate in the study.

Participants were able to communicate and understand the instructions of the study. They self-reported to be free of any pain relief medications 24 h prior and any caffeine products at least 2 h prior to the experiment, and to have had sufficient sleep the night before. Sufficient sleep means that participants did not express any complaints about sleep disturbances. We did not measure their sleep. All participants provided written consent, which was approved by the Institutional Review Board of Rambam Health Care Campus (Haifa, Israel).

Participants were categorized into two groups—sensory over responsiveness (SOR) group (n = 9, 1 male) and control group (n = 11, 3 males). The SOR group was comprised of those whose Sensory Responsive Questionnaire Intensity Scale (SRQ-IS; [43])-Aversive score exceeded 2 standard deviations from its mean. The control group was comprised of those with scores within the 2 SD from the mean. Note, the SRQ-IS is designed to clinically identify those with sensory modulation disorder and is comprised of Hedonic scores and Aversive scores [44]. The Aversive scores that were used as a criterion to categorize groups involve answering intensity levels (on a scale 1–5) on scenarios such as "Being in dark/unlit surroundings bothers me," and "Watching T.V./computer in a well-lit room bothers me." Further details of participant recruitment can be found in [34]. By using these scores, we operationalized each participant's perception of sensory experience.

2.2. Experiment

This was a block design experiment, whereby each participant performed all three conditions in blocks of trials. They sat comfortably in a quiet air-conditioned room under all 3 conditions. In the first condition, the participant was instructed to close his/her eyes and rest for 5 min. In the second and third condition, pain was administered for 5 min. Note, both conditions are identical and merely sequential in order. In each of these pain conditions, heat stimulus was applied to the participant's forearm with 8–12 s interval to simulate a pain experience. Specifically, the participant was applied with a heat stimulus by the Contact Heat-Evoked Potential Stimulator, which is a computerized thermal stimulator (Medoc Ltd. Advanced Medical Systems, Ramat Yishai, Israel). The temperature was tailored to everyone to evoke a peak pain magnitude of 50/100 (pain-50) on the numeric rating scale. Specifically, we gave 30 stimuli, ISI 8-10, baseline temperature 39 °C with destination pain 50 described in [42] +0.5 °C. After each stimulus, during ISI, subjects provided pain intensity and pain unpleasantness ratings, using the numerical rating scale. During the study, EEG signals were recorded with a 32-electrode cap (Easy Cap Q40; FMS Falk Minow Services, Herrsching, Germany) with the Quick Amp EEG System (Brain

Products GmbH, Munich, Germany). These signals were processed at 500 Hz sampling rate, with 0.15–100 Hz bandpass filter, and a notch filter at 50 Hz. The EEG signals were further preprocessed using the PrepPipeline toolbox [45], with which we referenced via a robust average reference procedure, where channels were iteratively referenced to the average signal, while bad channels, such as those showing extreme amplitudes (deviation z-score exceeds 5) or lacked correlation with any other channel (correlation less than 0.4), were excluded and interpolated in this process.

2.3. Data Analysis

2.3.1. Analyses in the Frequency Domain

For each condition, pairwise cross-coherence was computed using each of the 32 EEG channel waveforms (Figure 2A). Across the frequency range within the cross-coherence values, we extracted the maximal value within the beta and gamma bands (13–100 Hz), as this bandwidth showed to have a noticeable difference between the SOR and control groups (Figure 2B). Note, we had examined other bandwidths, as well as beta and gamma band separately, but did not find such a pattern. For that reason, we focused on the beta and gamma bands combined.

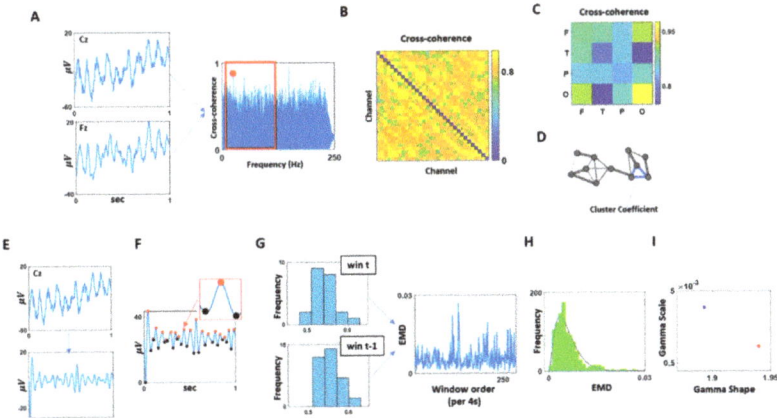

Figure 2. Data analytics pipeline. (**A**) For each pair of EEG channel combination, cross-coherence was computed, and its maximal value within the beta and gamma band (13–100 Hz) was extracted. (**B**) The maximal cross-coherence values obtained from (**A**) were used to construct an adjacency matrix of all EEG channel combinations. (**C**) EEG channel combinations were categorized by a combination of different scalp areas (F: frontal, T: temporal, P: parietal, O: occipital), and these categories' median of maximal cross-coherence values, as shown in (**B**), were computed and compared. (**D**) Based on the channel's adjacency matrix shown in (**B**), a network was constructed, where the nodes corresponded to each EEG channel, and the links corresponded to the maximal coherence values. As a measure of segregation of this network, cluster coefficients were computed and compared. (**E**) The channel with the highest cluster coefficient, computed at (**D**), was selected and its EEG waveform was band-pass filtered at 13–100 Hz. (**F**) The band-passed waveform was shifted up so that all values were positive. Then the spikes (maxima; denoted in red) and valleys (minima; denoted in black) were extracted to compute MMS (micro-movement spikes; standardized spike amplitudes), where the MMS is computed as dividing the spike value by the sum of the spike value and the average of the signal values between the two local minima as shown in Equation (2). (**G**) For each 4 s time window, MMS were gathered and plotted a histogram. For two consecutive time windows, the earth mover's distance (EMD) was computed and compiled across time for each condition (5 min duration). (**H**) Histogram of EMDs were plotted and fitted to a Gamma PDF. (**I**) The fitted Gamma parameters obtained at (**H**) were plotted on the Gamma parameter plane, and its parameters were compared across conditions and groups.

From the maximal cross-coherence values obtained, we built an adjacency matrix for each participant from each condition (Figure 2C). Based on this matrix, first, we categorized the channels by scalp areas—frontal (F), temporal (T), parietal (P), and occipital—and compared the median of maximal cross-coherence values between different combinations of scalp areas (Figure 2D).

Further, using the adjacency matrix, we built a network where the nodes correspond to a single EEG channel's activity, and edge corresponds to the maximal cross-coherence value between the two nodes. Here, network edges between a set of nodes form triangles, and the fraction of triangle numbers formed around each node is defined as the cluster coefficient. This is a measure of segregation within a network and is computed using the average intensity (geometric mean) of all triangles associated with each node using an algorithm by [46]. Equation (1) describes the computation, where N is the set of all nodes, C_i is the Cluster Coefficient of node i (out of n = 32 nodes); t_i is the geometric mean of triangle links formed around node i and k_i is the number of degrees (links) formed around node i. The median of these cluster coefficients from all EEG channel was then computed for each participant and compared across different groups and conditions using the Kruskal–Wallis nonparametric test.

$$C_i = \sum_{i \in N} \frac{t_i}{k_i(k_i - 1)} \qquad (1)$$

2.3.2. Analyses in the Temporal Domain

Among the 32 EEG channels, we selected a channel with the highest cluster coefficient, as it would be deemed a hub channel, and analyzed its temporal data. The location of the selected channel can be found in Figure A1. Specifically, we bandpass filtered the data at 13–100 Hz using IIR filter at 20th order (Figure 2E). Then we extracted the micro-movement spikes (MMS).

$$\text{MMS} = \frac{\text{local peak}}{\text{local peak} + \text{avg}(\text{activity}_{\text{mintomin}})} \qquad (2)$$

This standardization equation is commonly used to address allometric effects (Mosimann, 1970) that occur due to individual anatomical differences (Figure 2F).

Micro-movements spikes (MMS): To standardize the amplitudes of the data, we shifted the data up so that the minimum value of the waveform equals 0. Then, to compute a set of standardized spike amplitudes, we took each spike amplitudes from the filtered and shifted waveforms and divided this local peak by the sum of this raw spike amplitude value and the average of the signals sampled within the two adjacent minima surrounding that local spike, as shown in Equation (2).

To examine the change in stochastic variations of the signals over time, we extracted the MMS due to fluctuations in the signals' amplitude from each condition (of 5 min duration) and examined how the frequency distribution of these standardized spike amplitudes changed over time. Specifically, we segmented the data by 4 s time window, while sliding it with 50% overlap between consecutive windows. This allowed us to gather on average 100 spikes per window (the criteria to have proper statistical power for our 95% confidence in the empirical estimation.) For each time window, histograms of MMS peaks' amplitudes were plotted, binned from 0.5 to 0.7 with 0.02 intervals. Then, we used similarity metric that enables us to compare probability distributions pairwise and estimate differences in probability space. We obtained the earth mover's distance (EMD) [47–49] between 2 sequential windows' histograms to quantify the change in stochasticity (Figure 2G). The EMD (also known as the Kantarovich–Wasserstein distance [47,48,50,51]) is a distance metric that can quantify stochastic shifts in probability space. Previous work elaborates on the algorithm to compute this distance adapted to our biometrics [7]. The stochastic shifts in the EMD across the data set were thus examined, by obtaining the distribution of EMD values (Figure 2H) using Freedman–Diaconis binning rule [52] and fitting a Gamma probability distribution function (PDF) using maximum likelihood estimation with 95% confidence intervals (Figure 2I).

The Gamma PDF is defined by two parameters—the shape and the scale—and these parameters are informative to provide interpretations of stochastic features of a single participant by localizing the participant's signatures (empirically estimated) on the Gamma parameter plane (Figure 2I.) Then we can interpret this personalized signature in relation to other participants localized under similar conditions, and in relation to the baseline signature of the participant as we vary the conditions (e.g., from resting state to pain, to de-adaptation from pain).

The continuous family of Gamma probability distribution functions (PDF) ranges from exponential (shape equals 1, representing the case of the memory-less exponential distribution) to skewed, asymmetrical distributions with heavy tails, to Gaussian-like symmetric distributions (with higher shape values). By sampling over large numbers of nervous systems biorhythms sampled from the human population, across disorders of the nervous system, ages, and between sex, we have empirically found a power law relating the shape and the scale parameters. In this empirically found relation, as the shape values increase, the scale values decrease consistently with a tight linear fit on the log-log Gamma parameters' plane spanned by the values of the shape and scale. The scale values represent the noise to signal ratio, NSR (i.e., empirically estimated Gamma variance over the Gamma mean). Knowing one parameter (the shape) helps us infer the other (the scale), owing to this power-law relation. We have empirically found that processes with high noise (high scale value) and close to the random exponential distribution (small shape value) correspond to stochastic regimes of high uncertainty, leading to poor prediction of future events from present events. Likewise, processes with symmetric distributions (high shape values) and low NSR correspond to stochastic processes with high certainty, describing predictive performance with high accuracy. This has been the case for data related to central signals registered from EEG and resting-state fMRI processing, and for peripheral signals registering kinematics of different movement classes. This has also been the case for autonomic signals related to heart and breathing activities [53–56].

3. Results

3.1. SOR Participants Show Reduced Cortical Interactions within the Beta and Gamma Bands during Resting Condition

As a first step, between all pairs of channels, we obtained the cross-coherence measure and extracted the maximum for each comparison. We extracted this information within the beta and gamma bands (13–100 Hz). By categorizing the channel pairs by their corresponding scalp areas, we find an overall lower coherence among the SOR group than the control group. This is most noticeable from the interactions between temporal and frontal ($\chi(1,19) = 4.69$, $p = 0.03$), parietal and temporal ($\chi(1,19) = 4.05$, $p = 0.04$), and occipital and temporal areas ($\chi(1,19) = 4.37$, $p = 0.04$) (Figure 3A). Such reduced coherence among SOR were observed only during the resting condition, and not during the pain induced conditions, during which the coherence levels were similar between the two groups. From this, we find that reduced cortical interactions within the beta and gamma bands during resting condition is characteristic of SOR.

As a subsequent analysis in the frequency domain, we used the adjacency matrix of pairwise cross-coherence values to create a network graph and quantify the connectivity across all channels. We computed the clustering coefficient value for each channel and obtained the median to compare values between the two groups, controls and SOR.

During the resting condition, SOR showed lower clustering coefficients than the control group ($\chi(1,18) = 4.37$, $p = 0.04$), implying a more sparse connection across the scalp within the beta and gamma band. On the other hand, under the two pain conditions, the connectivity remained similar between the two groups (Figure 3B).

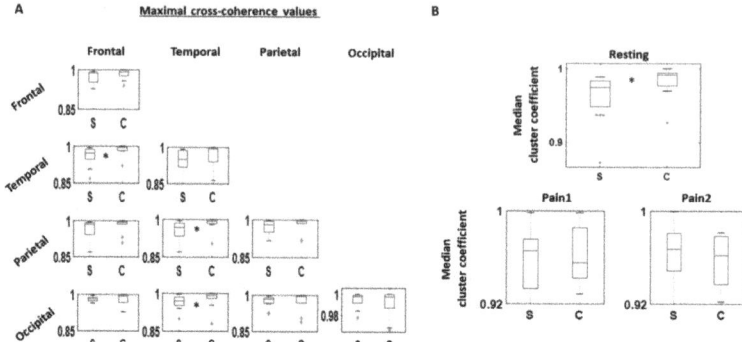

Figure 3. Cross-coherence between EEG channels. (**A**) 32 channels are categorized to one of these areas—Frontal, Temporal, Parietal, and Occipital—and maximal cross-coherence value examined within the beta and gamma band (13–100 Hz) for all channel pairs. Median values among the different channel pairs categorized by the scalp areas are then compared between SOR (S) and control (C) groups, where SOR exhibits lower values than the controls, particularly between frontal and temporal channels, parietal and temporal channels, and occipital and temporal channels. This pattern is found only during the resting condition. (**B**) Based on the adjacency matrix of maximal cross-coherence values, cluster coefficients are computed for all channels. The median of cluster coefficients is compared between the SOR and control groups for all three conditions. Cluster coefficient values are lower for SOR than the control group during the resting condition, but not significantly different when pain is induced.

3.2. Relative to Baseline, SOR Participants Show Higher Rates of Change in Stochastic Signatures than Controls

The temporal stochasticity of the most connected channel (i.e., channel with highest cluster coefficient) was examined by band-passing the time series through the beta and gamma band (13–100 Hz), extracting the MMS amplitudes, and building a stochastic trajectory on the Gamma plane. We then examine the first-order rate of change in Gamma parameter position, using the frequency histogram of the MMS peaks and computing the EMD between two consecutive histograms (PDFs.) This amounts to a "speed temporal profile" of the PDFs as they shift stochastic signatures per unit time on the Gamma parameter plane. Our unit time is 4 s time window, enough time to make an empirical estimation with statistical power and high confidence (based on frequency histograms derived from over 100 peaks.) The EMD values thus obtained per two consecutive time windows were then accumulated into a frequency histogram, and the distribution of EMDs compared between the two groups for each condition.

As shown in Figure 4A, in the resting condition, the SOR group showed a more symmetrical distribution of EMD values, reflected by its higher shape ($\chi(1,19) = 8.91$, $p < 0.01$), and lower scale fitted parameter values ($\chi(1,19) = 6.91$, $p < 0.01$) than the control group. As shown by the symmetry of EMD distribution from the SOR group, the MMS amplitudes of the cortical signal tends to be more predictive with reduced noise. Conversely, the typical individual from the control group tends to have an exponential-like distribution of EMD values, implying that their signals tend towards a memoryless regime, where the past is not informative to predict the future.

In the first pain condition, when the pain was induced for the first time, the SOR group and the control group started to show less distinction in their stochasticity. The typical individual from the control group did not change too much from the resting condition, where the EMD values were distributed closer to an exponential (memoryless) distribution. However, in this condition, the SOR group started to exhibit a pattern similar to the control group, shown by a reduced shape value and higher scale parameter values. Nevertheless the distinction is still statistically significant between the two groups for the shape ($\chi(1,19)$ = 4.85, p = 0.03) and borderline significant for the scale ($\chi(1,19)$ = 3.41, p = 0.06) parameter.

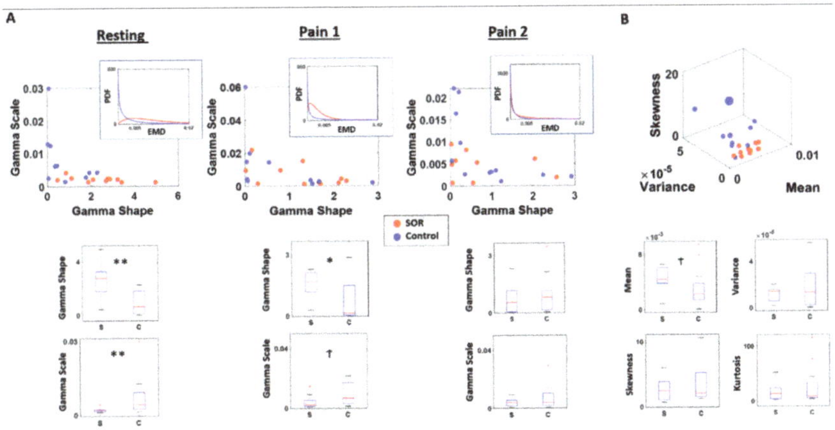

Figure 4. Differential localization in probability space and faster rate of change across pain conditions in SOR than controls. Stochastic shifts across time characterized by the distribution of EMDs between sequential time windows of MMS distributions reveal the departure of SOR from controls. (**A**) Distribution of EMDs obtained from sequential sliding windows of 4 s were examined and fitted a Gamma distribution. Under the resting state, SOR group tended to show a more symmetric (higher shape; more predictable) and less variable (lower scale; lower NSR) shifts in its EMD distributions. Under the first pain condition (Pain 1), the SOR group shifted distribution to a different regime tending to show less difference with the control group. Their PDF shifted to a less symmetric and less variable distribution; while the control group shifted to a lesser degree and mostly maintained its exponential distribution. Under the second pain condition (Pain 2), the SOR group showed even less difference with the control group, by exhibiting a more asymmetric (lower shape; more random) and more variable (higher scale; higher noise) pattern. (**B**) The distinction between the two groups can also be observed from the moments of EMD distributions, where the SOR tends to have a higher mean and a tighter range of variance and skewness than the control group. ** p < 0.01, * p < 0.05, † p < 0.10.

In the second pain condition, the SOR group and control group no longer exhibited their distinction with statistical significance, as quantified by the shape ($\chi(1,19)$ = 0.61, p = 0.43) and scale ($\chi(1,19)$ = 0.61, p = 0.43) values. At this point, both groups show their EMD values to be distributed closer to an exponential distribution, implying that their MMS amplitudes of the cortical signals have higher uncertainty, with higher noise and randomness relative to baseline.

At a different angle, when we also examine the empirical moments of the EMD distribution between the two groups, we found some distinction in the resting condition. In general, the SOR group tended to have a higher mean ($\chi(1,19)$ = 2.91, p = 0.09) EMD values implying higher rates of stochastic change from their baseline state, compared to controls. Although other moments were not statistically different in their values (variance $\chi(1,19)$ = 0.01, p = 0.94; skewness $\chi(1,19)$ = 0.85, p = 0.35; kurtosis $\chi(1,19)$ = 0.50, p = 0.48), within each condition, the variance and skewness tend to have a tighter range across individuals for the SOR than the control group (Figure 4B).

Given the significant differences in the rates of stochastic shift between controls and SOR relative to baseline and their non-significant statistical difference during pain and pain recovery conditions, and given the result that controls do not shift from the exponential regime during pain conditions, we can safely conclude that the EEG beta and gamma bands of the EEG signals from the SOR experienced significantly higher shifts at a faster rate than controls did when transitioning from condition to condition. Their stochastic signatures localize these two groups on different probability distributions and the shifts in probability space are larger in magnitude and rate for SOR.

3.3. Inventory Scores Agree with Stochastic Characterization of Brain EEG Signals' Fluctuations

With an aim to find correspondence between metrics obtained from different domains—temporal, frequency, and clinical inventory scores—we visualized these together as shown in Figure 5A for EMD fitted shape parameter, cluster coefficient (CC), and SRQ-IS score, and in Figure 5B for EMD fitted scale parameter, cluster coefficient, and SRQ-IS score. Overall, the EMD shape parameter has a strong relation with CC and the SRQ-IS scores, and thereby separate the SOR group from the control group well. On the other hand, EMD scale parameter has some relation to those metrics, but to a lesser degree.

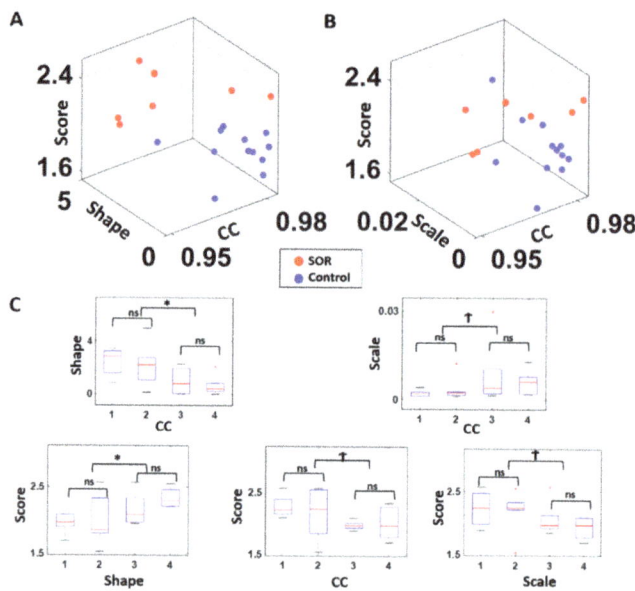

Figure 5. Congruence of clinical scores and stochastic signatures expressed in a parameter space spanned by score range, and stochastic signatures in the temporal, and frequency domains. (**A**) For each participant, the SRQ-IS was plotted on the z-axis (clinical score) along with the EMD's fitted shape parameter on the y-axis (temporal) and the median cluster coefficient (CC) value of cross-coherence networks on the x-axis (frequency). Combining these metrics across 3 domains shows a good separation between the two groups. (**B**) A similar plot was made as (**A**), but with the EMD's fitted scale parameter on the y-axis. Although the two groups show some separation, this visualization distinguishes the two groups slightly less than in (**A**), where the fitted Gamma shape parameter was utilized. (**C**) For statistical comparison, all participants were median ranked by cluster coefficients (CC; ranked in descending order) and expressed relative to the shape ((**C**) top-left) and scale ((**C**) top-right), with statistically significant differences between the extreme ranked quartiles in the shape parameter. The EMD's fitted shape and scale parameters and cluster coefficients ((**C**) bottom subpanels) were also categorized into 4 ordered-ranked groups, and the SQR-IS (score) were compared between the upper and lower 50 percentiles; and between the lowest quartile and 2nd lowest quartile; and between the highest quartile and the 2nd highest quartile. Noticeably, all metrics show statistically significant correspondence between each other at a coarse level (as the upper and lower 50 percentiles show differences) but do not correspond at a finer level (as shown by the similarity between the 1st and 2nd quartiles, and 3rd and 4th quartiles). * $p < 0.05$, † $p < 0.10$.

To examine the correspondence to a finer level (Figure 5C), we median ranked the participants by quartiles along the shape and scale parameters and along the CC values, and compared the quartile groups' inventory scores, CC, and Gamma parameter values using a non-parametric Kruskal–Wallis test. Specifically, we compared between the 1st and 2nd quartiles, between 3rd and 4th quartiles, and between the lower 50 percentile and the higher 50 percentile (i.e., the 1st and 2nd quartiles combined against the 3rd and 4th quartiles combined). In general, when comparing the lower and upper 50 percentiles, the Gamma shape parameter had a strong correspondence with CC ($\chi(1,19) = 6.43$, $p < 0.01$) and the inventory score ($\chi(1,18) = 4.55$, $p = 0.03$); and the Gamma scale parameter exhibited such relation, but to a lesser degree with CC ($\chi(1,19) = 3.61$, $p = 0.06$) and inventory score ($\chi(1,18) = 3.45$, $p = 0.06$). However, for both Gamma parameters, their statistical significance was only observed when comparing the lower and upper 50 percentile, which is roughly the separation of the SOR group against the control group. When we examine at a finer level, to compare within the SOR group and within the control group, such correspondence is hard to see for all 3 metrics.

4. Discussion

This work aimed at offering a new characterization of central signals from EEG activities registered during baseline state, and pain conditions in participants with SOR, relative to controls. We successfully reproduced previously published results including population-based statistical analyses in [34] whereby the baseline EEG activities of SOR during resting state significantly differed from controls. Further, we add new findings to the objective characterization of pain.

In the present analyses, we employed a personalized approach whereby we made use of the gross data (i.e., all fluctuations away from the empirically estimated mean of the person's data) that is usually discarded as noise. We characterized each participant's gross data by the MMS of EEG signals' amplitude, and empirically estimated the continuous family of probability distributions that best fitted these fluctuations for each participant in an MLE sense. We then uniquely localized each participant on a probability parameter space. Using this information, and a proper distance metric to measure change in probability space, we then tracked for each participant and for the entire cohort, the rates of change in stochastic shifts, when transitioning from resting state to pain 1 and to pain 2 conditions.

This individualized characterization of the brain EEG activity revealed two fundamental differences between SOR and control participants: (1) the distributions of the EMD signaling stochastic shifts was exponential in controls and tending to symmetric in SOR; (2) the shifts in the shape of this type of probability distribution in controls was not visible (i.e., they remained exponential) during the pain conditions, but significantly shifted from more to less symmetric shapes, to exponential, in SOR participants. Lastly, we found good correspondence between the clinical classification scores and the stochastic signatures that we empirically estimated for each participant, signaling that our personalized approach is not at odds with the clinical approach. This is important to augment the subjective inventories reflecting the person's self-perception of pain, with the objective biometrics quantifying the physical sensations of pain evoked by this experimental assay. The type of temperature-based manipulation used by the assay occurs at the periphery. Through afferent flow, the processing, transduction, and transmission of these signals from the peripheral to the central nervous systems give rise to physiological EEG signals reflecting the brain activities during these conditions. When the fluctuations in these probability distribution signatures are exponentially distributed, random memoryless, and with high NSR, the peripheral stimuli are not perceived as painful (controls cases). When the shifts in signals are distributed with quasi-symmetric shapes tending to the Gaussian distribution, the stimuli are perceived as a lingering sensation of discomfort and reported as pain (SOR cases.) As such, our work here offers a set of biometrics whereby the perception of pain levels coincides with the physiological (physical) sensation of bodily signals. Peripheral changes are centrally registered both at the level of the stochastic shifts in EEG signals and at the level that the person can consciously self-report.

The discovery that the baseline signatures in controls are exponential when the SOR signatures are Gaussian-like lends itself to the following interpretation (in light of what we know from reafferent signals in the resting state EEG activities of deafferented participant IW, who cannot sense movement): The controls' baseline activity with a random, memoryless regime that does not change much during pain conditions, implies that there is not enough buffering of the activity to sustain the sensory information and use it as an anchor to predict impending events (signal's fluctuations) in the pain condition. The control participant experiences the baseline and the pain in "the here and now" with a renewal process that is too random and variable (with high NSR) to systematically sustain a memory of the events and anticipate impending spiking activity in the context of pain. As such, the control participant does not reportedly sense pain, because this information does not shift stochastic signatures from baseline and at baseline, the information is just random background noise. In stark contrast, the SOR participant starts out at resting state with systematic signals that have higher shape values (more symmetric distributions) and lower scale values (lower NSR) implying higher statistical certainty. This higher certainty is amenable to build a more reliable predictive code whereby impending variations in the signals can be systematically anticipated, thus scaffolding the ability to build a memory buffer to consciously register the change from resting to pain state. In this sense, the physical pain at the periphery surfaces to consciousness as the brain activity seems to offer more awareness of change in SOR than in the controls' signals, which remain as random noise.

When transitioning from Pain1 ➔ Pain2 condition, the data from SOR participants shows a trend that approaches the controls. We interpret this as an adaptive phenomenon. As the system adapts to the lingering sensation of pain, the Pain1 ➔ Pain 2 case, the SOR activity returns to the exponential (random and memoryless) case whereby the person does not feel the lingering sensation of pain with the same intensity as it did in the Resting ➔ Pain 1 condition. The activity seemingly went back to a random memoryless state with no memory (no buffering of the activity long enough to bring it up to conscious perception) thus not sustaining the lingering sensation with the same intensity as in the initial block of the experiment. In this sense, the proposed stochastic-process interpretation of the pain sensation is to have these two opposing limiting states along a continuum (random memoryless vs. predictive) instantiated by the distribution of the signals and how they change from moment to moment. The EMD in this case provides information about the shifts of the frequency histograms representing probabilities derived from the signals' fluctuations. Of course, this is merely a proposition and will need validation with larger N, but we express this caveat in the section below, referring to these issues.

Our results of treating everyone (individually) as a random process and empirically characterizing the individual stochastic signatures and their rates of change during pain states, invites a new characterization of pain states in relation to resting states. This personalized characterization is also amenable to examine the cohort behavior and identify statistical self-groupings congruent with clinical scores. We see that the physical sensation of pain is perceived and reported by the person with SOR but not by the control participant, whose activities do not sustain, nor anticipate the pain state.

In summary, the changes in EEG MMS that we quantified in the beta and gamma band (13–100 Hz) may reflect the renewal processes in central neural processing that is continuously refreshed by the peripheral feedback from afferent signals. The activity of the gamma band alone (putatively related to attentional states) or of the beta band alone (putatively related to movement afference) will not produce these patterns. It is their combined activities that brings the signal that reflects their integration as the person reaches awareness of the lingering sensation of pain (Resting ➔ P1), or as the system deadapts from it in the second block (P1 ➔ P2).

A predictive shift in the MMS of this combined signal, as quantified by the EMD distribution, may imply that participants with SOR perceive a lingering effect of the painful experience. We propose it as a systematic predictive memory of it that is sustained long enough to bring it to awareness. This may be through increased certainty experienced by increasingly systematic prediction-confirmation loops, away from randomness. This interpretation, which is further supported by the congruence of our statistical inference with the clinical scores, warrants further investigation, given the critical need for objective characterizations of pain and the potential applications of these methods to scale up the results of this work.

Caveats and Limitations

Despite the clean new results and the congruence with the prior work based on the same data set, we caution that the modest size of the cohort limits our conclusions. The treatment of each participant as a random process guarantees the statistical power of each empirically estimated signature with 95% confidence interval. We ensured that the 4s-window with 50% overlap provided a continuous estimation with renewal of activity every 2 s comprising enough fluctuations to make a sound stochastic estimate and shift to the next point along the stochastic trajectory. However, the n of 21 participants, 9 with SOR is modest. We need a larger cohort. Further, the group was not balanced in sex and age. Ideally, we would like to sample larger numbers of males and females, but also examine transgender groups and groups with same-sex orientation. Lastly, it would be great to sample from other disorders of the nervous systems that also complain about issues with pain and temperature dysregulation.

5. Conclusions

Using this new approach, it will be possible to scale up our results from this modest cohort and ascertain subtypes of pain sensation. A positive note is that by integrating the complementary subjective and objective methods that we used here, we will attain much more than using only one method on its own right. In this sense, despite the caveats, we feel confident that the present methods have the potential to help us advance our understanding of the perception of physically induced pain—as registered by micro fluctuations in EEG brain signals.

Author Contributions: Conceptualization, J.R. and E.B.T.; methodology, J.R. and E.B.T.; software, J.R. and E.B.T.; validation, J.R.; formal analysis, J.R.; investigation, J.R. and E.B.T.; resources, E.B.T.; data curation, J.R., T.B.-S., Y.G., I.W.-F.; writing—original draft preparation, E.B.T.; writing—review and editing, J.R., T.B.-S., Y.G., I.W.-F.; visualization, J.R. and E.B.T.; supervision, E.B.T.; project administration, E.B.T. and T.B.-S.; funding acquisition, E.B.T. All authors have read and agreed to the published version of the manuscript.

Funding: This research was funded by The Nancy Lurie Marks Family Foundation Career Development Award to E.B.T and by the Fellowship of Excellence in Computational and Data Science by Rutgers Discovery Informatics Institute to J.R.

Institutional Review Board Statement: The study was conducted according to the guidelines of the Declaration of Helsinki and approved by the Rutgers University Institutional Review Board approved this de-identified data sharing. The IRB committee of Rambam Health Care Campus approved this study in 2013. The IRB number is 3075, The Israeli ministry of health # HT4858.

Informed Consent Statement: Informed consent was obtained from all subjects involved in the study.

Data Availability Statement: The data presented in this study are available on request from the corresponding author. The data are not publicly available due to health privacy issues.

Acknowledgments: We thank the participants and the personnel that carried on these experiments.

Conflicts of Interest: The authors declare no conflict of interest.

Appendix A

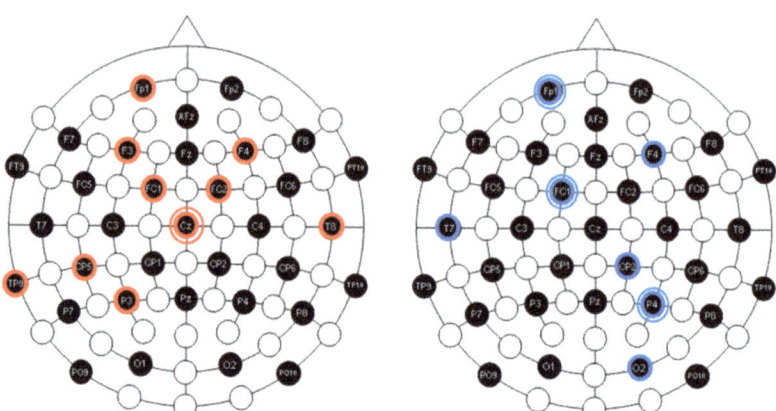

Figure A1. Location of channels with highest cluster coefficient. The hub channel (i.e., channel with highest cluster coefficient) is shown for SOR (red) and controls (blue). Each colored line represents a single participant's data. For example, if there are 2 circles surrounding a single channel, that means 2 participants had their hub channel positioned there. Overall, SOR hub channels tend to be positioned in the frontal and lateral area; and Control's hub channel tends to be distributed in the medial area. Notice that controls do not have any central lead (in contrast to SOR) and that controls have occipital lead (in contrast to SOR.) Notice that across the cohort, the maximal clustering coefficient leads in SOR are more distributed thank those in the controls.

References

1. Corniani, G.; Saal, H.P. Tactile innervation densities across the whole body. *J. Neurophysiol.* **2020**, *124*, 1229–1240. [CrossRef] [PubMed]
2. Torres, E.B.; Zipser, D. Reaching to Grasp with a Multi-Jointed Arm (I): Computational Model. *J. Neurophysiol.* **2002**, *88*, 2355–2367. [CrossRef] [PubMed]
3. Torres, E.B. Signatures of movement variability anticipate hand speed according to levels of intent. *Behav. Brain Funct.* **2013**, *9*, 10. [CrossRef]
4. Torres, E.B.; Denisova, K. Motor noise is rich signal in autism research and pharmacological treatments. *Sci. Rep.* **2016**, *6*, 37422. [CrossRef] [PubMed]
5. Torres, E.B. *Objective Biometric Methods for the Diagnosis and Treatment of Nervous System Disorder*; Elsevier: Amsterdam, The Netherlands, 2018; p. 580.
6. Caballero, C.; Mistry, S.; Torres, E.B. Age-Dependent Statistical Changes of Involuntary Head Motion Signatures across Autism and Controls of the ABIDE Repository. *Front. Integr. Neurosci.* **2020**, *14*, 23. [CrossRef]
7. Torres, E.B.; Caballero, C.; Mistry, S. Aging with Autism Departs Greatly from Typical Aging. *Sensors* **2020**, *20*, 572. [CrossRef]
8. Torres, E.B.; Brincker, M.; Isenhower, R.W.I.; Yanovich, P.; Stigler, K.A.; Nurnberger, J.I.; Metaxas, D.N.; José, J.V. Autism: The micro-movement perspective. *Front. Integr. Neurosci.* **2013**, *7*, 32. [CrossRef]
9. Torres, E.B. Two classes of movements in motor control. *Exp. Brain Res.* **2011**, *215*, 269–283. [CrossRef]
10. Torres, E.B.; Yanovich, P.; Metaxas, D.N. Give spontaneity and self-discovery a chance in ASD: Spontaneous peripheral limb variability as a proxy to evoke centrally driven intentional acts. *Front. Integr. Neurosci.* **2013**, *7*, 46. [CrossRef]
11. Vallbo, A.B.; Johansson, R.S. Properties of cutaneous mechanoreceptors in the human hand related to touch sensation. *Hum. Neurobiol.* **1984**, *3*, 3–14.
12. Kandel, E.R. *Principles of Neural Science*, 5th ed.; McGraw-Hill: New York, NY, USA, 2013; Volume 1, p. 1709.
13. Witney, A.G.; Wing, A.; Thonnard, J.-L.; Smith, A.M. The cutaneous contribution to adaptive precision grip. *Trends Neurosci.* **2004**, *27*, 637–643. [CrossRef] [PubMed]
14. Panek, I.; Bui, T.; Wright, A.T.B.; Brownstone, R.M. Cutaneous afferent regulation of motor function. *Acta Neurobiol. Exp.* **2014**, *74*, 158–171.
15. Tsakiris, M. My body in the brain: A neurocognitive model of body-ownership. *Neuropsychologia* **2010**, *48*, 703–712. [CrossRef] [PubMed]
16. McGlone, F.; Wessberg, J.; Olausson, H. Discriminative and Affective Touch: Sensing and Feeling. *Neuron* **2014**, *82*, 737–755. [CrossRef]

17. Torres, E.B.; Whyatt, C. *Autism: The Movement Sensing Perspective*; CRC Press/Taylor & Francis Group: Boca Raton, FL, USA, 2018.
18. Gomez-Mayordomo, V.; Palacios-Ceña, M.; Guerrero-Peral, Á.; Fuensalida-Novo, S.; Fernández-de-las-Peñas, C.; Cuadrado, M.L. Widespread Hypersensitivity to Pressure Pain in Men With Cluster Headache During Pro-longed Remission Is Not Related to the Levels of Depression and Anxiety. *Pain Pract.* **2020**, *20*, 147–153. [CrossRef] [PubMed]
19. Arroyo-Fernandez, R.; Bravo-Esteban, E.; Domenech-Garcia, V.; Ferri-Morales, A. Pressure-Induced Referred Pain as a Biomarker of Pain Sensitivity in Fibromyalgia. *Pain Physician* **2020**, *23*, E353–E362.
20. Fardo, F.; Vinding, M.C.; Allen, M.; Jensen, T.S.; Finnerup, N.B. Delta and gamma oscillations in operculo-insular cortex underlie innocuous cold thermosensation. *J. Neurophysiol.* **2017**, *117*, 1959–1968. [CrossRef]
21. Giehl, J.; Meyer-Brandis, G.; Kunz, M.; Lautenbacher, S. Responses to tonic heat pain in the ongoing EEG under conditions of controlled attention. *Somatosens. Mot. Res.* **2013**, *31*, 40–48. [CrossRef]
22. Chen, A.C.; Rappelsberger, P.; Filz, O. Topology of EEG coherence changes may reflect differential neural network activation in cold and pain perception. *Brain Topogr.* **1998**, *11*, 125–132. [CrossRef]
23. Backonja, M.; Howland, E.W.; Wang, J.; Smith, J.; Salinsky, M.; Cleeland, C.S. Tonic changes in alpha power during immersion of the hand in cold water. *Electroencephalogr. Clin. Neurophysiol.* **1991**, *79*, 192–203. [CrossRef]
24. Bockadia, H.; Cole, J.; Torres, E.B. Neural Connectivity Evolution during Adaptive Learning with and without Proprioception. In Proceedings of the 7th International Symposium on Movement and Computing, New Jersey, NJ, USA, 15–17 July 2020; ACM: New Jersey, NJ, USA, 2020.
25. Cole, J.D.; Merton, W.L.; Barrett, G.; Katifi, H.A.; Treede, R.-D. Evoked potentials in a subject with a large-fibre sensory neuropathy below the neck. *Can. J. Physiol. Pharmacol.* **1995**, *73*, 234–245. [CrossRef] [PubMed]
26. Cole, J. *Pride and a Daily Marathon*, 1st ed.; MIT Press: Cambridge, MA, USA, 1995; 194p.
27. Cole, J. Rehabilitation after sensory neuronopathy syndrome. *J. R. Soc. Med.* **1998**, *91*, 30–32. [CrossRef] [PubMed]
28. Cole, J.D.; Sedgwick, E.M. The perceptions of force and of movement in a man without large myelinated sensory afferents below the neck. *J. Physiol.* **1992**, *449*, 503–515. [CrossRef] [PubMed]
29. Brincker, M.; Torres, E.B. Noise from the periphery in autism. *Front. Integr. Neurosci.* **2013**, *7*, 34. [CrossRef] [PubMed]
30. Brincker, M.; Torres, E.B. *Chapter 1—Why Study Movement Variability in Autism?: The Movement Sensing Perspective*; Torres, E.B., Whyatt, C., Eds.; CRC Press/Taylor & Francis Group: Boca Raton, FL, USA, 2018.
31. Alliance of Psychoanalytic Organizations. *Psychodynamic Diagnostic Manual (PDM)*; Alliance of Psychoanalytic Organizations: Baltimore, MD, USA, 2006.
32. Bar-Shalita, T.; Granovsky, Y.; Parush, S.; Weissman-Fogel, I. Sensory Modulation Disorder (SMD) and Pain: A New Perspective. *Front. Integr. Neurosci.* **2019**, *13*, 27. [CrossRef]
33. Bar-Shalita, T.; Vatine, J.-J.; Parush, S. Sensory modulation disorder: A risk factor for participation in daily life activities. *Dev. Med. Child Neurol.* **2008**, *50*, 932–937. [CrossRef]
34. Granovsky, Y.; Weissman-Fogel, I.; Bar-Shalita, T. Resting-State Electroencephalography in Participants with Sensory Overresponsiveness: An Exploratory Study. *Am. J. Occup. Ther.* **2019**, *73*, 1–11. [CrossRef]
35. Edinoff, A.; Sathivadivel, N.; McBride, T.; Parker, A.; Okeagu, C.; Kaye, A.D.; Kaye, A.M.; Kaye, J.S.; Kaye, R.J.; Sheth, M.M.; et al. Chronic Pain Treatment Strategies in Parkinson's Disease. *Neurol. Int.* **2020**, *12*, 61. [CrossRef]
36. Failla, M.D.; Gerdes, M.B.; Williams, Z.J.; Moore, D.J.; Cascio, C.J. Increased pain sensitivity and pain-related anxiety in individuals with autism. *PAIN Rep.* **2020**, *5*, e861. [CrossRef]
37. Abplanalp, S.J.; Mueser, K.T.; Fulford, D. The role of physical pain in global functioning of people with serious mental illness. *Schizophr. Res.* **2020**, *222*, 423–428. [CrossRef]
38. Summers, J.; Shahrami, A.; Cali, S.; D'Mello, C.; Kako, M.; Palikucin-Reljin, A.; Savage, M.; Shaw, O.; Lunsky, Y. Self-Injury in Autism Spectrum Disorder and Intellectual Disability: Exploring the Role of Reactivity to Pain and Sensory Input. *Brain Sci.* **2017**, *7*, 140. [CrossRef] [PubMed]
39. Torres, E.B.; Isenhower, R.W.; Nguyen, J.; Whyatt, C.; Nurnberger, J.I.; Jose, J.V.; Silverstein, S.M.; Papathomas, T.V.; Sage, J.; Cole, J. Toward Precision Psychiatry: Statistical Platform for the Personalized Characterization of Natural Be-haviors. *Front. Neurol.* **2016**, *7*, 8. [CrossRef] [PubMed]
40. Torres, E.B. *Systems and Methods for Tracking Neurodevelopment Disorders*; Google Patents, USPTO, Ed.; Rutgers State University of New Jersey: New Jersey, NJ, USA, 2019; p. 27.
41. Torres, E.B. *Methods for the Diagnosis and Treatment of Neurological Disorders*; Google Patents, USPTO, Ed.; Rutgers State University of New Jersey: New Jersey, NJ, USA, 2018; p. 38.
42. Weissman-Fogel, I.; Granovsky, Y.; Bar-Shalita, T. Sensory Over-Responsiveness among Healthy Subjects is Associated with a Pronociceptive State. *Pain Pr.* **2018**, *18*, 473–486. [CrossRef] [PubMed]
43. Bar-Shalita, T.; Seltzer, Z.; Vatine, J.-J.; Yochman, A.; Parush, S. Development and psychometric properties of the Sensory Responsiveness Questionnaire (SRQ). *Disabil. Rehabil.* **2009**, *31*, 189–201. [CrossRef] [PubMed]
44. Bar-Shalita, T.; Vatine, J.-J.; Parush, S.; Deutsch, L.; Seltzer, Z. Psychophysical correlates in adults with sensory modulation disorder. *Disabil. Rehabil.* **2011**, *34*, 943–950. [CrossRef]
45. Bigdely-Shamlo, N.; Mullen, T.; Kothe, C.; Su, K.-M.; Robbins, K.A. The PREP pipeline: Standardized preprocessing for large-scale EEG analysis. *Front. Neuroinform.* **2015**, *9*, 120. [CrossRef]

46. Onnela, J.-P.; Saramäki, J.; Kertész, J.; Kaski, K. Intensity and coherence of motifs in weighted complex networks. *Phys. Rev. E* **2005**, *71*, 065103. [CrossRef]
47. Arjovsky, M.; Chintala, S.; Bottou, L. Wasserstein Generative Adversarial Networks. In Proceedings of the 34th International Conference on Machine Learning, Sydney, Australia, 6–11 August 2017.
48. Stolfi, J.; Guibas, L.J. The earth mover's distance as a metric for image retrieval. *Int. J. Comput. Vis.* **2000**, *40*, 99–121.
49. Rubner, Y.; Guibas, L.J.; Tomasi, C. The earth mover's distance, multi-dimensional scaling, and color-based image retrieval. In Proceedings of the ARPA Image Understanding Workshop, New Orleans, LA, USA, 11–14 May 1997.
50. McClelland, J.; Koslicki, D. EMDUniFrac: Exact linear time computation of the unifrac metric and identification of differentially abundant organisms. *J. Math. Biol.* **2018**, *77*, 935–949. [CrossRef]
51. Monge, G. Memoire sur la theorie des deblais et des remblais. In *Histoire de l' Academie Royale des Science; Avec Les Memoired de Mathematique et de Physique*; De L'imprimerie Royale: Paris, France, 1781.
52. Freedman, D.; Diaconis, P. On the histogram as a density estimator: L theory. *Probab. Theory Relat. Fields* **1981**, *57*, 453–476. [CrossRef]
53. Ryu, J.; Torres, E.B. The Autonomic Nervous System Differentiates between Levels of Motor Intent and End Effector. *J. Pers. Med.* **2020**, *10*, 76. [CrossRef] [PubMed]
54. Ryu, J.; Vero, J.; Dobkin, R.D.; Torres, E.B. Dynamic Digital Biomarkers of Motor and Cognitive Function in Parkinson's Disease. *J. Vis. Exp.* **2019**. [CrossRef] [PubMed]
55. Ryu, J.; Torres, E.B. Characterization of Sensory-Motor Behavior under Cognitive Load Using a New Statistical Platform for Studies of Embodied Cognition. *Front. Hum. Neurosci.* **2018**, *12*, 1–19. [CrossRef] [PubMed]
56. Ryu, J.; Vero, J.; Torres, E.B. Methods for Tracking Dynamically Coupled Brain-Body Activities during Natural Movement. In Proceedings of the MOCO '17: 4th International Conference on Movement Computing, London, UK, 28–30 June 2017; ACM: London, UK, 2017.

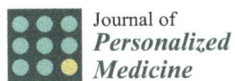

Article

A Child's Perception of Their Developmental Difficulties in Relation to Their Adult Assessment. Analysis of the INPP Questionnaire

Alina Demiy [1], Agata Kalemba [1,*], Maria Lorent [1], Anna Pecuch [1,3], Ewelina Wolańska [1,2], Marlena Telenga [1] and Ewa Z. Gieysztor [1,3]

[1] Student Research Group of the Developmental Disorders of Children and Youth, Department of Physiotherapy, Faculty of Health Sciences, Medical University, 50-367 Wroclaw, Poland; alina.demiy@student.umed.wroc.pl (A.D.); maria.lorent@student.umed.wroc.pl (M.L.); anna.pecuch@student.umed.wroc.pl (A.P.); ewelina.wolanska@student.umed.wroc.pl (E.W.); marlena.telenga@student.umed.wroc.pl (M.T.); ewa.gieysztor@umed.wroc.pl (E.Z.G.)

[2] Division Pediatric Propedeutics and Rare Disorders, Department of Pediatrics, Faculty of Health Sciences, Medical University, 50-367 Wroclaw, Poland

[3] Laboratory of Clinical Bases of Physiotherapy, Department of Physiotherapy, Faculty of Health Sciences, Medical University, 50-367 Wroclaw, Poland

* Correspondence: agata.kalemba@student.umed.wroc.pl

Received: 5 August 2020; Accepted: 5 September 2020; Published: 5 October 2020

Abstract: This study involved a comparison of the perception of developmental difficulties in a child by the parents, the teacher, and through the child's self-assessment. Based on the Institute for Neuro-Psychological Psychology (INPP) questionnaire according to S. Goddard Blythe, three groups were examined: schoolchildren, parents, and teachers. Each of them answered a set of 21 questions and assessed the degree of occurrence of a given difficulty for the child on a scale from 0 to 4. The questions concerned psychomotor problems related to balance, motor coordination and concentration, as well as school skills. In total, 49 questionnaires from children and parents and 46 from teachers were used for the study. The mean answer to each question was calculated within the following groups: child–parent, child–teacher, and parent–teacher. The sum of the children's answer points was significantly higher than the sum of the parents' answer points ($p = 0.037$). Children assessed their developmental difficulties more strongly than teachers, but this difference was not statistically significant. The individual difficulties of the children were assessed significantly more seriously or more gently than by the National Scientific Conference "Human health problems—causes, present state, ways for the future" speeches by 44 teacher participants on 5 June 2020. Parents and teachers also assessed the children's difficulties significantly differently ($p = 0.044$). The biggest difference in answers concerned the question of maintaining attention. The obtained results indicate a significant difference in the perception of difficulties occurring in the same child by the teacher and the parent. The child's behavior in school and home environments may be different and, depending on the requirements, assessed differently. Children perceive their difficulties much more seriously than adults. Talking and the support of adults can make it easier for a child to overcome developmental difficulties.

Keywords: children; adult; difficulties; disorders; coordination; focus

1. Introduction

The appearance of symptoms such as problems with maintaining balance; coordination problems; difficulty with jointing together elements of running, jumping, throwing, and catching a ball; time–space orientation disorder; deep sensibility or kinesthesia (awareness of the arrangement of the body in space and ability to repeat a set motor pattern) in a schoolchild is a clear sign of developmental difficulties that should be considered by parents or legal guardians. Other indications include issues with reading, writing, and mathematical abilities, such as counting and understanding of instructions [1]. All of the aforementioned symptoms increase the risk of dyslexia and can be the reason for psychomotor and social problems in adult life [2,3]. There are preliminary screening tests that enable early detection of problems connected to learning and behavioral or emotional disorders in schoolchildren. These include, among others, the Institute for Neuro-Psychological Psychology (INPP) questionnaire by Goddard Blythe, which allows a profound examination of children in terms of the presence of psychomotor disorders, which, in turn, can be a sign of neuromotor immaturity [4,5]. The use of a questionnaire allows the selection of children who have trouble at school and children who have motoric problems, which indicate disintegrated primitive reflexes [6]. Research with the use of the aforementioned questionnaire was conducted by Grzywniak. According to the author, a child aged 6 or 7 years old gains the neuropsychological maturity for school learning through a correct development and the integration of the primary reflex within the central nervous system [2,4]. The methods of evaluation of retained reflexes became the research objects of not only Goddard Blythe but also of Masgutova who developed a rehabilitative and therapeutic system, Masgutova neurosensorimotor reflex integration (MNRI), with a view to helping patients with neurological and cognitional disorders [5]. Both authors in their methods acknowledge the importance of the incorrect work of structures responsible for the equilibrium and coordinative abilities of the child (cerebellum and central nervous system) in contrast with neonatal reflex [1].

The use of the INPP questionnaire can determine which children have school and motor problems, indicating disintegrated primary reflexes.

Research concerning the perception of difficulties in children is extremely important for both the parent and teacher perspective, and most importantly the children themselves. An adult becomes a witness of the everchanging influence of the environment, that is the school or home, on the behavior of a schoolchild. The foregoing problem arises because of many factors, e.g., the parental attitude, overprotectiveness of the parents or a liberal upbringing style, peer contact, emotional experiences, teacher competences, and the methods of knowledge transfer. Different attitudes will be observed by a parent in a house where the child feels much more at ease and has a greater sense of security and acceptance and a possibility to release emotions in contrast with teacher observations in the school environment where there are top-down rules and time frames regarding the length of the lessons or breaks. With the use of the screening test and observation, the teacher is able to recognize the children with psychomotor disorders [1]. The early pedagogical diagnosis gives the opportunity to take further educational and, if there is such a need, therapeutic steps [4].

The aim of this study was to compare the perception of a child's developmental difficulties by the parents, a teacher, and through the child's self-assessment based on an analysis of the INPP questionnaire.

2. Materials and Methods

2.1. Examined Group

A total of 68 children took part in the research. For comparison, a number of questionnaires were completed; 49 were filled out by children, 49 by parents (72%), and 44 by teachers (74%). A greater number of questionnaires was taken into consideration for the possibility of comparison depending on the analyzed group. Each pupil was rated thrice—by a parent, a teacher, and through the pupil's self-assessment.

The first treatment group counted 49 children (21 girls and 28 boys). The average age was 8 years. The youngest pupil was 6 years old, and the oldest was 12 years old (SD = 1.63; MED = 8.0; MOD = 6). All of the participants were elementary students. The second group was formed of parents, and the third of teachers.

2.2. Questionnaire

The research was conducted with the use of the INPP screening test by S. Goddard Blythe. It comprises 21 questions for which the answers are given on a 5-grade scale (0–4) where 4 means that the disorder is present to a great extent and 0 means a lack of the disorder [7–9].

In the questionnaire, each of the groups had to determine on a scale from 0 to 4 the degree of difficulty with which the child copes in day-to-day life. Among them, concentration problems; problems with sitting still, writing, or reading; easy distraction; and motor problems such as swimming, bike riding, or coordination can be distinguished.

Moreover, every child's result was summed up and categorized into levels, where the larger the sum of the point, the greater the disorder. The aforementioned scale can be seen in Table 1.

Table 1. The scale of disorder assessment.

Sum	Level	Degree of Disorder
0	0	no disorder
1–21	1	present to a minimum degree
22–42	2	present to a moderate degree
43–63	3	present to a great degree
64–84	4	present at a very high intensity

2.3. Statistical Methods

Statistical analysis was performed using IBM SPSS Statistics version 25 (IBM Corp., Armonk, NY, USA). Means, standard deviation, and medians were calculated. The Mann–Whitney U test was used to compare the two groups in terms of quantitative/ordinal variables. The level $\alpha = 0.05$ or $\alpha = 0.01$ was used for comparisons. The effect size was calculated using eta-squared for the Mann–Whitney U test.

3. Results

The results were analyzed in three subgroups: child–parent (Table 2), child–teacher (Table 3), and parent–teacher (Table 4). Tables 2–4 show the distribution of the average of particular answers to questions between the groups. Statistically significant differences are highlighted in red. In the child–teacher comparison, 10 of the answers show this feature. Similarly, in the parent–teacher group, the answers vary significantly in 10 cases. In the last child–parent column, there are six differences in grading particular difficulties that are statistically significant

Table 5 shows a comparison between the average sums of results and the sum of levels, and the calculated average score in the subgroups. The number of given answers differs significantly. It is the most noticeable in the parent–teacher subgroup where the averages and the division into levels are substantially apart. The parents often assessed the children's troubles at the first level. Eight pupils more were classified as that level by the parents than those classified as that level by the teachers. The teachers scored the children's troubles higher, and the children were classified as the second level more by the teachers than by the parents. The difference in the sum of the points is 6.16 (0.57 for the child–teacher subgroup; 5.32 for child–parent). In this group, there is also the greatest difference between the levels, that being 0.38 (child–teacher 0.08; child–parent 0.26). In the remaining groups, the answers are the same or differ insignificantly in at least two aspects.

Table 2. The distribution of responses in the child–parent group.

Questionnaire	Children (n = 40)			Parents (n = 40)			U	p	η^2
	M	Me	SD	M	Me	SD			
1. Inability to sit still	1.2	1	1.2	1.1	1	1.2	786	0.45	0.00
2. Attention problems	1.3	1	1.3	1.1	1	1.1	753	0.33	0.00
3. Easy to distract	1.6	1	1.4	1.4	1	1.1	740	0.28	0.00
4. Coordination problems	1.0	0	1.4	0.8	0	1.1	780	0.35	0.00
5. Incorrect grip	0.9	0	1.3	0.7	0	1.1	744	0.30	0.00
6. Incorrect sitting posture	1.0	1	1.2	1.1	1	1.1	739	0.28	0.00
7. Difficulty catching the ball	1.2	1	1.2	0.8	0	1.2	660	0.09	0.02
8. Difficulty learning to swim	1.4	1	1.5	0.8	0	1.1	642	0.06	0.03
9. Diffiiculty riding a bike	0.5	0	1.2	0.2	0	0.8	701	0.17	0.01
10. Travel sickness	1.1	0	1.5	0.5	0	1.0	638	0.06	0.03
11. Reading problems	1.4	1	1.4	0.8	0	1.1	589	0.02	0.05
12. Writing problems	1.2	1	1.2	0.9	0.5	1.1	697	0.16	0.01
13. Rewriting problems	0.9	0.5	1.2	0.7	0	1.1	718	0.22	0.01
14. Math problems	1.1	1	1.2	0.5	0	1.0	546	0.00	0.08
15. Spelling problems	1.4	1	1.4	1.1	1	1.2	713	0.16	0.01
16. Rearranging numbers or letters	0.7	0	1.0	1.0	1	1.2	692	0.15	0.01
17. Difficulty reading the time	1.5	1	1.6	1.1	0	1.4	669	0.08	0.02
18. Difficulty multi-tasking	0.9	0.55	1.0	0.9	0	1.2	818	0.49	0.00
19. Recurring headaches	1.0	1	1.1	0.2	0	0.7	437	0.00	0.15
20. Frequent fatigue	1.1	1	1.1	0.6	0	1.0	570	0.01	0.06
21. Clear agitation	1.2	1	1.3	1.0	1	1.1	767	0.37	0.00
Sum	23.3	23	13.2	17.3	16	12.1	681	0.05	0.02
Level	1.6	2	0.6	1.4	1	0.7	616	0.04	0.04

* Statistically significant values are marked in red.

Table 3. The distribution of responses in the child–teacher group.

Questionnaire	Children (n = 44)			Teachers (n = 44)			U	p	η^2
	M	Me	SD	M	Me	SD			
1. Inability to sit still	1.18	1	1.17	1.52	1	1.62	909	0.31	0.00
2. Attention problems	1.34	1	1.22	2.57	3	1.44	506	0.00	0.15
3. Easy to distract	1.66	1	1.41	2.57	3	1.44	637	0.00	0.09
4. Coordination problems	0.78	0	1.19	0.25	0	0.94	725	0.02	0.05
5. Incorrect grip	0.75	0	1.14	1.34	1	1.24	680	0.01	0.07
6. Incorrect sitting posture	1.07	1	1.25	1.43	1	1.42	836	0.14	0.01
7. Difficulty catching the ball	1.18	1	1.23	0.80	0	1.19	854	0.05	0.01
8. Difficulty learning to swim	1.43	1	1.55	0.09	0	0.60	471	0.00	0.20
9. Diffiiculty riding a bike	0.57	0	1.23	0.09	0	0.60	795	0.07	0.02
10. Travel sickness	1.23	0	1.57	0.32	0	1.03	610	0.00	0.10
11. Reading problems	1.25	1	1.28	1.43	2	1.39	905	0.30	0.00
12. Writing problems	1.05	1	1.16	1.45	1	1.25	782	0.06	0.03
13. Rewriting problems	0.89	1	1.19	1.30	1	1.19	745	0.03	0.04
14. Math problems	1.12	1	1.19	1.20	1	1.11	945	0.36	0.00
15. Spelling problems	1.46	1	1.28	1.32	1	1.20	945	0.36	0.00
16. Rearranging numbers or letters	0.68	0	0.93	0.64	1	0.81	958	0.47	0.00
17. Difficulty reading the time	1.46	1	1.53	0.25	0	0.89	514	0.00	0.16
18. Difficulty multi-tasking	0.82	1	0.99	1.50	1	1.34	868	0.04	0.01
19. Recurring headaches	0.87	1	1.05	0.09	0	0.60	474	0.00	0.19
20. Frequent fatigue	1.14	1	1.12	0.98	0	1.21	861	0.15	0.01
21. Clear agitation	1.18	1	1.30	1.52	1	1.70	926	0.36	0.00
Sum	23.1	23	12.6	22.70	22	13.30	1003	0.27	0.00
Level	1.61	2	0.65	1.90	2	0.73	794	0.07	0.02

* Statistically significant values are marked in red.

Table 4. The distribution of responses in the parent–teacher group.

Questionnaire	Parents (n = 38)			Teachers (n = 38)			U	p	η^2
	M	Me	SD	M	Me	SD			
1. Inability to sit still	1.13	1	1.23	1.66	1	1.60	591	0.09	0.03
2. Attention problems	1.11	1	1.03	2.68	3	1.42	284	0.00	0.27
3. Easy to distract	1.32	1	1.09	2.68	3	1.42	329	0.00	0.22
4. Coordination problems	0.76	0	1.08	0.29	0	1.01	496	0.01	0.07
5. Incorrect grip	0.61	0	1.00	1.40	1	1.31	462	0.00	0.10
6. Incorrect sitting posture	1.08	1	1.12	1.40	1	1.37	640	0.20	0.01
7. Difficulty catching the ball	0.84	0	1.15	0.87	0	1.26	715	0.47	0.00
8. Difficulty learning to swim	0.79	0	1.14	0.11	0	0.65	463	0.00	0.10
9. Diffiiculty riding a bike	0.21	0	0.81	0.11	0	0.65	685	0.35	0.00
10. Travel sickness	0.51	0	1.02	0.37	0	1.10	602	0.14	0.02
11. Reading problems	0.79	0	1.04	1.55	2	1.45	517	0.02	0.06
12. Writing problems	1.00	1	1.16	1.53	2	1.31	557	0.04	0.04
13. Rewriting problems	0.76	0	1.15	1.37	1	1.26	504	0.01	0.07
14. Math problems	0.58	0	1.08	1.32	1	1.14	431	0.00	0.12
15. Spelling problems	1.21	1	1.28	1.29	1.5	1.29	697	0.40	0.00
16. Rearranging numbers or letters	1.05	1	1.18	0.66	1	0.85	604	0.11	0.02
17. Difficulty reading the time	1.11	0	1.45	0.26	0	0.95	485	0.01	0.08
18. Difficulty multi-tasking	0.90	0	1.25	1.66	1	1.36	462	0.00	0.10
19. Recurring headaches	0.24	0	0.68	0.11	0	0.65	649	0.22	0.01
20. Frequent fatigue	0.55	0	0.95	0.92	0	1.22	613	0.13	0.02
21. Clear agitation	1.00	1	1.09	1.45	1	1.64	648	0.22	0.01
Sum	17.53	16.5	12.17	23.66	22	13.91	503	0.01	0.07
Level	1.29	1	0.65	1.71	2	0.73	489	0.01	0.08

* Statistically significant values are marked in red.

Table 5. The average sum of results and levels.

	Child	Teacher	Parent	Teacher	Child	Parent
Average sum of results	23.3	22.73	17.5	23.66	20.16	14.84
Level 0 *	0	0	2	0	6	10
Level 1	22	19	25	17	22	26
Level 2	19	23	9	19	18	11
Level 3	3	0	2	0	3	2
Level 4	0	2	0	2	0	0
Average levels	1.57	1.65	1.32	1.70	1.36	1.1

* Degrees of disorders are described as "levels".

3.1. Child–Teacher Subgroup

In order to compare the answers in the child–teacher group in detail, 44 questionnaires were analyzed. The results are presented in Figures 1 and 2.

The charts show the layout of the children's and teachers' answers. There are clear differences between the perception of the problems that the child struggles with (Figure 1), especially in questions 1, 2, and 3. They touch upon the abilities concerning difficulties with sitting still and keeping attention and the child's ability to stay focused.

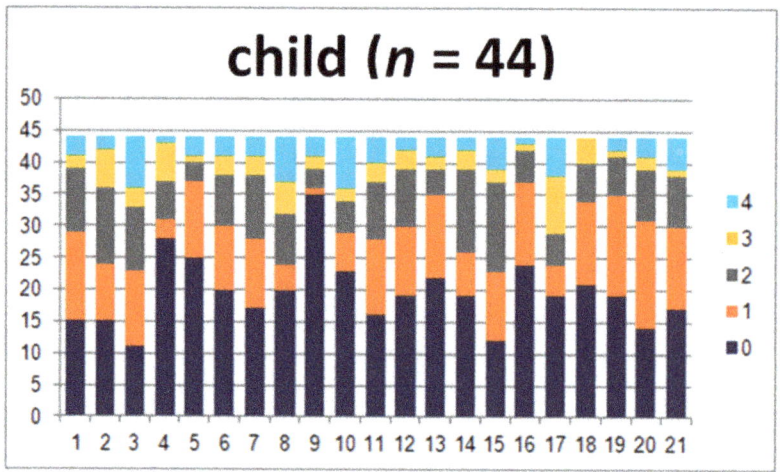

Figure 1. Answers given by the examined children.

The teachers marked levels 3 and 4, which are "present to a great degree" and "present at a very high intensity", more frequently, while the children were more likely to give 0, 1, or 2 points (Figure 2). The opposite was observed for questions 4, 5, 8, 9 10, 17, 18, and 19, where teachers marked 0. The questions concerned motor abilities, coordination, motion sickness, the ability to read the analogue clock, and headaches. All of the aforementioned differences are statistically significant ($p \leq 0.02$). Differences in answers to question 1 are not statistically significant. Moreover, the comparison of the sum of the points and levels is also not significant ($p \geq 0.05$).

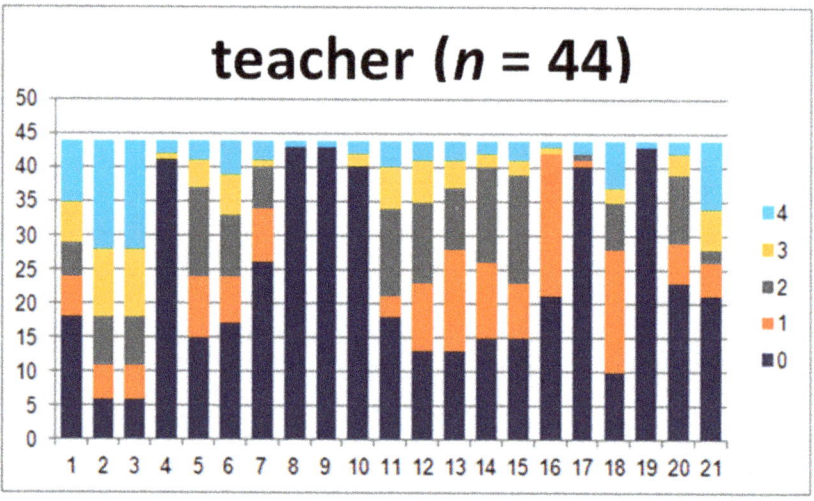

Figure 2. Answers given by the teachers.

3.2. Parent–Teacher Subgroup

In this group, there were 37 analyzed questionnaires.

In the comparison of the parent–teacher group's answers, there are differences between the answers to questions 2, 3, 4, and 8, where the teachers marked many more 4s than the parents (Figure 3). Those questions were related to motor coordination.

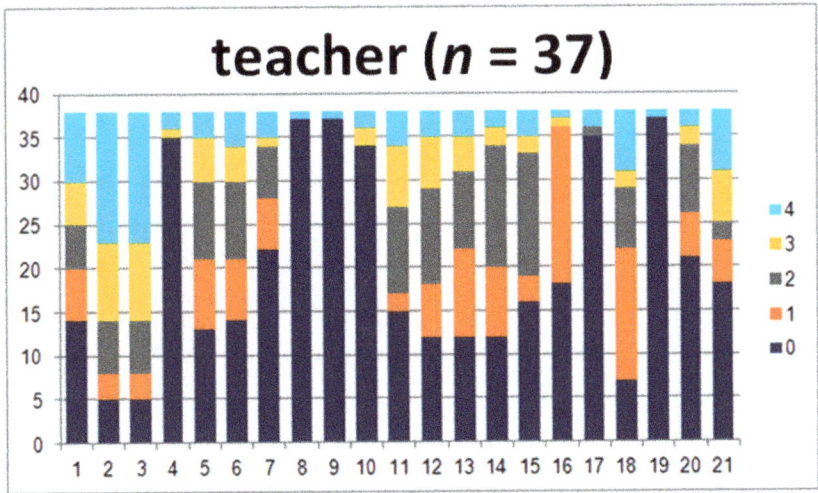

Figure 3. Answers given by the teachers.

For the question concerning reading the time, the teachers marked 0 most of the time, in contrast to parents who marked the 0–3 answers (Figure 4). In questions 11, 13, 14, and 18, the parents marked lower answers (0 and 1) much more frequently than the teachers. These questions concerned the issues of writing, rewriting, and mathematical abilities. Question number 18 touched upon headaches. All of the parameters and the comparison of the sum of points and levels show great statistical importance.

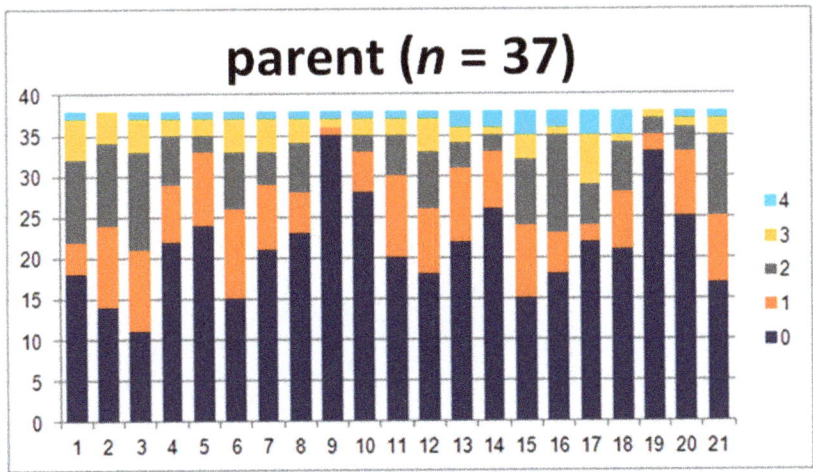

Figure 4. Answers given by parents of examined children.

3.3. Child–Parent Subgroup

In this group, there were 49 analyzed questionnaires.

In the child–parent group, the answers differ the most for questions 17, 18, 19, and 20 (19 and 20, $p < 0.05$), where the parents more commonly gave answers of 0 (Figure 5). The questions concerned reading the time, maintaining attention, headaches, and fatigue. Parents seldomly marked 4 (present at a very high intensity). Furthermore, there are statistically important differences when it comes to questions 8, 10, 11, and 14. These questions touched upon swimming, motion sickness, reading, and mathematical abilities, respectively.

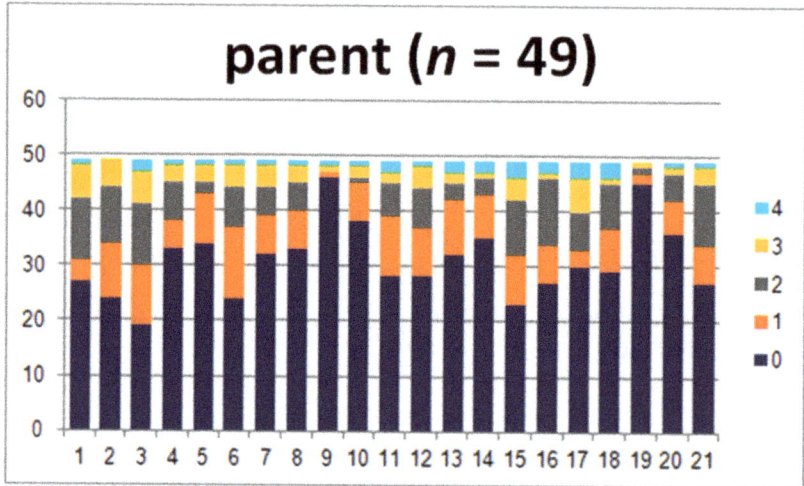

Figure 5. Answers given by parents of examined children.

The children's answers indicated that they have more difficulties with the aforementioned areas than their parents acknowledge (Figure 6). The comparison between the average sums of the points and levels shows great statistical significance ($p = 0.04$ and $p = 0.03$).

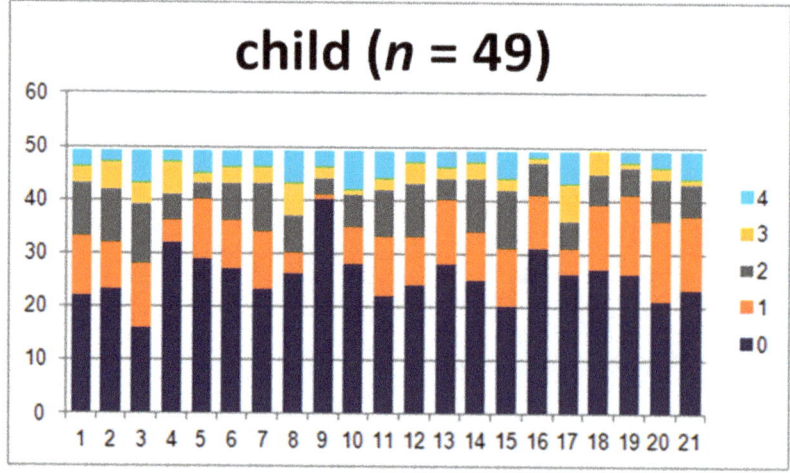

Figure 6. Answers given by examined children.

4. Discussion

The results of our research show that the answers in the parent–teacher group differed substantially in many aspects. The biggest difference was found for the answers given to the question concerning keeping attention, where the provided scales differ by 2 degrees. The results present a significant difference in the way that parents and teachers perceive a child's abilities. The difference of the teacher's and the parent's assessment where the child's answer is similar to the teacher's answer might be a result of a parent's limited awareness concerning the child, who is in a situation that demands focused attention during the class. However, the similarity between the child's and the parent's answers and substantially different teacher's answers might suggest that the teacher perceives the child to be in a difficult situation in the school environment. Different scores in the answers may also reflect the different expectations of the teacher, the child, and the parent. The difference might moreover suggest that the child behaves differently at school than he/she behaves at home. Significant differences appeared in the answers to the questions concerning the child's ability to catch a ball and the frequency of headaches. There was an incompatibility between the child's answer and the parent's answer concerning this issue. The children more often graded themselves higher in the answer to the question about catching the ball and lower when it comes to the answer concerning headaches. This might indicate the children's understated self-esteem and concealment of experiencing pain such as headaches, or it might suggest a lack of knowledge about how to qualify the frequency of their condition.

Similar research was previously conducted involving parent–teacher groups. There were also studies conducted with the use of other tests in a form of the questionnaires SRD-6, SPE_R, and the SPE IBE scale. The results of our study, however, showed that the teachers' observations are far more adequate than the data obtained by the use of the questionnaires mentioned above [1]. However, the INPP questionnaire focuses in particular on the children's difficulties, and it is proven to be an accurate and precise research tool [6]. Furthermore, there are studies that compare groups of children with groups of adults in general, for instance, children who are hospitalized, the nurses who are taking care of them, and the children's parents. These studies show that the children, though being under their parents' custody by law, should have the possibility to be consulted about and take an active part in adjusting the treatment they are undergoing, and they should be allowed to receive the information concerning their medical condition [10,11].

The differences in the perception of children's problems can lead to misunderstanding and create a stressful situation between parents and teachers. However, it could be reduced by analyzing the results of the research conducted with the use of the INPP questionnaire [4]. This allows us to initially discover the children's difficulties. With the use of the questionnaire, both the parents and the teachers are able to check which aspects of their children's life they should focus on more and whether the child is in a need of deeper analyses and further diagnosis. This tool can easily limit the problems that the child deals with and suggest therapeutic steps that will inhibit the progress of the problem in the future. The therapeutic activity and further diagnosis can show the child's autism disorders, which also are the cause of a child's problems at school and at home [12]. The observation and the reduction of a risk of further progress of dyslexia, problems reading and writing, and other symptoms of language disorders, at an early stage, can eliminate negative consequences that would appear later on [1]. The difficulties might be caused by the survival of the primitive reflexes [6]. They might indicate that the child suffers from mental problems [13]. They could also be an effect of the collision between home and school environment [14]. The atmosphere of home and the atmosphere of school differ substantially. They consist of different components, such as peers, teachers, parents, siblings who simultaneously influence the child's behavior [15]. To engage in a dialogue about the differences in perceiving children's difficulties enables us to make better decisions concerning the form of help that the child should receive.

Moreover, other factors that influence the rate of a child's difficulties should be taken into consideration too. Some other decisive factors that influence the child's difficulties include financial situation; parents' educational background; living conditions; access to knowledge, science, and information; and state of health [16]. All of them should be analyzed in a dialogue between the teacher, the parent, and possibly the child [10,11].

The main limitation of this study is that small groups were used for the INPP test. Future work could involve a larger group of children with neurological disorders, thus providing information about the children's and adults' perception of the children's developmental difficulties [1]. Future study could also include a sociological interview to determine the parents' wealth and education.

The conversation about developmental problems between children and the people who support their development should lead to developing the best tactic on how to act in school and home environments. The cooperation between parents and teachers is necessary in order to achieve maximum results while taking into account the child's individual needs too. This also enables objective comparison of information provided by both of these sources.

5. Conclusions

The presented research concerning parents' and teachers' perceptions of children and the children's self-assessment enabled us to draw the following conclusions:

1. Teachers notice children's problems with concentration and distraction during the classes substantially more often than the children themselves.

2. Teachers notice writing and copying problems and issues with math skills more often than parents.

3. Children notice their own physical coordination problems and trouble with concentration more often than parents do.

4. Children are perceived differently by their parents, their teachers, and by themselves. Something that is perceived as troublesome by children is not always perceived as problematic by parents or teachers.

The presented conclusions might provide an important reference both for parents and teachers. The integration and support for both of these communities is the key to success in the proper perception of a child in daily life [17].

Author Contributions: Concept and study design, A.P., E.W., M.T., E.Z.G.; data collection and compilation, A.D., A.G., M.L., A.P., E.W., M.T., E.Z.G.; data analysis and interpretation, A.D., A.K., M.L., E.Z.G.; writing the article, A.K., M.L.; critically reviewing the article, E.Z.G.; approval of the final version of the article, A.D., A.K., M.L., A.P., E.W., M.T., E.Z.G. All authors have read and agreed to the published version of the manuscript.

Funding: The publication was prepared under the project financed from the funds granted by the Ministry of Science and Higher Education in the "Regional Initiative of Excellence" program for the years 2019–2022, project number 016/RID/2018/19 and amount of funding 11 998 121.30 PLN.

Conflicts of Interest: The authors declare no conflict of interest.

References

1. Wiejak, K.; Krasowicz-Kupis, G.; Awramiuk, E. Linguistic determinants of early reading and writing skills based on the teacher's assessment using the IBE Educational Forecasting Scale. *Educ. Psychol.* **2017**, *11*, 41–63.
2. Bogdanowicz, M. Specific difficulties in reading and writing—Developmental dyslexia. In *Speech Therapy: Questions and Answers*; Gałkowski, T., Jastrzębowska, G., Eds.; University of Opole: Opole, Poland, 1999; pp. 815–859.
3. Bogdanowicz, M. *Risk of Dyslexia. Problem and Diagnosis*; Harmonia Publishing House: Gdańsk, Poland, 2002.
4. Grzywniak, C. Research on neuropsychological maturity for school learning. *Rep. Own Res. Men Disabil. Soc.* **2015**, *2*, 67–83.
5. Pecuch, A.; Kołcz-Trzęsicka, A.; Żurowska, A.; Paprocka-Borowicz, M. Psychomotor disorders assessment in 4–6 year-old children with INPP test battery. *Nurs. Public Health* **2018**, *8*, 11–20. [CrossRef]
6. Gieysztor, E.; Sadowska, L.; Choińska, A. The degree of primitive reflexes integration as a diagnostic tool to assess the neurological maturity of healthy preschool and early school age children. *Nurs. Public Health* **2017**, *7*, 5–11. [CrossRef]
7. Goddart-Blythe, S. The role of primitive survival reflexes in the development of the visual system. *J. Beh. Opt.* **1995**, *6*, 31–35.
8. Goddard-Blythe, S. *Reflexes, Learning and Behavior: A Window into the Child's Mind*; Fern Ridge Press: Eugene, OR, USA, 2005.

9. Goddard-Blythe, S. *Attention, Balance and Coordination: The A.B.C. of Learning Success*; Wiley: Hoboken, NJ, USA, 2009.
10. Coyne, I. Consultation with children in hospital: Children, parents' and nurses' perspectives. *J. Clin. Nurs.* **2006**, *15*, 61–71. [CrossRef] [PubMed]
11. Coyne, I. Children's participation in consultations and decision-making at health service level: A review of the literature. *Int. J. Nurs. Stud.* **2008**, *45*, 1682–1689. [CrossRef] [PubMed]
12. Crane, L.; Batty, R.; Adeyinka, H.; Goddard, L.; Henry, L.A.; Hill, E.L. Autism Diagnosis in the United Kingdom: Perspectives of Autistic Adults, Parents and Professionals. *J. Autism. Dev. Disord.* **2018**, *48*, 3761–3772. [CrossRef] [PubMed]
13. Soneson, E.; Childs-Fegredo, J.; Anderson, J.K.; Stochl, J.; Fazel, M.; Ford, T.; Humphrey, A.; Jones, P.B.; Howarth, E. Acceptability of screening for mental health difficulties in primary schools: A survey of UK parents. *BMC Public Health* **2018**, *18*, 1404. [CrossRef] [PubMed]
14. Trusz, S. *Cognitive and Social Development of a Child in the Light of Interpersonal Expectations of Parents and Teachers*; Institute of Educational Sciences, Pedagogical University of Cracow: Cracow, Poland, 2011.
15. Sikorska, I. *"The Diversity of Contexts of the Social Development of a Child" Department of Developmental and Educational Psychology Im. Stefan Szuman*; Jagiellonian University Cracow, Developmental Psychology: Cracow, Poland, 2005.
16. Frydrychowicz, A.; Misiorna, E.; Kozłowska, E.; Pietrzak-Kurzac, M.; Rusiak, P.; Szczepkowska-Szcześniak, K. Teacher's advisor for six-year-olds: Methodological materials for teachers developed as a result of the project "Study of school readiness of six-year-olds" implemented at the Methodological Center of Psychological and Pedagogical Assistance. In *Development and Assessment of Reading Skills of Six-Year-Old Children*; Methodological Center for Psychological and Pedagogical Assistance: Warsaw, Poland, 2006.
17. Peterson, J.; Bruce, J.; Patel, N.; Chamberlain, L.J. Parental Attitudes, Behaviors, and Barriers to School Readiness among Parents of Low-Income Latino Children. *Int. J. Env. Res. Public Health* **2018**, *15*, 188. [CrossRef] [PubMed]

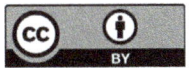

© 2020 by the authors. Licensee MDPI, Basel, Switzerland. This article is an open access article distributed under the terms and conditions of the Creative Commons Attribution (CC BY) license (http://creativecommons.org/licenses/by/4.0/).

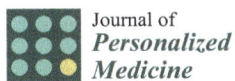

Article
Reframing Psychiatry for Precision Medicine

Elizabeth B. Torres [1,2,3]

1. Department of Psychology, Rutgers University, New Brunswick, NJ 08854, USA; ebtorres@psychology.rutgers.edu; Tel.: +1-(011)-858-445-8909; Fax: +1-(011)-732-445-2987
2. Center for Cognitive Science (RUCCS), Rutgers University, New Brunswick, NJ 08854, USA
3. Computer Science, Center for Biomedicine Imaging and Modelling (CBIM), Rutgers University, New Brunswick, NJ 08854, USA

Received: 19 July 2020; Accepted: 16 September 2020; Published: 25 September 2020

Abstract: The art of observing and describing behaviors has driven diagnosis and informed basic science in psychiatry. In recent times, studies of mental illness are focused on understanding the brain's neurobiology but there is a paucity of information on the potential contributions from peripheral activity to mental health. In precision medicine, this common practice leaves a gap between bodily behaviors and genomics that we here propose to address with a new layer of inquiry that includes gene expression on tissues inclusive of brain, heart, muscle-skeletal and organs for vital bodily functions. We interrogate gene expression on human tissue as a function of disease-associated genes. By removing genes linked to disease from the typical human set, and recomputing gene expression on the tissues, we can compare the outcomes across mental illnesses, well-known neurological conditions, and non-neurological conditions. We find that major neuropsychiatric conditions that are behaviorally defined today (e.g., autism, schizophrenia, and depression) through DSM-observation criteria have strong convergence with well-known neurological conditions (e.g., ataxias and Parkinson's disease), but less overlap with non-neurological conditions. Surprisingly, tissues majorly involved in the central control, coordination, adaptation and learning of movements, emotion and memory are maximally affected in psychiatric diagnoses along with peripheral heart and muscle-skeletal tissues. Our results underscore the importance of considering both the brain–body connection and the contributions of the peripheral nervous systems to mental health.

Keywords: autism; schizophrenia; mental depression; ataxia; fragile X; Parkinson's disease; mitochondria; gene expression; tissues; neurological disorders; nervous systems disorders

1. Introduction

Modern medicine is at an inflexion point [1], whereby advances in computational methods, wearable sensing technology and open access to Big Data are reshaping the ways in which we inform basic science and rapidly translate our knowledge to actionable treatments. Psychiatry is one of those medical fields that is rapidly evolving, while adapting traditional models to help advance the main goal of helping patients improve their quality of life. Along those lines, computational psychiatry [2], a nascent subfield within psychiatry, is merging methods from Computational Neuroscience with clinical approaches through successful collaborations. These new developments are bound to open new frontiers in therapeutic treatments. Further, as part of a more general effort in the medical field, precision medicine (PM) [1] has emerged as a new platform to combine expertise from multiple layers of the knowledge network in order to ultimately design personalized targeted treatments (Figure 1A). Integrating the personalized concept of PM with the new advances in computational psychiatry could give us a new way to approach mental illness and help patients cope with lifelong changing needs.

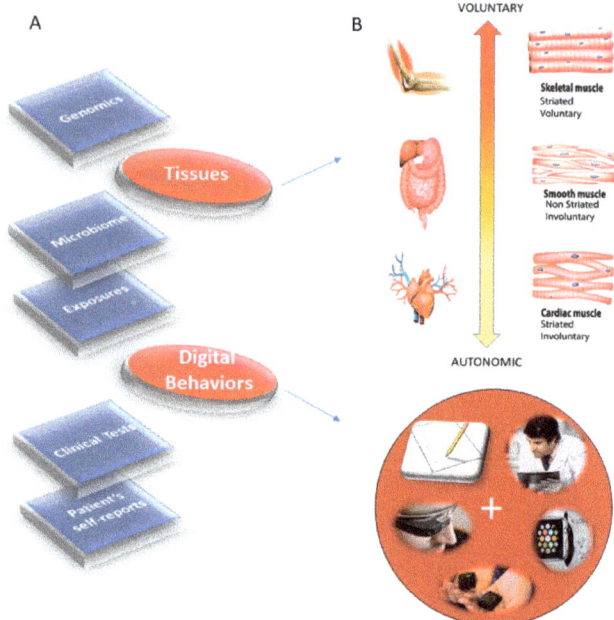

Figure 1. Roadmap to implement the precision medicine model for diagnoses and treatments of mental illnesses. (**A**) PM's interconnected knowledge network can contribute information about the individual's medical history, behaviors, environment, microbiome, and genetic makeup. Importantly, the new proposed layer of *digitized behaviors* leveraging the wearable biosensors revolution can transform medicine by creating truly personalized assessments. Additionally, the layer of behaviors can be connected to nervous system functioning via fundamental levels of neuromotor control that span along a phylogenetically orderly taxonomy. (**B**) This proposed taxonomy is based on levels of maturation in autonomous neuromotor control, linked to three fundamental muscle types: autonomic (by cardiac muscles), involuntary (by smooth muscles) and voluntary (by skeletal muscles). By linking the fundamental muscle types to the levels of control in the nervous systems, digital behaviors can then be mapped to bodily autonomy, bodily autonomy mapped to muscle types and muscle types mapped to genes/proteins. Any measure of treatment effectiveness for mental illnesses can then map back to improvements in observable behaviors embedded in activities of daily social life.

The task ahead is challenging because there is no proper roadmap to connect the layers of the knowledge network in PM and produce personalized diagnoses and measures of treatment outcomes that truly separate disease progression from treatment effectiveness according to age and development. Part of the problem is that most brain science has focused on experimental assays and methods that curtail natural movements. As such, our knowledge about the dynamics of natural behaviors is very limited, particularly in reference to those aspects of behavior that remain hidden to the naked eye of the clinician trained to observe specific expected behavioral landmarks of a psychiatric disorder conceived exclusively as a mental illness. In so doing, the clinically trained eye may miss important information that is perhaps common across different disorders of the nervous systems and rather relevant to help improve the patient's quality of life. For example, motor coordination and volitional control are critical ingredients of autonomy in any natural behavior underlying activities of daily living. Yet, these are not considered part of the diagnostics criteria for mental illnesses such as autism, schizophrenia and depression, as per the Diagnostics Statistical Manual (DSM-5) [3] (and see Supplementary Materials).

Research on the underlying neurobiology of mental illnesses has revealed their associated genetics [4] and/or helped characterize patterns of brain activity in response to external stimuli [5] (while curtailing naturalistic bodily motions to avoid instrumentation artifacts in imaging data or in EEG, MEG, etc.). This central approach to brain science has left us with a paucity of information about the possible contributions to mental illness from the peripheral nervous systems, and from vital organs important for autonomous living. The peripheral activity, however, continuously feeds back to the brain via afferent (body-to-brain) channels and is, in turn, dynamically updated through efferent (brain-to-body) activity, self-generated by the system itself. This recursive loop, whereby re-entrant information that is partly self-produced by the organism and partly influenced by external environmental conditions, would provide important clues about truly evolving dynamics and stochastic (variability) across all-natural behaviors. Approaching the problem through this lens could bring a new quantifiable layer of granularity to basic research. This would include the design of age-appropriate metrics reflecting the development of the organism as it ages and as it copes with a disorder [6,7]. The micro- and macro-motion data from the nervous systems biorhythms is the low hanging fruit that we can easily attain by leveraging the wearable sensors revolution. Further, because these quantifiable digitized activities and signals therein are partly self-generated, self-monitored and self-corrected by and within the nervous systems, this quantitative approach has the potential to take us from a purely correlational science to a science that is based on causal relations between nervous system activities and external/contextual stimuli. In this sense, the new proposed approach to mental illness is amenable to intervene and modify the system with well-informed, near-optimal means capable of improving its performance.

Micro- and macro-motions that underly all aspects of human behavior depend on the intactness of fundamental tissues, many of which have already been characterized in genomics according to cell types [8]. Here, we propose to combine micro-level underlying aspects of behavior with the current genomics knowledge to inform psychiatry of possible ways to improve quantification of nervous system activities. Ultimately, we seek to compile this information to help build accommodations and support for the patient population, while reconceptualizing mental illness as a physically quantifiable disorder of *the nervous systems*.

The nervous systems already offer a taxonomy of function and control that is phylogenetically ordered and well organized along several axes. Some of these axes are accessible today with non-invasive means and, as such, we can obtain signals and build computational models to understand mechanisms and translate them to actionable societal solutions. One possible orderly structure is suggested in Figure 1B, where we propose to map levels of neuromotor control (voluntary, involuntary, and autonomic) to fundamental types of muscles (skeletal, smooth, and cardiac) linked to commonly sampled tissues in genomic datasets. Combining information about gene expression on tissues that involve key components of the central nervous systems (the brain and the spinal cord), key organs for vital bodily functions (including smooth muscle lining internal organs), muscle-skeletal tissues and nerves, and cardiac tissues (for autonomic heart functioning), we explore the effects of removing disease-associated genes, on the overall remaining genome expression on these tissues. As a first step in this exercise, we reasoned that the genes associated with a given disorder ought to be important in the functioning of certain systems, which in turn depend on certain tissues. We also reasoned that such stochastic variations and combinations could be measured relative to the presence of all genes and to the absence of genes across neurological or non-neurological conditions.

What is the tissue distribution of gene expression in neuropsychiatric disorders such as autism, schizophrenia, and depression in relation to well-characterized neurological conditions? Is there convergence in the remaining gene expression on the tissues upon removal of the genes associated with that disease? Furthermore, how would the gene expression change across the tissues in non-neurological conditions such as various forms of cancer, immunodeficiencies, endocrine system deficiencies and so forth? How would it change in acquired disorders such as Post Traumatic Stress Syndrome (PTSD), currently diagnosed through observation?

Take autism for example. Autism is an umbrella term for a very heterogeneous set of neurodevelopmental disorders, but no gold-standard criteria include core neurological symptoms that could help us create early accommodations and support for the nascent nervous systems of the infant (during pre-cognitive stages of neurodevelopment). The rule of thumb is to assume that the child has odd, socially inappropriate behaviors and that they should be modified through operant and cognitive conditioning techniques—often translated from lab animals to human babies, without any type of collaboration with other fields studying infant development. Current methods of diagnoses and treatments in autism are not based on normative neurodevelopmental data charts to understand age-dependent departures from typical neurodevelopment. Without any systematic way to build age-appropriate metrics in order to capture highly non-linear, stochastic patterns and rates of change in the (rather accelerated) infant neurodevelopment, entire generations of infants, children and adolescents have been exposed to such means of behavioral treatments and no information can tie these back to the underlying genomic pool of this population.

In schizophrenia, delusions, avolition and catatonia are at the core of the disorder, but as in autism above, no criteria in the DSM highlight the profound somatic sensory-motor issues that have been found in patients [9]—even without the use of psychotropic medications known to alter motility. Interestingly, historical accounts of psychiatry (in pre-Freudian times) show the reliance on motor aspects of the behaviors that defined several mental illness from a neurological perspective [10].

Depression is also currently treated purely as a mental illness, but it may be important to understand potential contributions to various forms of depression, from the peripheral nervous systems and from the body in general. Genetic information may give us a way to link tissues affected in these neuropsychiatric conditions with those affected in neurological conditions, for which treatments and interventions of various forms may be effective. These may be in the form of drugs, or in the form of physical, mindfulness and occupational therapies aimed at helping support the person's bodily autonomy and overall increase the chances for independent living.

We here offer a new lens to help balance psychiatric with neurological criteria derived from genomic information specific to each disorder. In a first (crude) step of many to come, we start by comparing well-known neuropsychiatric and neurological conditions, the results from eliminating the genes associated with each disorder and quantifying the degree of convergence in the maximally affected tissues, in relation to those resulting from eliminating the genes associated with non-neurological conditions. We focus our discussion on possible ways to continue this path of inquiry and highlight current caveats for future improved iterations of the proposed methods.

2. Materials and Methods

We combine the datasets from genes associated with mental illnesses with well-known neurological disorders and with illnesses that are not directly associated with the nervous systems. We also include genes associated with manifestations of acquired Post-Traumatic Stress Syndrome Disorder (PTSD). Among mental illnesses defined by the DSM-5, we include autism, schizophrenia and mental depression of different types, (e.g., general, bipolar and unipolar). Among neurological conditions, we include ataxias (e.g., cerebellar, spinocerebellar, progressive, and gait) and Parkinson's disease. Among non-neurological disorders, we include colon cancer, breast cancer, diabetes, congenital heart disease, hematologic neoplasm, and various autoimmune disorders (lupus systemic erythematosus, psoriasis, and irritable bowel syndrome).

We use the genes, gene expression, and tissues from the Genotype-Tissue Expression project, GTEx pPortal human RNA-seq (Transcripts Per Million (TPM), see Appendix A for note in TPM) as reference specifically using the files denoted in Appendix B. In autism, we use the gene scoring module of the Simons Foundation Autism Research Initiative (SFARI) scored according to evidence from the literature. We also use ataxia genes, the X genes and the FX genes taken from various literature reviews [11,12]. Furthermore, we use genes associated with mitochondrial disorders [13] and genes identified in Parkinson's disease, taken from [14–19]. Besides the autism SFARI genes and the genes reported in literature reviews, we take the genes associated with autism, schizophrenia and depression reported in https://www.disgenet.org/home/ along with other genes from the above-mentioned non-neurological disorders. The latter will inform us of fundamental differences in gene expression between these diseases and those which affect neuromotor control and basic functioning, as mediated by interactions between the brain and the peripheral nervous systems (including the autonomic nervous system).

The SFARI autism categories that we used were those reported as of 03-04-2020. Quoting from their site:

- CATEGORY 1 Genes in this category are all found on the SPARK gene list. Each of these genes has been clearly implicated in Autism Spectrum Disorders, ASD—typically by the presence of at least three de novo likely-gene-disrupting mutations being reported in the literature—and such mutations identified in the sequencing of the SPARK cohort are typically returned to the participants. Some of these genes meet the most rigorous threshold of genome-wide significance; all at least meet a threshold false discovery rate of <0.1.
- CATEGORY 2 Genes with two reported de novo likely-gene-disrupting mutations. A gene uniquely implicated by a genome-wide association study, either reaching genome-wide significance or, if not, consistently replicated and accompanied by evidence that the risk variant has a functional effect.
- CATEGORY 3 Genes with a single reported de novo likely-gene-disrupting mutation. Evidence from a significant but unreplicated association study, or a series of rare inherited mutations for which there is not a rigorous statistical comparison with controls.
- SYNDROMIC The syndromic category includes mutations that are associated with a substantial degree of increased risk and consistently linked to additional characteristics not required for an ASD diagnosis. If there is independent evidence implicating a gene in idiopathic ASD, it will be listed as "#S" (e.g., 2S, 3S). If there is no such independent evidence, the gene will be listed simply as "S".

The GTEx dataset is as the 06-05-2017 v8 release. For every gene in autism, ataxia, X, FX, mitochondrial diseases, Parkinson's disease, and the non-neurological diseases, we first confirmed the presence of the gene in the GTEx dataset and then incorporated it into the analyses.

The genes from the DisGeNet portal were found by interrogation of their dataset under disease type and saving the outcome to excel files containing all pertinent information. All sample files used in our analyses are provided in Supplementary Materials.

2.1. Count Normalization

The GTEx matrix of RNA-seq genes along the rows (56,146) × the tissues (54) along the columns was transposed (54 × 56,246), such that we expressed each tissue as a function of the gene expression denoted by the count (TPM). Each individual count value was then normalized using Equation (1).

$$Normalized\ Count = \frac{count_i}{count_i + \frac{Avrg_{Global}Count}{Max_{Global}Count}} \quad (1)$$

Here, $count_i$ is the count value of the gene$_i$, $Avrg_{Global}Count$ is the overall average of the matrix of values taken along the columns and the rows. $Max_{Global}Count$ is the maximum count value, also taken globally across the matrix values. Figure 2 shows the original count numbers (Figure 2A) and the normalized version (coined micro-movement spikes (MMS)) in Figure 2B. Figure 2C shows the MMS derived from the fluctuations in counts normalized by Equation (1), while Figure 2D shows the histograms of the peaks (marked in red dots) for different tissues and genes scored by the SFARI.

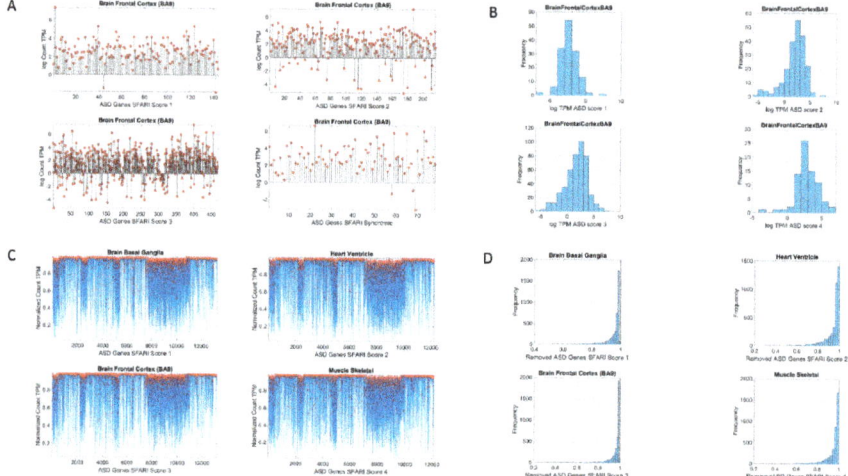

Figure 2. Analytical methods. (**A**) Sample raw data consisting of the log count (TPM) for different scored genes expressed in the brain frontal cortex (Brodmann Area 9). (**B**) Histograms of the log count TPM for each case in (**A**). (**C**) Upon removal of the Simons Foundation Autism Research Initiative (SFARI) autism genes, we obtain micro-fluctuation spikes in the normalized count, with deviations taken relative to empirically estimated mean, global averaged count, and global maximal count in Equation (1). (**D**) Histograms of the normalized micro-fluctuation spikes.

2.2. Gene Removal

For each of the disorders of interest in Appendix B Table A1 (mental illness and neurological) and Table A2 (non-neurological), we remove the genes associated with each condition from the human GTEx dataset. These disease-gene associations are as reported in the various databases (the SFARI, DisGeNet https://www.disgenet.org/home/ and the literature meta reviews). We then treat the resulting count series as a random process. We use the exponential distribution to characterize it and to assess the differential expression across the tissues relative to non-removal in the original human genome.

The question that we ask is: given the known neurological phenotypes, is there convergence between the most-affected tissues upon associated gene removal and the changes in the tissues that will be obtained by the removal of genes associated with mental illnesses? Furthermore, is there convergence with the outcome from removing the genes associated with non-neurological illnesses? Appendix B Tables A1 and A2 show the number of genes removed in each respective case as well as the source of the reported genes associated with each condition/disease.

2.3. Stochastic Analyses

Since the count values for each tissue can be conceived as a random series of numbers, we use maximum likelihood estimation (MLE) to model the numbers representing the counts, as generated by the exponential distribution using Equation (2)

$$y = \lambda e^{-\lambda x} \tag{2}$$

Here, x represents the normalized count value (as per Equation (1)) and y represents the value from the exponential distribution. We seek the value of the rate parameter λ to model this random counting process, which we use to represent the gene expression in the tissue. To that end, we estimate the likelihood $L(\lambda|x_1, x_2, \ldots, x_n)$ where the series of counts x_i, with i ranging from 1 to n, represent the normalized counts (according to Equation (1)) across all genes for one tissue. Appendix B shows the steps to find λ. Further, this is computed for each of the 54 tissues. We then rank the departure of λ (resulting from gene removal) from the λ obtained for the full human genome (see below). This is explained in Figure 3.

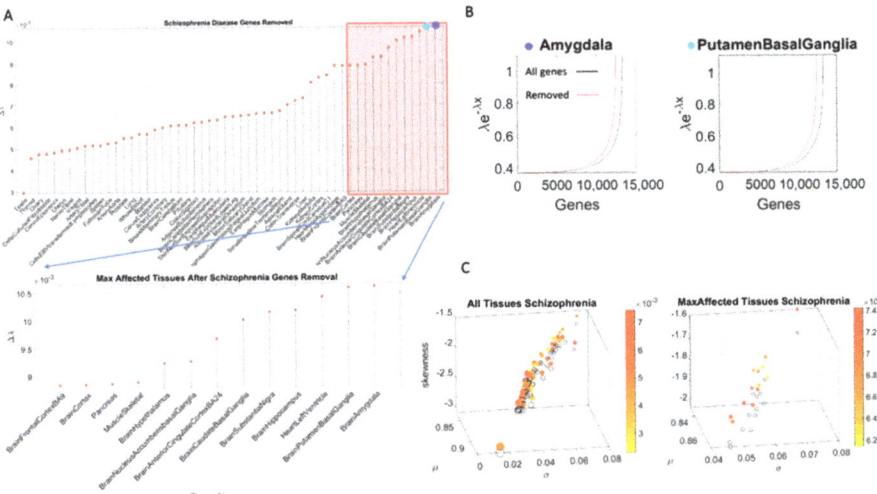

Figure 3. Sample metrics used for the stochastic analyses of a data sample (using 2697 schizophrenia-associated genes reported in DisGenNet portal and in the literature). (**A**) Effect of removing the schizophrenia genes from the GTEx human genome set expressed across 54 tissues. Tissues are sorted in ascending order, by the absolute difference Δλ between gene expression on the 54 tissues before and after removal. The red square highlights the top 13 median-ranked tissues shown in the panel below and the dark and light blue circles mark the top two tissues affected (the brain amygdala and brain putamen in the basal ganglia. (**B**) The exponential distribution curve is fit to the sorted normalized count representing the gene's expression in TMP on the top median-ranked affected tissues (as in Figure 2C, taking the peaks highlighted in red and fitting the exponential distribution to the frequency histogram, as in Figure 2D) before (black line) and after (red line) the removal of the genes associated with the disease. The absolute value difference between the curves is the Δλ used to rank the tissues by the effect size. (**C**) The fitting of the gamma distribution yields the shape and scale parameters used to compute the gamma moments. The axes represent the mean, the variance, and the skewness of the distribution of the normalized values and the color map represents the Earth Mover's Distance values measuring the difference between the resulting exponential frequency histograms in (**B**). The size of the circle is proportional to the kurtosis and the color-filled circles represent the tissue (54 in the left panel) with the original gene expression from GTEx (our reference template) vs. the open circles representing the stochastic shift, i.e., upon the removal of the genes associated with the disease in DisGenNet. The right panel contains the top-ranked tissues (13) according to the median values of the Δλ.

2.4. Stochastic Analyses—Visualization of Change Relative to the Normative Data of the Full Human Genome

Using MLE, we also obtain for each of the 54 tissues, the frequency histograms of the normalized counts across all genes and fit the continuous gamma family of probability distributions with shape (a) and scale (b) values in order to obtain the gamma moments and plot them on a parameter space. We do this to visualize the spread of the tissues and their shift upon gene removal. To that end, we plot the mean, the variance, and the skewness across the x, y and z axes, respectively. We plot the size of the marker representing the tissue proportional to the kurtosis value, and we color the marker based on the change relative to the original genome count (i.e., containing all the genes, without removal).

To measure the stochastic shift between the tissues from the full genome and those upon removal of the genes identified with each known neurological condition, we take the absolute difference between the MLE λ for the full GTEx genome and that for the genome upon removal of the genes associated with each condition, disorder or disease, as shown in Figure 3.

We median rank the Δλ for each tissue, sorting Δλ in ascending order across the 54 tissues. Then we create four median-ranked blocks and plot the maximally affected block of tissues (Figure 3A). The highest-ranked group is then compared across all conditions—mental illness vs. those neurologically defined vs. those non-neurologically defined. We annotate the neurological functions that such tissues are known to maximally disrupt. Further, we determine whether there is convergence between the tissue outcome in mental illnesses, upon removing the associated genes from the human genome-tissue model, and the outcome upon removing those genes tied to the other known disorders of the nervous systems. We repeat this interrogation process using the genes associated with disorders in the DisGeNet portal, including autism, schizophrenia, depression, the neurological disorders in Appendix B Table A1, and the non-neurological disorders in Appendix B Table A2.

To assess tissue outcome upon removal of genes associated with various non-neurological diseases, we follow these procedures and compare these to the above results. These diseases include colon cancer, breast cancer, psoriasis, diabetes, congenital heart disease, hematologic neoplast and systemic lupus. Appendix B Table A2 describes the number of genes associated with each of these diseases and the sources.

We also examine other mental illnesses described by the DSM. These include schizophrenia, depression, unipolar depression, and bipolar depression. We determine whether there are tissues that overlap with those affected in the neurological disorders. Lastly, we examine mitochondria-related disorders and PTSD using these methods. We reasoned that these may be disorders that have potentially affected tissues across a broader range of functions, including those from the brain and other bodily organs.

3. Results

3.1. Autism, Ataxia and FX Have Convergence in Maximally Affected Tissues by the Removal of Associated Genes

The maximally affected tissues upon gene removal, according genes stochastic expression (count in Transcripts Per Million (TPM)), are depicted in Appendix B Table A3. Tissue gene expression was modelled by the exponential distribution $y = \lambda e^{-\lambda x}$, with x as the gene combination expressed in the tissues, and λ as the exponential rate parameter. The Δλ between the neurotypical template case from the GTEx portal (containing all genes) and the modeled disorder case (upon removal of the SFARI genes) provides a sense of the departure from the normative case. This difference, taken for the removal of the SFARI genes, is depicted in Figure 4A, with samples of maximally affected tissues in Figure 4B that are known to be critical for motor control, regulation, adaptation/learning, and coordination.

The Δλ median ranking quantified the difference between neurotypical tissue gene expression vs. tissue gene expression upon removal of the genes corresponding to the disorders in question, with four groups ordered by the size of Δλ. This λ quantity was first obtained relative to the neurotypical population tissues, i.e., including all the counts (gene expression) from all genes, in order to model an exponential process. The computation of λ using maximum likelihood estimation (MLE) is explained in Appendix A. It does not assume any order of the counts, but rather seeks to identify the resulting λ for each tissue, treating the gene count (expression) as a random, memoryless stochastic process. Typically, the exponential distribution is used to model times between events, but here we used it to model the fluctuations in the values of the counts across the genes, as they randomly fluctuate their expression across each of the 54 tissues reported in the GTEx portal. We note this to underscore that the results spontaneously self-emerge from the random combination of the genes involved (with and without removal), rather than from the clinical criteria used to denote gene relevance to autism, or the evidence from the literature used to determine their association. There is in fact no scoring of such relevance for the genes associated with the other neurological disorders under consideration (e.g., ataxias and Parkinson's disease) or for the autistic disorders reported in the DisGenNet portal. Using those genes instead of the SFARI genes reveals tissues in Appendix B Table A4, where we report the convergence.

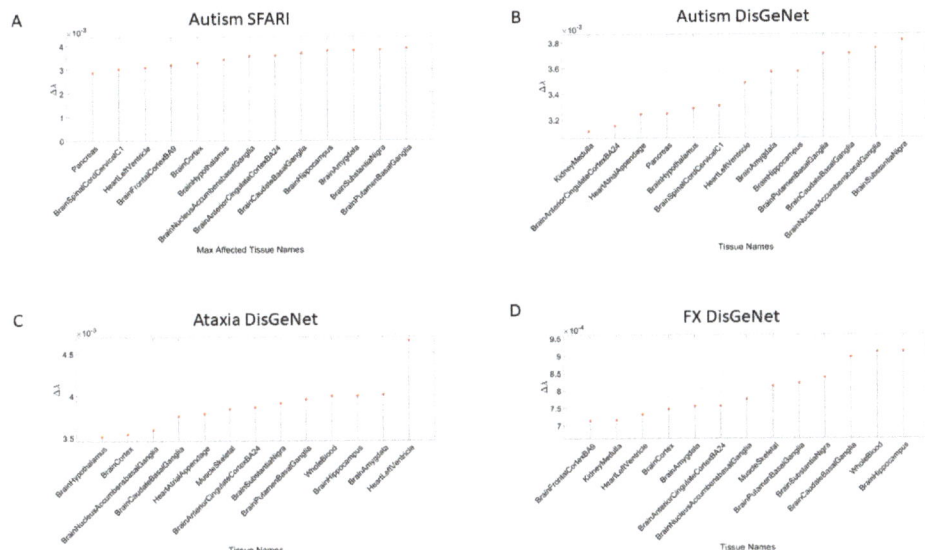

Figure 4. Convergence between autism and known neurological disorders shown by comparison of maximally affected tissues after removing genes associated with the disorder in autism (from the SFARI), autistic disorders (**A**,**B**) (from the DisGeNet portal) vs. ataxia (**C**) and fragile X (**D**) (See Appendix B Tables A3 and A4).

Removal of the SFARI genes, ranked by change in gene expression, reveals brain tissues linked to the CNS, in brain subcortical tissues linked to motor control (basal ganglia, striatum), memory (hypocampus), emotions (amygdala) and regulation (hypothalamus); and the spinal cord. This is also generally the case for the removal of the DisGeNet genes associated with autistic disorders and with FX and ataxia. Congruent with the outcome from the removal of the SFARI genes from the GTEx genome, the DisGeNet gene removal also affected the tissues associated with CNS function. Important tissues for systemic organ functioning such as those containing smooth muscles, cardiac and skeletal muscles in the taxonomy proposed in Figure 1B were also affected (commonly) across these disorders. Figure 4 shows a summary of the results, visualizing the stochastic shifts. Appendix B Tables A3 and A4 show the tissues ranked in descending order and color coded according to CNS (brain and spinal cord in blue), heart related (pink), muscle-skeletal (green), and peripheral vital organs (gray). Most tissues in autism and the neurological disorders are from the CNS, followed by PNS-related tissues in the heart and muscle-skeletal and with vital organs towards the end of the $\Delta \lambda$ ranking.

Supplementary Figures S1–S3 show these results separately for each neurological condition. We note in Supplementary Materials that removal of the SFARI autism syndromic genes from the GTEx genome reveals maximal differences in tissues of organs with smooth and cardiac muscles linked to involuntary and autonomic function in the proposed taxonomy of Figure 1B.

Removal of the overlapping SFARI genes and neurological disorders also reveal brain tissues linked to motor control, memory, emotions, and regulation. This is depicted in Figure 4. Given the congruence between the tissues maximally affected by removing the SFARI autism genes from the GTEx database and those from the neurological conditions, we next ascertain the extent to which these genes overlap with those used from ataxias in the literature. To that end, we divide them into the autosomal dominant, the autosomal recessive and the X-chromosome genes. Figure 5A shows the result upon removal of overlapping genes between the SFARI autism set and ataxias (dominant and recessive and X-chromosome sets) from the literature. Appendix B Table A3, Column 3 lists the tissues, while Appendix B Table A5 also has the scoring from the SFARI autism genes. Supplementary Materials Table S2 lists the phenotypic information of the disorders associated with these genes, as described by the clinical literature. Figure 5B lists the PD gene that overlaps with the SFARI autism genes, also depicted in Appendix B Table A5 along with the score ranking from the SFARI portal.

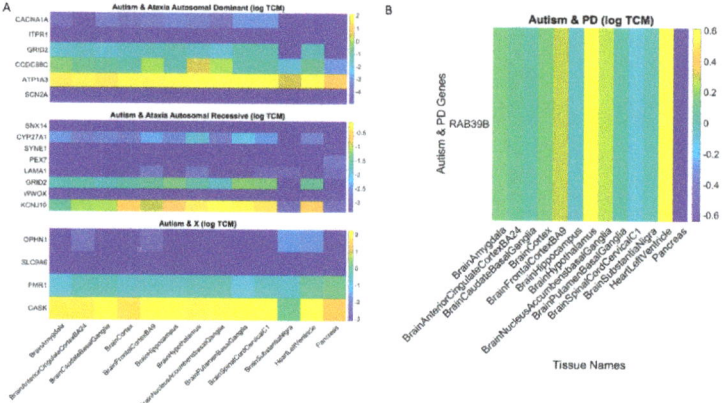

Figure 5. Gene expression on maximally affected tissues (color bar coded in log TPM) upon removal of overlapping genes between the SFARI autism set and ataxias (dominant and recessive and X-chromosome sets) from the literature (**A**) and (**B**) from Parkinson's disease. The horizontal axis lists the tissue names and the vertical axis lists the gene names.

We note that removing this subset of 14 overlapping genes from the SFARI autism set (Appendix B Table A5) does not change the primary result, whereby the most-affected tissues upon removal of the SFARI autism set from the GTEx dataset are those associated with subcortical brain structures critical for motor control, adaptation/learning, regulation, coordination and autonomic function as well as memory and emotion. This is shown in Figure 5A,B and in the third column of Appendix B Table A3. In Figure 4D, we also plot the top-ranked tissues affected by the removal of the FX genes reported in the DisGeNet portal from the GTEx dataset. Supplementary Figures S19–S22 further provide details on X-chromosome genes in Figure 5A implicated in autism according to the SFARI genes portal.

The result that convergence in the ranked descending order of the CNS (brain and spinal cord tissues), followed by heart-related tissues, muscle-skeletal tissue and lastly peripheral vital organs for systemic functioning in the SFARI autism and well-known neurological disorders from the literature is also congruent with the results using the genes associated with these conditions in the DisGeNet portal. There, we interrogated autistic disorders, ataxias and fragile X, confirming the overlap in genes, their expression on the 54 tissues of the GTEx database and the orderly levels of tissues maximally affected by the removal of the associated genes. We grouped the tissues by CNS, heart, muscle-skeletal and peripheral vital organs to follow the proposed taxonomy of Figure 1B.

In the remaining sections of this paper, we consistently use this tissue grouping to simplify visualization of the Appendix B tables and data presentation. Figure 6 shows the results for different types of ataxias and FX, while Appendix B Table A6 summarizes the top-ranked affected tissues in different types of ataxias. These are color coded according to the tissue grouping, approximating the taxonomy proposed in Figure 1B.

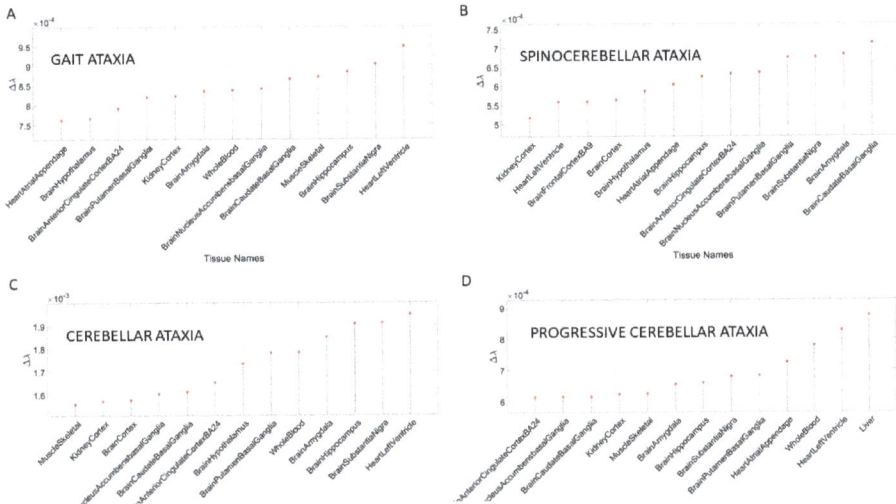

Figure 6. Different types of ataxia showing the top Δλ-ranked tissues, also shown in Appendix B Table A7. (**A**) Gait ataxia; (**B**) spinocerebellar ataxia; (**C**) cerebellar ataxia; (**D**) progressive cerebellar ataxia.

3.2. Removal of Genes Associated with Schizophrenia and Multiple Forms of Mental Depression Reveals Convergence with Neurological Disorders

The removal of the DisGeNet genes associated with mental illnesses such as schizophrenia, depression, bipolar depression and unipolar depression from the normative GTEx genome resulted in convergence of maximally affected tissues involved in the CNS, especially those brain regions necessary for neuromotor control, memory, and emotion. This is depicted in Appendix B Table A7 and Figure 7. Several of these tissues were also found to be affected upon removal of the SFARI genes and the genes associated in DisGeNet with autistic disorders. Furthermore, these are maximally affected tissues in the well-known neurological conditions depicted in Figures 4 and 5 and Appendix B Tables A3–A5.

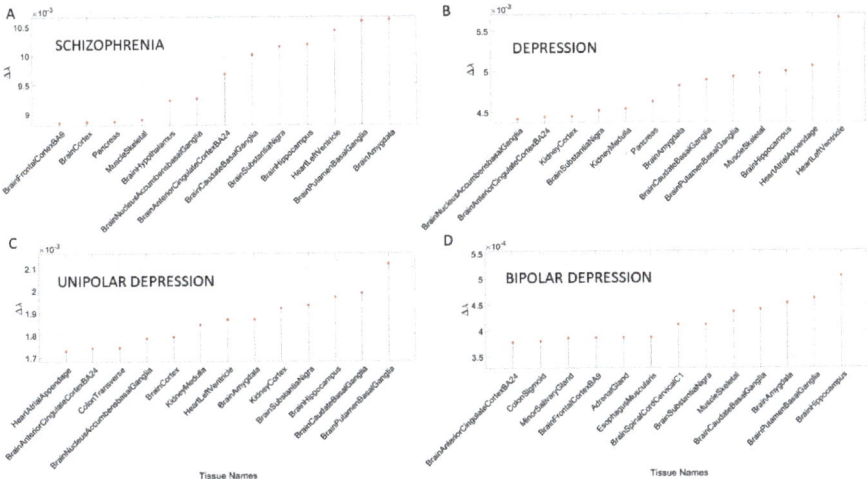

Figure 7. Maximally affected tissues in schizophrenia (**A**) and depression (**B**), and in different types of depression (unipolar (**C**) and bipolar (**D**)) shown in Appendix B Table A7.

3.3. Removal of Genes Associated with Non-Neurological Disorders Reveals Other Non-CNS Tissues

In addition to the examination of mental illnesses and neurological disorders, we also interrogated the GTEx genome upon removal of genes associated with various non-neurological disorders. These included various forms of cancers, inflammatory and autoimmune disorders and other tissues related to the heart, the circulatory and the endocrine systems. Appendix B Tables A8 and A9 summarize the results of this interrogation and Figures 8 and 9 show the Δλ-ranking graphs.

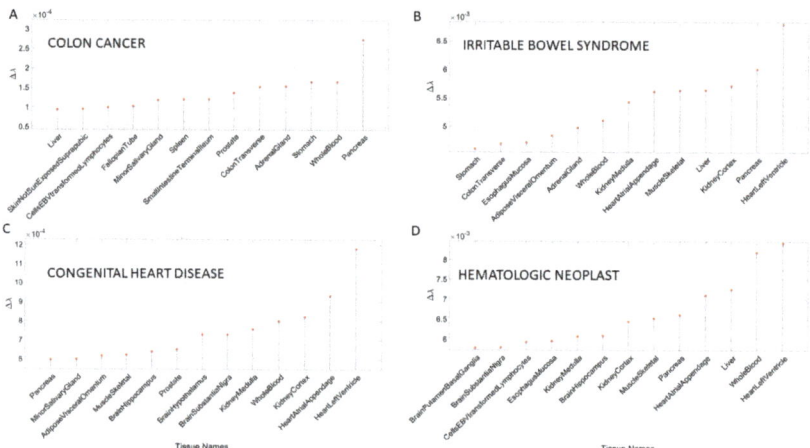

Figure 8. Maximally affected tissues in a sample non-neurological diseases of Appendix B Table A8 reveal primarily non-CNS tissues involving peripheral vital organs for systemic functioning, followed by heart-related and muscle-skeletal tissues. As before, the interrogation of the GTEx genome is based on the genes associated with diseases in the DisGeNet portal. (**A**) Colon cancer; (**B**) irritable bowel syndrome; (**C**) congenital heart disease and (**D**) hematologic neoplast. Color code as in previous tables.

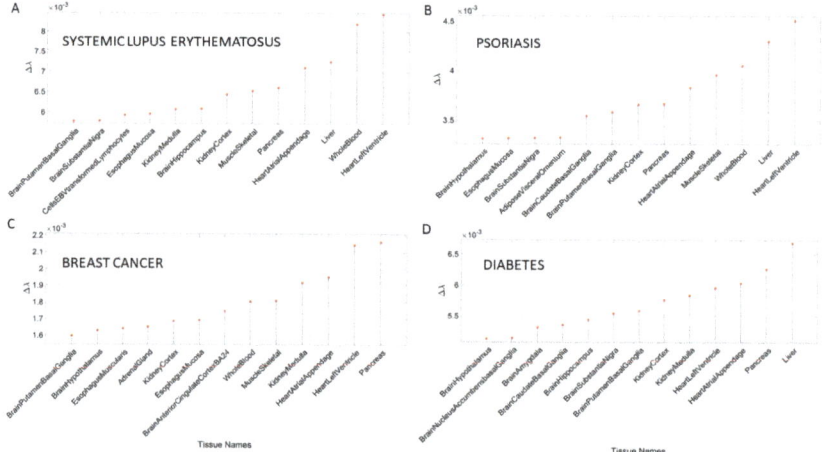

Figure 9. Maximally affected tissues in non-neurological diseases. (**A**) Systemic Lupus Erythematosus; (**B**) Psoriasis; (**C**) Breast Cancer; (**D**) Diabetes. These are depicted in Appendix B Table A10 median-ranked according to the Δλ values obtained from the absolute difference between the tissues according to the full genome in the GTEx database and the GTEx genome without the genes associated with each disease, according to the queries to the DisGeNet portal.

The results of the maximally affected tissues upon the removal of the genes associated with these non-neurological disorders revealed a very different picture than those upon removal of the genes associated with the mental illnesses (autism, schizophrenia and the depressions) and those associated with the known neurological conditions (the various forms of ataxia, FX and Parkinson's disease). Namely, the CNS-related tissues were less affected in these non-neurological diseases than those related to the PNS (muscle-skeletal and ANS heart), and those linked to peripheral bodily organs were the most visibly affected. The exception was diabetes, maximally affected tissues in peripheral organs, but also CNS and PNS tissues in the tail of the top $\Delta\lambda$-ranked tissues. We next interrogate the genome in relation to mitochondrial disorders of several kinds and acquired PTSD.

3.4. Removal of Genes Associated with Mitochondrial Diseases Reveals that Heart-Related Tissues Are Maximally Affected but PTSD Is Mixed

Removal of genes associated with mitochondrial disorders of various types from the GTEx genome, according to the genes in the DisGeNet portal, reveal a mixture of tissues associated with peripheral vital organs for systemic functions, heart-related and muscle-skeletal- and CNS-related tissues. The top half of the highest-ranked tissues in mitochondrial disease shows affected tissues related to the heart, muscle-skeletal and peripheral organs, while the bottom half shows more involvement of brain-related tissues in subcortical regions of motor control. In contrast, mitochondrial myopathies show a predominance of CNS-related tissues, including the brain and spinal cord, with top $\Delta\lambda$-ranked tissues related to the heart and muscle-skeletal tissues. Mitochondrial encephalopathy, lactic acidosis, and stroke-like episodes (MELAS) show a predominance of tissues associated with peripheral vital organs for systemic function and heart-related tissues. Only two brain regions for motor control and emotion are present in the bottom-ranked tissues of the most-affected tissues.

The case of acquired PTSD also reveals a mixture of tissues from brain, heart, and peripheral organs. There, we see maximally affected tissues linked to subcortical regions of the brain involved in motor control, adaptation, learning, and coordination intermixed with tissues linked to peripheral bodily organs (like the kidneys) and the autonomic systems' heart. Furthermore, we also see tissues linked to the hypothalamus, a regulatory brain structure. Figure 10 shows the graphs of the $\Delta\lambda$ difference, which was median ranked, as in the previous cases, for these disorders.

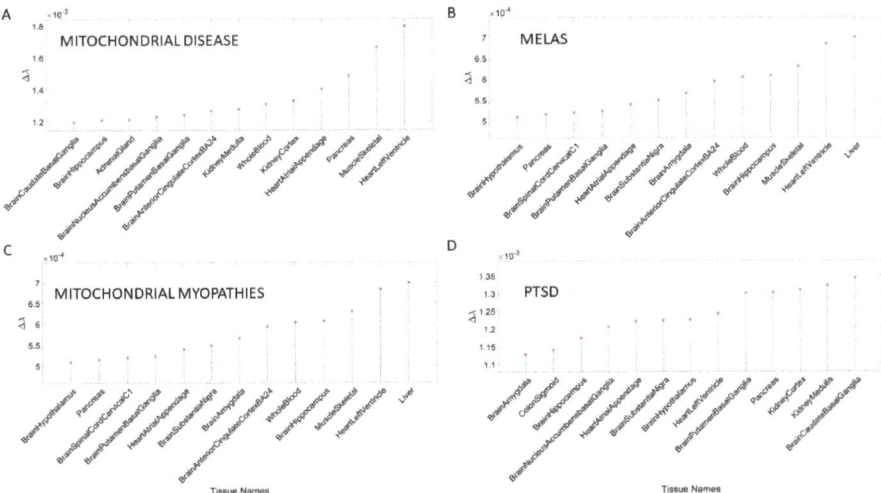

Figure 10. Maximally affected tissues in mitochondrial diseases (**A–C**) and in PTSD (**D**) of Appendix B Table A10, shown in graphical form according to the $\Delta\lambda$ values.

We summarize the results across all 54 tissues (in alphabetical order from left to right) in Figure 11. Here, a color map depicts the values of Δλ normalized for each disease (along the rows) across the tissues (columns) by dividing by the maximum Δλ value of each row. The patterns reveal that the maximally affected tissues (upon genes removal) are common to both neurological disorders and mental illnesses. They correspond to the brain tissues involved in motor control, adaptation, and learning (basal ganglia, striatum, substantia nigra), tissues in involved in emotion (amygdala), memory (hippocampus) and systemic regulation (hypothalamus). They also reveal that whole blood tissue is not as affected in the mental illnesses as in the neurological disorders (marking a point of divergence that warrants further investigation). Heart-related tissues and muscle-skeletal tissues are also shared between these mental illnesses and neurological disorders when the genes specific to each disorder are removed from the GTEx genome. Interestingly, the pancreas is an example of a peripheral bodily organ with tissues that are commonly affected across most of the disorders and diseases interrogated here. Yet they have lower weight the neurological disorders compared to the non-neurological diseases under examination.

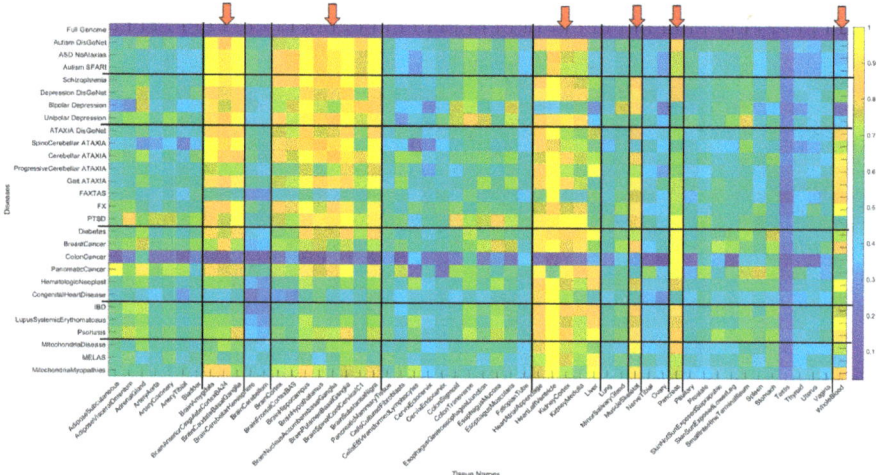

Figure 11. Summary of disorders/diseases (27 rows) x tissues (54 columns) in alphabetical order. Entries are Δλ (difference with respect to the gene expression values from the full GTEx genome) values normalized by the maximum across the tissues for each row (disorder/disease). The first row is the 0–Δλ difference reference from the full genome. Red arrows mark the maximally affected tissues across all diseases, showing mental illnesses on the top, followed by neurological disorders, then non-neurological, including several types of cancer, autoimmune disorders, and diabetes. Black lines delineate blocks of diseases (along rows) and blocks of gene expression on tissues (along columns).

The non-neurological diseases reveal less involvement of the CNS-related tissues but highly overlap with the heart and muscle-skeletal tissues. Tissues linked to the kidneys, liver and pancreas are also maximally affected by genes' removal in these diseases. Colon cancer shows an interesting pattern whereby the pancreas reveals maximal normalized Δλ values. Figure 12 summarizes the patterns in binary form by turning ON (yellow) values above 0.8 considered high and OFF those below (blue). This cut off is chosen to further highlight overlap and differences across diseases based on high Δλ.

The patterns revealed by the high values of the normalized Δλ quantity, show convergence of maximally affected brain tissues in mental illnesses with the neurological disorders but not with the non-neurological disorders (except for diabetes which does affect some brain regions.) The mitochondrial diseases do not show the same intensity of the CNS-related Δλ values as the mental illnesses and the neurological disorders, but they do share the heart and muscle-skeletal patterns with all the examined diseases and disorders. This is interesting, given that some of the children with various forms of mitochondrial disorders may receive diagnoses of autism. In summary, there is clear overlap between mental illness and neurological disorders, suggesting involvement of the central nervous systems in both. We also see major contributions from the peripheral nervous systems, particularly the heart, the muscle-skeletal tissues and, to a lesser degree, tissues of peripheral organs. The latter are most affected in the non-neurological diseases. Figure 13 shows the most-affected tissue in each disease/disorder (also depicted in Appendix B Table A11).

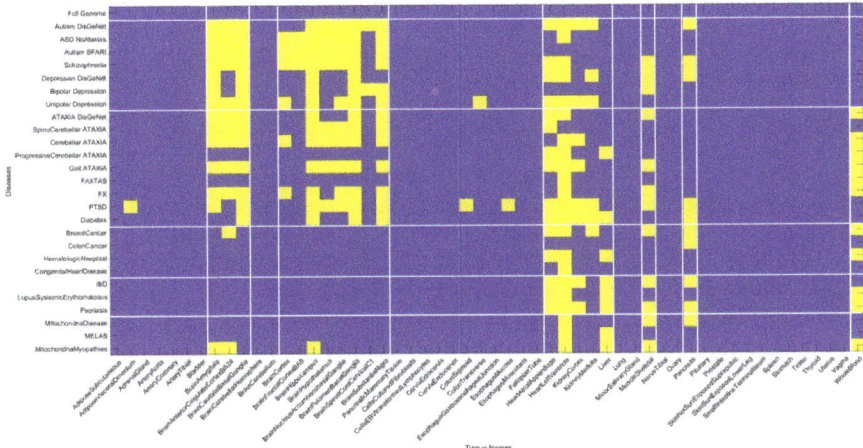

Figure 12. Binary version of the matrix in Figure 11 upon thresholding by a high normalized $\Delta\lambda$ value of 0.8 shows that the overlap across mental illnesses, neurological disorders and non-neurological diseases is primarily in the heart tissues, the muscle-skeletal tissues and organs such as the pancreas, liver, and kidney. Whole blood tissue is shared between neurological and non-neurological disorders but not present in the mental illnesses. Brain tissues are shared between mental illnesses and neurological disorders.

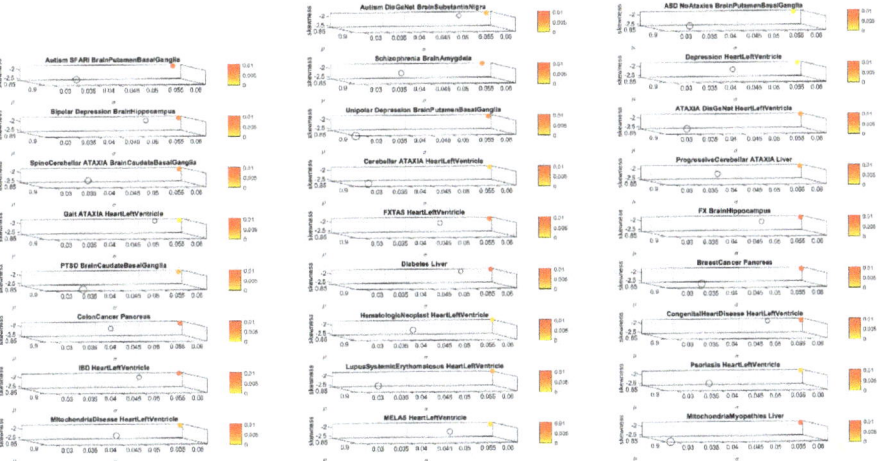

Figure 13. Stochastic shift of gene expression on tissue after gene removal for each disease/disorder under consideration (colored circle) relative to the gene expression on that tissue using the full genome

in GTEx (open circles). The most-affected tissue in each disorder/disease under consideration was selected according to the maximum $\Delta\lambda$ value, the absolute difference between the empirically estimated λ using MLE of the exponential distribution rate parameter for the full GTEx genome and for the genome minus the genes associated with each disease/disorder. Since the exponential distribution is a particular case of the continuous gamma family of probability distributions (when the gamma shape parameter is 1), we also used MLE to estimate the shape and scale gamma parameters and the four gamma moments, plotted here in a five-dimensional parameter space. Along the x axis, we plot the empirically estimated gamma mean; along the y axis, we plot the gamma variance; along the z axis, we plot the gamma skewness and the kurtosis is used to represent the size of the marker (more kurtotic distributions have higher value, i.e., larger circle). The fifth dimension is the color representing the $\Delta\lambda$ (see also Figure 3C, visualizing one single disease and all 54 tissues or summarizing the top 13 median-ranked tissues as those most affected).

4. Discussion

This work interrogated the human genome by removing genes associated with various diseases and comparing the outcome from the remaining gene expression on 54 tissues commonly examined in the GTEx portal. These tissues involve parts of the central nervous systems (the brain and the spinal cord) and parts of the peripheral nervous systems (the muscle-skeletal tissue and the heart tissues as part of the autonomic nervous system), which we grouped in Figure 1B. Other tissues are from peripheral vital organs for systemic bodily functions (whole blood, pancreas, liver, kidneys, lungs, etc.).

We compared mental illnesses such as autism, schizophrenia, and various types of mental depression (including unipolar and bipolar), with well-known neurological disorders such as different types of ataxias, fragile X and Parkinson's disease. We found convergence between the tissues maximally affected by the removal of disease-associated genes across these mental illnesses and neurological disorders. CNS-related tissues in subcortical regions of the brain related to motor control, motor learning, motor coordination, and motor adaptation, as well as memory and emotion, were predominantly maximally affected by the corresponding gene removal across both the mental illnesses and the neurological disorders. This convergence demonstrates overlap between psychiatric and neurological conditions with specific involvement of motor, memory, emotional and regulatory axes. In autism and FX, we obtained congruent results on maximally affected tissues. The results were consistent using removal of the genes from the SFARI autism database and using the genes upon querying the DisGeNet portal. In addition to the genes reported by querying DisGeNet, we also used the genes reported in the literature for schizophrenia and depression, and for Parkinson's disease. We found congruence in all cases.

To further test our hypothesis that these mental illnesses are *disorders of the nervous systems* and that removing the gene pool associated with them gives rise to overlapping tissues related to CNS functioning, we also queried DisGeNet about other non-neurological diseases. We found that in such cases, the predominance of maximally affected tissues was on tissues associated with peripheral vital bodily organs related to the disease, such as pancreas, kidney, liver, and colon transverse in colon cancer. Furthermore, several of these diseases had maximally affected heart-related tissues and whole blood. Other cases also revealed a predominance of peripheral organs. We lastly, interrogated the genome in relation to mitochondrial diseases and acquired PTSD. In these cases, we hypothesized and confirmed a mixture of tissues related to peripheral organs (for mitochondrial diseases) and the CNS (for PTSD).

In the case of mitochondrial diseases, the heart-related tissues were revealed as the most affected along with muscle-skeletal tissue. Furthermore CNS-related tissues were more affected by gene removal in mitochondrial myopathies (i.e., the amygdala and the anterior cingulate cortex), as compared to MELAS or mitochondrial disease. The common thread across all three types of mitochondrial-related disorders was the heart-related tissues. The case of acquired PTSD showed a mixture of CNS-related tissues, tissues related to bodily peripheral organs, and heart-related tissues. The kidney and pancreas were also affected in PTSD. When we examined the maximum $\Delta\lambda$ for each disorder/disease under examination, we found that the basal ganglia was maximally affected in autism, unipolar depression, spinocerebellar ataxia, and PTSD), while the heart left ventricle tissue was maximally affected in depression, ataxia, cerebellar ataxia, gait ataxia and fragile X tremor ataxia syndrome (FXTAS). This result indicates overlap between the psychiatric mental illnesses and the neurological disorders. It also shows the importance of examining mental illnesses in a more systemic way that includes the autonomic nervous system of the PNS.

This test on non-neurological illnesses served as a control to show that removal of the genes associated with each disorder did have specificity with the disorder and yet a very different outcome when comparing the mental illnesses to the non-neurological disorders. Among the top tissues affected across non-neurological diseases, the pancreas was maximally affected by the removal of disease-associated genes in breast and colon cancer, while the liver was maximally affected in diabetes. The heart left ventricle was maximally affected across autoimmune disorders such as psoriasis, lupus systemic erythematosus, and irritable bowel disease (IBD). The heart was also maximally affected in hematologic neoplast, congenital heart disease, mitochondrial disease and MELAS, in contrast to the mitochondrial myopathies which showed the liver as the maximally affected tissue.

This exercise demonstrated that despite the stochastic nature of gene expression, upon removal and random recombination, there is convergence across psychiatric and neurological disorders, thus potentially rendering both as *disorders of the nervous systems*. In both cases, we found a strong prevalence of the CNS, but also found important differences in tissues from the PNS, including the heart and the muscle-skeletal tissues involved in both mental illnesses and neurological disorders. Because of these convergences, and the fact that there are treatments and accommodations to help persons with neurological disorders, it may be possible to leverage some of those types of bodily-based supports to help persons with mental illnesses. Behaviors that are described by observation to define mental illnesses can now be connected with underlying tissues involved in voluntary, involuntary, and autonomic function across the CNS and the PNS and mapped to the genome, thus closing the present gap between behaviors and genomics in the precision medicine knowledge network. In this sense, the present methods offer a new way to interrogate the genome and link tissues with behavioral phenotyping.

A surprising finding here is the potential contributions of peripheral structures and organs to mental illness. Tissues of the autonomic nervous systems were maximally impacted by the removal of the genes associated with these mental illnesses, as was the muscle-skeletal tissue among the top-ranked illnesses. Tissues associated with subcortical brain regions necessary for motor control, learning, adaptation, and coordination (basal ganglia and striatum) were highly impacted by the removal of the genes in both mental illnesses and neurological disorders, along with those tissues important for memory (hippocampus), emotion (amygdala) and regulation (hypothalamus). Surprisingly, we did not see cerebellum-related tissues among the most affected by the removal of the genes (even in ataxias) where we do know that the cerebellum plays a large role [20–23]. This was also the case in autism, where we know the cerebellum has been implicated [24,25].

Lastly, the autoimmune disorders that we examined had very different brain tissue patterns from the mental illnesses and neurological conditions but shared the heart-related tissues and the muscle-skeletal tissue. In this sense, the contributions from the peripheral systems to mental illnesses and to autoimmune disorders seem important. However, blood tissue marked a departure of neurological disorders from mental illnesses, as it was maximally affected in neurological disorders but not in the mental illnesses. Overall, these gene removals revealed surprising results that invite rethinking how we may want to describe, diagnose, and treat mental illnesses in general.

Caveats and Future Directions

Although we found evidence that the mental illnesses and neurological disorders have remarkable overlap in the types of brain tissues that are maximally affected by the removal of their corresponding associated genes, we recognize that gene removal is a crude way to interrogate the human genome and its expression of the 54 tissues of the GTEx database. Future work will aim at developing more sophisticated methods to explore gene overexpression and to build simulations of the use of these methods in, e.g., combination with dynamic transcriptome evolution during neuronal differentiation in the development of cell lines from induced pluripotent stem cells. This will be important to move beyond a static approach and be able to assess asynchronous gene expression behaviors over time when cell lines differentiate into neuronal types. Full transcriptome dynamic interrogation longitudinally, over time, is now possible using these stochastic analyses in combination with the various data repositories featuring disease-associated genes.

The present work merely scratches the surface on possible new ways to interrogate the human genome in relation to diseases of all types (not just mental or neurological) in order to possibly build comparative models of outcomes *in tissues* that can be related to behavioral phenotypic manifestations of the clinical disorder. In this sense, the work presented here can help bridge the gap between behavioral description of a mental illness, or a neurological disorder, and its genetic underpinnings via the affected tissues. Combining this approach with the new wave of digital biomarkers that describe human behavior digitally at a microscopic level [9,26–29], using objective means and a finer level of granularity beyond naked eye detection, could help us redefine many psychiatric disorders and medical conditions under the precision medicine paradigm.

5. Conclusions

We here offer a new roadmap to reframe psychiatry using the precision medicine paradigm. The new stochastic approach can initiate the steps to connect behavioral phenotypic description from clinical observation and digital characterizations therein, with the underlying neurobiology of mental illnesses. Borrowing knowledge from neurology and brain science, it will be possible to shift psychiatry from an art to a quantitative objective science under the tenets of precision medicine by integrating all layers of the knowledge network. This would help design personalized targeted treatments utilizing the person's genome, localizing the most-affected tissues defining central nervous system functions and distinguishing those from tissues related to vital organs for systemic functions. This new approach could potentially mark the beginning of a transformative era in mental health.

6. Patents

E.B.T. holds the US Patent "Methods and Systems for the Diagnoses and Treatments of Nervous Systems Disorders" combined in this paper as micro-movement spikes (MMS) data type and continuous gamma probability distribution family empirical estimation.

Supplementary Materials: The following are available online at http://www.mdpi.com/2075-4426/10/4/144/s1, Figure S1: Outcome of genes' expression on most affected tissues upon removing the Ataxia genes from the normative data., Figure S2: Outcome of genes' expression on most affected tissues upon removing the FX and PD genes from the normative data., Figure S3: Outcome of genes' expression on most affected tissues upon removing the Mitochondrial disease genes from the normative data, Figure S4: Outcome of genes' expression on most affected tissues upon removing genes based on SFARI Autism scores., Figure S5: Information on gene CACNA1C common to the SFARI Autism set and the Ataxia Autosomal Dominant genes reported in the literature., Figure S6: Information on gene SCN2A common to the SFARI Autism set and the Ataxia Autosomal Dominant genes reported in the literature, Figure S7: Information on gene ATP1A3 common to the SFARI Autism set and the Ataxia Autosomal Dominant genes reported in the literature., Figure S8: Information on gene CCDC88C common to the SFARI Autism set and the Ataxia Autosomal Dominant genes reported in the literature., Figure S9: Information on gene ITPR1 common to the SFARI Autism set and the Ataxia Autosomal Dominant genes reported in the literature., Figure S10: Information on gene KCNJ10 common to the SFARI Autism set and the Ataxia Autosomal Recessive genes reported in the literature., Figure S11: Information on gene WWOX common to the SFARI Autism set and the Ataxia Autosomal Recessive genes reported in the literature., Figure S12: Information on gene GRID2 common to the SFARI Autism set and the Ataxia Autosomal Recessive genes reported in the literature., Figure S13: Information on gene LAMA1 common to the SFARI Autism set and the Ataxia Autosomal Recessive genes reported in the literature., Figure S14: Information on gene PEX7 common to the SFARI Autism set and the Ataxia Autosomal Recessive genes reported in the literature., Figure S15: Information on gene SYNE1 common to the SFARI Autism set and the Ataxia Autosomal Recessive genes reported in the literature., Figure S16: Information on gene CYP27A1 common to the SFARI Autism set and the Ataxia Autosomal Recessive genes reported in the literature., Figure S17: Information on gene SNX14 common to the SFARI Autism set and the Ataxia

Autosomal Recessive genes reported in the literature., Figure S18: Information on gene RAB39B common to the SFARI Autism set and the Ataxia Autosomal Recessive genes reported in the literature., Figure S19: Information on gene CASK common to the SFARI Autism set and the X-Chromosome genes reported in the literature., Figure S20: Information on gene FMR1 common to the SFARI Autism set and the X-Chromosome genes reported in the literature., Figure S21: Information on gene SLC9A6 common to the SFARI Autism set and the X-Chromosome genes reported in the literature., Figure S22: Information on gene OPHN1 common to the SFARI Autism set and the X-Chromosome genes reported in the literature., Table S1: Genes common to the SFARI Autism set and the Ataxias and PD-early onset literature.

Funding: This research was funded by the New Jersey Governor's Council for Medical Research and Treatments of Autism and by the generosity of the Nancy Lurie Marks Family Foundation.

Acknowledgments: I thank the SFARI, GTex and DisGeNet researchers for the curation and maintenance of their genes module and the compilation of the literature database supporting these repositories.

Conflicts of Interest: The author declares no conflict of interest. The funders had no role in the design of the study; in the collection, analyses, or interpretation of data; in the writing of the manuscript, or in the decision to publish the results.

Appendix A

TPM explanation from the site: "Transcripts Per Million (TPM) is a normalization method for RNA-seq, should be read as for every 1,000,000 RNA molecules in the RNA-seq sample, x came from this gene/transcript. For each transcript in the gene model, the number (raw count) of reads mapped is divided by the transcript's length, giving a normalized transcript-level expression. The distribution of ambiguous reads (between transcripts of the same gene, or between different genes) is handled by OmicSoft's RSEM implementation. The sum of ALL normalized transcript expression values is divided by 1,000,000, to create a scaling factor. Each transcript's normalized expression is divided by the scaling factor, which results in the TPM value. Gene-level TPM's are calculated by summing up the transcript-level TPM for each gene. In this scaling, the sum of all TPMs (transcript-level or gene-level) should always equal 1,000,000. For cells that have approximately the same number of transcripts-per-cell, the TPM expression values can be compared between these cells to estimate relative abundance. For a given sample, TPM values will linearly scale with FPKM values for genes or transcripts, but FPKM will not add up to 1,000,000, so TPM can also be thought as FPKM, scaled to sum to 1,000,000".

Derivation of Maximum Likelihood Estimation of the rate parameter in the Exponential Distribution:

We estimate the likelihood $L(\lambda|x_1, x_2, \ldots, x_n)$, where x_i is the series of counts representing the gene expression on each given tissue and i ranges from 1 to n, the number of genes.

$$\begin{aligned} L(\lambda|x_1, x_2, \ldots, x_n) &= \lambda e^{-\lambda x_1} \lambda e^{-\lambda x_2} \ldots \lambda e^{-\lambda x_n} \\ &= \lambda^n \left(e^{-\lambda x_1} e^{-\lambda x_2} \ldots e^{-\lambda x_n} \right) \\ &= \lambda^n \left(e^{-\lambda(x_1 + x_2 + \ldots + x_n)} \right) \end{aligned} \tag{A1}$$

To obtain the maximum likelihood, we take the derivative of the likelihood in Equation (A1) and set it to 0 (since the derivative is 0 at the maximum likelihood value).

$$\frac{d}{d\lambda} L(\lambda|x_1, x_2, \ldots, x_n) = \frac{d}{d\lambda} \lambda^n \left(e^{-\lambda(x_1 + x_2 + \ldots + x_n)} \right) \tag{A2}$$

We take the log here because the derivative of the function and the derivative of the log of the function equals 0 at the same point. So, for the purposes of finding where the derivative is 0, the original function in Equation (A2) and the log of it are interchangeable.

$$\begin{aligned} \frac{d}{d\lambda} \log\left(\lambda^n \left(e^{-\lambda(x_1+x_2+\ldots+x_n)}\right)\right) &= \frac{d}{d\lambda} \log \lambda^n + \log\left(e^{-\lambda(x_1+x_2+\ldots+x_n)}\right) \\ \frac{d}{d\lambda} n \log \lambda - \lambda(x_1 + x_2 + \ldots + x_n) &= 0 \\ n \frac{1}{\lambda} - (x_1 + x_2 + \ldots + x_n) &= 0 \\ \lambda &= \frac{n}{(x_1 + x_2 + \ldots + x_n)} \end{aligned} \tag{A3}$$

Further, with this result in Equation (A3), we can obtain the maximum likelihood estimate of each λ_j, given all the 56,146 genes expressed with some random value for each of the $j = 1 : 54$ tissues.

Appendix B

Table A1. Gene distributions used in the removal process and literature sources.

Neurological	Number of Genes	Source
Parkinson's disease	17	Lit Review [14,16–19]
Ataxia Autosomal Recessive	70	Lit Review [11,12]
Ataxia Autosomal Dominant	46	Lit Review [11,12]
X-chromosome	6	Lit Review [11,12]
Fragile X (SFARI scores)	73 [1] (17,11,30,15)	SFARI Genes Module
Fragile X Syndrome	194	DisGeNet
FXTAS	62	DisGeNet
Ataxia	813	DisGeNet
cerebellar Ataxia	421	DisGeNet
gait Ataxia	159	DisGeNet
Progressive cerebellar Ataxia	134	DisGeNet
Spinocerebellar Ataxia	145	DisGeNet
Neuropsychiatric (DSM)	**Number of Genes**	**Source**
autism (SFARI scores)	906 [1] (144,216,468,78)	SFARI Genes Module
Autistic Disorder	1043	DisGeNet
schizophrenia	2697	Lit Review [30–35] and DisGeNet
Mental depression	1468	DisGeNet
depression Unipolar	641	DisGeNet
depression Bipolar	116	DisGeNet

[1] SFARI scores for autism and FX genes were also used to assess each scored module separately. FXTAS stands for fragile X tremor ataxia syndrome.

Table A2. Genes associated with non-neurological diseases.

Non-Neurological	Number of Genes	Source
Colon Cancer	3669	DisGeNet
Diabetes Mellitus (non-insulin dependent)	3134	DisGeNet
Estrogen Receptor-Positive Breast Cancer	510	DisGeNet
Congenital Heart Disease	267	DisGeNet
Hematologic Neoplasm	827	DisGeNet
Systemic Lupus Erythematosus	1883	DisGeNet
Psoriasis	1308	DisGeNet
Irritable Bowel Syndrome	1483	DisGeNet
Mixed	**Number of Genes**	**Source**
Mitochondria	41	Lit Review [13]
Mitochondrial Myopathies	121	DisGeNet
Mitochondrial Diseases	284	DisGeNet
MELAS Syndrome	81	DisGeNet
PTSD	418	DisGeNet

MELAS (a form of dementia) stands for mitochondrial encephalopathy, lactic acidosis, and stroke-like episodes.

The data file name from the GTEx portal https://www.GTExportal.org/home/datasets used in this paper is GTEx_Analysis_2017-06-05_v8_RNASeQCv1.1.9_gene_median_tpm.gct.csv (accessed on 18 September 2020).

The data file name from the SFARI genes is located at https://gene.sfari.org/database/human-gene/ and named SFARI-Gene_genes_03-04-2020release_03-05-2020export.csv (accessed on 18 September 2020).

Table A3. The 13 top median-ranked tissues in descending order of Δλ value, the most-affected tissues upon removal of the SFARI genes (906) linked to autism from the human GTEx database in column 1. Ataxias, X-chromosome, fragile X, Parkinson's disease and mitochondrial disease extracted from the literature and column 3 is the same as in column 1 while removing from the SFARI autism set 14 genes that overlap with ataxias and PD (see those genes listed in Supplementary Table S2). Tissues are grouped by CNS (brain and spinal cord in blue); muscle-skeletal (green), heart (pink) and peripheral organs (gray). SFARI autism (11/13 (84.6%) CNS, 1/13 (7.6%) heart and 1/13 (7.6%) peripheral organ); neurological disorders (10/13 (76.9%) CNS, 2/13 heart (15.3%) and 1/13 (7.6%) muscle-skeletal); SFARI autism without the overlapping genes from the neurological disorders (11/13 (76.9%) CNS, 1/13 (7.6%) heart and 1/13 (7.6%) peripheral organs).

SFARI Autism	Ataxias, X, FX, PD, Mitochondria	SFARI Autism without Overlapping Ataxia, PD Genes
Putamen Basal Ganglia	Hippocampus	Putamen Basal Ganglia
Substantia Nigra	Amygdala	Substantia Nigra
Amygdala	Substantia Nigra	Amygdala
Hippocampus	Heart Left Ventricle	Hippocampus
Caudate Basal Ganglia	Whole Blood	Caudate Basal Ganglia
Anterior Cingulate Cortex	Muscle Skeletal	Nucleus Accumbent Basal Ganglia
Nucleus Accumbent Basal Ganglia	Nucleus Accumbent Basal Ganglia	Anterior Cingulate Cortex
Hypothalamus	Putamen Basal Ganglia	Hypothalamus
Brain Cortex	Anterior Cingulate Cortex	Brain Cortex
Frontal Cortex	Brain Cortex	Frontal Cortex
Heart Left Ventricle	Hypothalamus	Spinal Cord
Spinal Cord	Heart Atrial Appendage	Heart Left Ventricle
Pancreas	Caudate Basal Ganglia	Kidney Cortex

Table A4. Most-affected tissues upon removal of the DisGeNet genes associated with autistic disorders (1043) from the human GTEx database (column 1); ataxia (813 genes) in DisGeNet (column 2) and FX (194 genes) in DisGeNet (column 3). Convergence between autism and neurological disorders is noted in the shaded tissues color coded as in Table A4, based on CNS, heart, and peripheral organs.

DisGeNet Autistic Disorders	DisGeNet Ataxia	FX DisGeNet
Substantia Nigra	Heart Left Ventricle	Hippocampus
Nucleus Accumbent Basal Ganglia	Amygdala	Whole Blood
Caudate Basal Ganglia	Hippocampus	Caudate Basal Ganglia
Putamen Basal Ganglia	Whole Blood	Substantia Nigra
Hippocampus	Putamen Basal Ganglia	Putamen Basal Ganglia
Amygdala	Substantia Nigra	Muscle Skeletal
Heart Left Ventricle	Anterior Cingulate Cortex	Nucleus Accumbent Basal Ganglia
Spinal Cord	Muscle Skeletal	Anterior Cingulate Cortex
Hypothalamus	Heart Atrial Appendage	Amygdala
Pancreas	Caudate Basal Ganglia	Brain Cortex
Heart Atrial Appendage	Nucleus Accumbent Basal Ganglia	Heart Left Ventricle
Anterior Cingulate Cortex	Brain Cortex	Kidney Medulla
Kidney Medulla	Hypothalamus	Frontal Cortex

Table A5. Overlapping genes between ataxias (dominant and recessive genes) and Parkinson's disease with the genes from the SFARI portal. Scores in parenthesis refer to the scoring of the gene according to the SFARI site (see Methods for explanation on each category). Syndromic is (4). Supplementary Figures S5–S18 provide the GTEx violin plots of these gene expressions in the top-ranked tissues unveiled by our analyses. Supplementary Table S2 compiles additional information on the genes from various sources in the clinical literature.

SFARI Autism and Ataxia Dominant	SFARI Autism and Ataxia Recessive	SFARI Autism and (Early Onset) PD
CACNA1C (1)	KCNJ10 (2)	RAB39B (3)
SCN2A (1)	WWOX (2)	
ATP1A3 (3S)	GRID2 (3)	
CCDC88C (3)	LAMA1 (3)	
ITPR1 (3)	PEX7 (3)	
	SYNE1 (3S)	
	CYP27A1 (4)	
	SNX14 (4)	

Table A6. Most-affected tissues upon removal of the DisGeNet genes associated with different types of ataxias, color coded by CNS (brain and spinal cord), heart-related, muscle-skeletal, and peripheral vital organ for systemic functioning. Predominance of CNS is evident, followed by heart-related and muscle-skeletal and peripheral organs.

Gait Ataxia	Spinocerebellar Ataxia	Cerebellar Ataxia	Progressive-C Ataxia
Heart Left Ventricle	Caudate Basal Ganglia	Heart Left Ventricle	Liver
Substantia Nigra	Brain Amygdala	Substantia Nigra	Heart Left Ventricle
Hippocampus	Substantia Nigra	Hippocampus	Whole Blood
Muscle Skeletal	Putamen Basal Ganglia	Amygdala	Heart Atrial Appendage
Caudate Basal Ganglia	N Accumbens BG	Whole Blood	Putamen Basal Ganglia
N Accumbens BG	Ant Cingulate Cortex	Putamen Basal Ganglia	Substantia Nigra
Whole Blood	Hippocampus	Hypothalamus	Hippocampus
Brain Amygdala	Heart Atrial Appendage	Ant Cingulate Cortex	Brain Amygdala
Kidney Cortex	Hypothalamus	Caudate Basal Ganglia	Muscle Skeletal
Putamen Basal Ganglia	Brain Cortex	N Accumbens BG	Kidney Cortex
Ant Cingulate Cortex	Frontal Cortex	Brain Cortex	Caudate Basal Ganglia
Hypothalamus	Heart Left Ventricle	Kidney Cortex	N Accumbens BG
Heart Atrial Appendage	Kidney Cortex	Muscle Skeletal	Ant Cingulate Cortex

Table A7. Most-affected tissues upon removal of the DisGeNet genes associated with schizophrenia (2697) from the human GTEx database; depression genes (1468); unipolar depression genes (641); and bipolar depression genes (116). Convergence between schizophrenia and depression is high, with maximally affected CNS tissues (10/13), followed by heart-related and muscle-skeletal tissues. Unipolar and bipolar depression also show systemic effect of vital peripheral organs (N stands for Nucleus, Ant for Anterior, and BG for Basal Ganglia).

Schizophrenia	Depression	Unipolar Depression	Bipolar Depression
Amygdala	Heart Left Ventricle	Putamen Basal Ganglia	Hippocampus
Putamen Basal Ganglia	Heart Atrial Appendage	Caudate Basal Ganglia	Putamen Basal Ganglia
Heart Left Ventricle	Hippocampus	Hippocampus	Amygdala
Hippocampus	Muscle Skeletal	Substantia Nigra	Caudate Basal Ganglia
Substantia Nigra	Putamen Basal Ganglia	Kidney Cortex	Muscle Skeletal
Caudate Basal Ganglia	Caudate Basal Ganglia	Amygdala	Substantia Nigra
Ant Cingulate Cortex	Amygdala	Heart Left Ventricle	Spinal Cord
N Accumbens BG	Pancreas	Kidney Medulla	Esophagus Muscularis
Hypothalamus	Kidney Medulla	Brain Cortex	Adrenal Gland
Muscle Skeletal	Substantia Nigra	N Accumbens BG	Frontal Cortex
Pancreas	Kidney Cortex	Colon Transverse	Minor Salivary Gland
Brain Cortex	Ant Cingulate Cortex	Ant Cingulate Cortex	Colon Sigmoid
Frontal Cortex	N Accumbens BG	Heart Atrial Appendage	Ant Cingulate Cortex

Table A8. Most-affected tissues upon removal of the DisGeNet genes associated with colon cancer (3669) from the human GTEx database; irritable bowel syndrome genes (1483); congenital heart disease genes (267); and hematologic neoplast genes (827). Color code as in previous tables.

Colon Cancer	Irritable Bowel Syndrome	Congenital Heart Disease	Hematologic Neoplast
Pancreas	Heart Left Ventricle	Heart Left Ventricle	Heart Left Ventricle
Whole Blood	Pancreas	Heart Atrial Appendage	Whole Blood
Stomach	Kidney Cortex	Kidney Cortex	Liver
Adrenal Gland	Liver	Whole Blood	Heart Atrial Appendage
Colon Transverse	Muscle Skeletal	Kidney Medulla	Pancreas
Prostate	Heart Atrial Appendage	Substantia Nigra	Muscle Skeletal
Small Intestine T	Kidney Medulla	Hypothalamus	Kidney Cortex
Spleen	Whole Blood	Prostate	Hippocampus
Minor Salivary Gland	Adrenal Gland	Hippocampus	Kidney Medulla
Fallopian Tube	Adipose Viseral Oment	Muscle Skeletal	Esophagus Mucosa
EBT Lymphocytes	Esophagus Mucosa	Adipose Visceral O	EBT Lymphocytes
SkinNoSunExposed S	Colon Transverse	Minor Salivary Gland	Substantia Nigra
Liver	Stomach	Pancreas	Putamen Basal Ganglia

Table A9. Most-affected tissues upon removal of the DisGeNet genes associated with lupus systemic erythematosus (1883) from the human GTEx database; psoriasis genes (1308); breast cancer (510); and diabetes genes (3134). The top half of the highest-ranked tissues show no convergence with CNS-related tissues found in the mental illnesses and neurological disorders interrogated in this work. Instead, heart-related tissue, muscle-skeletal tissue and tissues related to peripheral vital organs for systemic functioning are found. The bottom half of the top Δλ-ranked tissues are a mixture of tissues in peripheral bodily organs and brain-related tissues. The latter are from motor control, coordination, and adaptation subcortical areas and from emotion, memory, and regulatory areas. Color code as in previous tables.

Systemic Lupus Erythematosus	Psoriasis	Breast Cancer	Diabetes
Heart Left Ventricle	Heart Left Ventricle	Pancreas	Liver
Whole Blood	Liver	Heart Left Ventricle	Pancreas
Liver	Whole Blood	Heart Atrial Appendage	Heart Atrial Appendage
Heart Atrial Appendage	Muscle Skeletal	Kidney Medulla	Heart Left Ventricle
Pancreas	Heart Atrial Appendage	Muscle Skeletal	Kidney Medulla
Muscle Skeletal	Pancreas	Whole Blood	Kidney Cortex
Kidney Cortex	Kidney Cortex	Ant Cingulate Cortex	Putamen Basal Ganglia
Hippocampus	Putamen Basal Ganglia	Esophagus Mucosa	Substantia Nigra
Kidney Medulla	Caudate Basal Ganglia	Kidney Cortex	Hippocampus
Esophagus Mucosa	Adipose Visceral O	Adrenal Gland	Caudate Basal Ganglia
EBT Lymphocytes	Substantia Nigra	Esophagus Muscularis	Amygdala
Substantia Nigra	Esophagus Mucosa	Hypothalamus	N Accumbens BG
Putamen Basal Ganglia	Hypothalamus	Putamen Basal Ganglia	Hypothalamus

Table A10. Most-affected tissues upon removal of the DisGeNet genes associated with mitochondrial disease (284) from the human GTEx database; mitochondrial myopathies genes (121); mitochondrial encephalopathy, lactic acidosis, and stroke-like episodes (MELAS) (81); Post-Traumatic Stress Disorder genes (418).

Mitochondrial Disease	Mitochondrial Myopathies	MELAS	PTSD
Heart Left Ventricle	Liver	Heart Left Ventricle	Caudate Basal Ganglia
Muscle Skeletal	Heart Left Ventricle	Liver	Kidney Medulla
Pancreas.	Muscle Skeletal	Kidney Cortex	Kidney Cortex
Heart Atrial Appendage	Hippocampus	Pancreas	Pancreas
Kidney Cortex	Whole Blood	Heart Atrial Appendage	Putamen Basal Ganglia
Whole Blood	Ant Cingulate Cortex	Kidney Medulla	Heart Left Ventricle
Kidney Medulla	Brain Amygdala	Putamen Basal Ganglia	Hypothalamus
Ant Cingulate Cortex	Substantia Nigra	Esophagus Mucosa	Substantia Nigra
Putamen Basal Ganglia	Heart Atrial Appendage	Brain Amygdala	Heart Atrial Appendage
N Accumbens BG	Putamen Basal Ganglia	Adipose Visceral Omen	N Accumbens BG
Adrenal Gland	Spinal Cord	Artery Coronary	Hippocampus
Hippocampus	Pancreas	Stomach	Colon Sigmoid
Caudate Basal Ganglia	Hypothalamus	Colon Traverse	Amygdala

Table A11. Most-affected tissue in each disease/disorder according to the maximum $\Delta\lambda$ value (See Figure 13 in the main text).

Disease/Disorder	Maximally Affected Tissue
Autism DisGeNet	BrainSubstantiaNigra
ASD NoAtaxias	BrainPutamenBasalGanglia
Autism SFARI	BrainPutamenBasalGanglia
Schizophrenia	BrainAmygdala
Depression DisGeNet	HeartLeftVentricle
Bipolar Depression	BrainHippocampus
Unipolar Depression	BrainPutamenBasalGanglia
ATAXIA DisGeNet	HeartLeftVentricle
SpinoCerebellar ATAXIA	BrainCaudateBasalGanglia
Cerebellar ATAXIA	HeartLeftVentricle
ProgressiveCerebellar ATAXIA	Liver
Gait ATAXIA	HeartLeftVentricle
FAXTAS	HeartLeftVentricle
FX	BrainHippocampus
PTSD	BrainCaudateBasalGanglia
Diabetes	Liver
BreastCancer	Pancreas
ColonCancer	Pancreas
HematologicNeoplast	HeartLeftVentricle
CongenitalHeartDisease	HeartLeftVentricle
IBD	HeartLeftVentricle
LupusSystemicErythomatosus	HeartLeftVentricle
Psoriasis	HeartLeftVentricle
MItochondriaDisease	HeartLeftVentricle
MELAS	HeartLeftVentricle
MitochondriaMyopathies	Liver

References

1. Hawgood, S.; Hook-Barnard, I.G.; O'Brien, T.C.; Yamamoto, K.R. Precision medicine: Beyond the inflection point. *Sci. Transl. Med.* **2015**, *7*, 300ps17. [CrossRef]
2. Adams, R.A.; Huys, Q.J.M.; Roiser, J.P. Computational psychiatry: Towards a mathematically informed understanding of mental illness. *J. Neurol. Neurosurg. Psychiatry* **2016**, *87*, 53–63. [CrossRef]

3. American Psychiatric Association. *Diagnostic and Statistical Manual of Mental Disorders*, 5th ed.; American Psychiatric Association: Arlington, VA, USA, 2013.
4. Ferraro, N.M.; Strober, B.J.; Einson, J.; Abell, N.S.; Aguet, F.; Barbeira, A.N.; Brandt, M.; Bucan, M.; Castel, S.E.; Davis, J.R.; et al. Transcriptomic signatures across human tissues identify functional rare genetic variation. *Sci. Mag.* **2020**, *369*, eaaz5900.
5. Torres, E.; Denisova, K. Motor noise is rich signal in autism research and pharmacological treatments. *Sci. Rep.* **2016**, *6*, 37422. [CrossRef]
6. Torres, E.; Caballero, C.; Mistry, S. Aging with Autism Departs Greatly from Typical Aging. *Sensors* **2020**, *20*, 572. [CrossRef] [PubMed]
7. Caballero, C.; Mistry, S.; Torres, E. Age-dependent statistical changes of involuntary head motion signatures across autism and controls of the ABIDE repository. *Front. Integr. Neurosci.* **2020**, *14*, 1–14. [CrossRef] [PubMed]
8. Kim-Hellmuth, S.; Aguet, F.; Oliva, M.; Muñoz-Aguirre, M.; Kasela, S.; Wucher, V.; Castel, S.E.; Hamel, A.R.; Viñuela, A.; Roberts, A.L.; et al. Cell type–specific genetic regulation of gene expression across human tissues. *Sci. Mag.* **2020**, *369*, eaaz8528. [CrossRef] [PubMed]
9. Nguyen, J.; Majmudar, U.; Papathomas, T.V.; Silverstein, S.; Torres, E.; Thomas, V.P. Schizophrenia: The micro-movements perspective. *Neuropsychologia* **2016**, *85*, 310–326. [CrossRef]
10. Rogers, D.M. *Motor Disorder in Psychiatry: Towards A Neurological Psychiatry*; J. Wiley & Sons.: Chichester, UK; New York, NY, USA, 1992; Volume viii, p. 159.
11. Bird, T.D. *Hereditary Ataxia Overview, in GeneReviews((R))*; Adam, M., Ardinger, H.H., Pagon, R.A., Wallace, S.E., Bean, L.J.H., Stephens, K., Amemiya, A., Eds.; University of Washington: Seattle, WA, USA, 1998.
12. Jayadev, S.; Bird, T.D. Hereditary ataxias: Overview. *Genet. Med.* **2013**, *15*, 673–683. [CrossRef]
13. Chinnery, P.F. *Mitochondrial Disorders Overview, in GeneReviews((R))*; University of Washington: Seattle: Seattle, WA, USA, 1993.
14. Domingo, A.; Westenberger, A.; Lee, L.V.; Brænne, I.; Liu, T.; Vater, I.; Rosales, R.; Jamora, R.D.G.; Pasco, P.M.; Paz, E.M.C.-D.; et al. New insights into the genetics of X-linked dystonia-parkinsonism (XDP, DYT3). *Eur. J. Hum. Genet.* **2015**, *23*, 1334–1340. [CrossRef]
15. Klein, C.; Westenberger, A. Genetics of Parkinson's disease. *Cold Spring Harb. Perspect. Med.* **2012**, *2*, a008888. [CrossRef]
16. Scott, W.K.; Nance, M.A.; Watts, R.L.; Hubble, J.P.; Koller, W.C.; Lyons, K.; Pahwa, R.; Stern, M.B.; Colcher, A.; Hiner, B.C.; et al. Complete genomic screen in Parkinson disease: Evidence for multiple genes. *JAMA* **2001**, *286*, 2239–2244. [CrossRef]
17. Hicks, A.; Petursson, H.; Jonsson, T.; Stefansson, H.; Jóhannsdóttir, H.S.; Sainz, J.; Frigge, M.L.; Kong, A.; Gulcher, J.; Stefansson, K.; et al. A susceptibility gene for late-onset idiopathic Parkinson's disease. *Ann. Neurol.* **2002**, *52*, 549–555. [CrossRef] [PubMed]
18. Valente, E.M.; Brancati, F.; Ferraris, A.; Bsc, E.A.G.; Davis, M.B.; Breteler, M.M.; Gasser, T.; Bonifati, V.; Bentivoglio, A.R.; de Michele, G.; et al. PARK6-linked parkinsonism occurs in several European families. *Ann. Neurol.* **2002**, *51*, 14–18. [CrossRef]
19. Kay, D.M.; Zabetian, C.P.; Factor, S.A.; Nutt, J.G.; Samii, A.; Griffith, A.; Bird, T.D.; Kramer, P.; Higgins, D.S.; Payami, H. Parkinson's disease and LRRK2: Frequency of a common mutation in U.S. movement disorder clinics. *Mov. Disord.* **2006**, *21*, 519–523. [CrossRef] [PubMed]
20. Soong, B.W.; Morrison, P.J. Spinocerebellar ataxias. *Handb. Clin. Neurol.* **2018**, *155*, 143–174.
21. Fujioka, S.; Sundal, C.; Wszolek, Z.K. Autosomal dominant cerebellar ataxia type III: A review of the phenotypic and genotypic characteristics. *Orphanet J. Rare Dis.* **2013**, *8*, 14. [CrossRef] [PubMed]
22. Sailer, A.; Houlden, H. Recent advances in the genetics of cerebellar ataxias. *Curr. Neurol. Neurosci. Rep.* **2012**, *12*, 227–236. [CrossRef]
23. Mariotti, C.; di Donato, S. Cerebellar/spinocerebellar syndromes. *Neurol. Sci.* **2001**, *22* (Suppl. 2), S88–S92. [CrossRef]
24. Mosconi, M.W.; Wang, Z.; Schmitt, L.M.; Tsai, P.T.; Sweeney, J.A. The role of cerebellar circuitry alterations in the pathophysiology of autism spectrum disorders. *Front. Neurosci.* **2015**, *9*, 296. [CrossRef]
25. Mostofsky, S.H.; Powell, S.K.; Simmonds, D.J.; Goldberg, M.C.; Caffo, B.; Pekar, J.J. Decreased connectivity and cerebellar activity in autism during motor task performance. *Brain* **2009**, *132*, 2413–2425. [CrossRef] [PubMed]

26. Ryu, J.; Vero, J.; Dobkin, R.D.; Torres, E.B. Dynamic digital biomarkers of motor and cognitive function in parkinson's disease. *J. Vis. Exp.* **2019**, *149*, e59827. [CrossRef] [PubMed]
27. Wu, D.; José, J.V.; Nurnberger, J.I.; Torres, E. A Biomarker Characterizing Neurodevelopment with applications in Autism. *Sci. Rep.* **2018**, *8*, 614. [CrossRef]
28. Torres, E.; Vero, J.; Rai, R. statistical platform for individualized behavioral analyses using biophysical micro-movement spikes. *Sensors* **2018**, *18*, 1025. [CrossRef] [PubMed]
29. Torres, E.; Brincker, M.; Isenhower, R.W.I.; Yanovich, P.; Stigler, K.A.; Nurnberger, J.I.; Metaxas, D.N.; José, J.V. Autism: The micro-movement perspective. *Front. Integr. Neurosci.* **2013**, *7*, 32. [CrossRef]
30. Salleh, M.R. The genetics of schizophrenia. *Malays. J. Med. Sci.* **2004**, *11*, 3–11.
31. Schizophrenia Working Group of the Psychiatric Genomics Consortium; Ripke, S.; Neale, B.M.; Corvin, A.; Walters, J.; Farh, K.-H.; Holmans, P.; Lee, P.; Bulik-Sullivan, B.; Collier, D.A.; et al. Biological insights from 108 schizophrenia-associated genetic loci. *Nature* **2014**, *511*, 421–427.
32. Kotlar, A.V.; Mercer, K.B.; Zwick, M.E.; Mulle, J.G. New discoveries in schizophrenia genetics reveal neurobiological pathways: A review of recent findings. *Eur. J. Med. Genet.* **2015**, *58*, 704–714. [CrossRef]
33. Fabbri, C.; Serretti, A. Role of 108 schizophrenia-associated loci in modulating psychopathological dimensions in schizophrenia and bipolar disorder. *Am. J. Med. Genet. B Neuropsychiatr. Genet.* **2017**, *174*, 757–764. [CrossRef]
34. Forsyth, J.K.; Asarnow, R.F. Genetics of childhood-onset schizophrenia 2019 update. *Child Adolesc. Psychiatr. Clin. N. Am.* **2020**, *29*, 157–170. [CrossRef]
35. Zamanpoor, M. Schizophrenia in a genomic era: A review from the pathogenesis, genetic and environmental etiology to diagnosis and treatment insights. *Psychiatr. Genet.* **2020**, *30*, 1–9. [CrossRef] [PubMed]

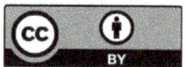

© 2020 by the author. Licensee MDPI, Basel, Switzerland. This article is an open access article distributed under the terms and conditions of the Creative Commons Attribution (CC BY) license (http://creativecommons.org/licenses/by/4.0/).

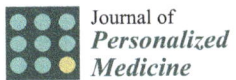

Article

Precision Telemedicine through Crowdsourced Machine Learning: Testing Variability of Crowd Workers for Video-Based Autism Feature Recognition

Peter Washington [1], Emilie Leblanc [2], Kaitlyn Dunlap [2], Yordan Penev [2], Aaron Kline [2], Kelley Paskov [3], Min Woo Sun [3], Brianna Chrisman [1], Nathaniel Stockham [4], Maya Varma [5], Catalin Voss [5], Nick Haber [6] and Dennis P. Wall [2,3,*]

[1] Department of Bioengineering, Stanford University, 443 Via Ortega, Stanford, CA 94305, USA; peterwashington@stanford.edu (P.W.); briannac@stanford.edu (B.C.)
[2] Department of Pediatrics (Systems Medicine), Stanford University, 1265 Welch Rd., Stanford, CA 94305, USA; emilie.leblanc@stanford.edu (E.L.); kaiti.dunlap@stanford.edu (K.D.); ypenev@stanford.edu (Y.P.); akline@stanford.edu (A.K.)
[3] Department of Biomedical Data Science, Stanford University, 1265 Welch Rd., Stanford, CA 94305, USA; kpaskov@stanford.edu (K.P.); minwoos@stanford.edu (M.W.S.)
[4] Department of Neuroscience, Stanford University, 213 Quarry Rd., Stanford, CA 94305, USA; stockham@stanford.edu
[5] Department of Computer Science, Stanford University, 353 Jane Stanford Way, Stanford, CA 94305, USA; mvarma2@stanford.edu (M.V.); catalin@cs.stanford.edu (C.V.)
[6] School of Education, Stanford University, 485 Lasuen Mall, Stanford, CA 94305, USA; nhaber@stanford.edu
* Correspondence: dpwall@stanford.edu

Received: 29 June 2020; Accepted: 10 August 2020; Published: 13 August 2020

Abstract: Mobilized telemedicine is becoming a key, and even necessary, facet of both precision health and precision medicine. In this study, we evaluate the capability and potential of a crowd of virtual workers—defined as vetted members of popular crowdsourcing platforms—to aid in the task of diagnosing autism. We evaluate workers when crowdsourcing the task of providing categorical ordinal behavioral ratings to unstructured public YouTube videos of children with autism and neurotypical controls. To evaluate emerging patterns that are consistent across independent crowds, we target workers from distinct geographic loci on two crowdsourcing platforms: an international group of workers on Amazon Mechanical Turk (MTurk) (N = 15) and Microworkers from Bangladesh (N = 56), Kenya (N = 23), and the Philippines (N = 25). We feed worker responses as input to a validated diagnostic machine learning classifier trained on clinician-filled electronic health records. We find that regardless of crowd platform or targeted country, workers vary in the average confidence of the correct diagnosis predicted by the classifier. The best worker responses produce a mean probability of the correct class above 80% and over one standard deviation above 50%, accuracy and variability on par with experts according to prior studies. There is a weak correlation between mean time spent on task and mean performance ($r = 0.358$, $p = 0.005$). These results demonstrate that while the crowd can produce accurate diagnoses, there are intrinsic differences in crowdworker ability to rate behavioral features. We propose a novel strategy for recruitment of crowdsourced workers to ensure high quality diagnostic evaluations of autism, and potentially many other pediatric behavioral health conditions. Our approach represents a viable step in the direction of crowd-based approaches for more scalable and affordable precision medicine.

Keywords: crowdsourcing; machine learning; diagnostics; telemedicine; autism; pediatrics

1. Introduction

Autism spectrum disorder (ASD or autism) is a developmental delay with a continuously rising prevalence in the United States [1,2]. Access to care can be limited, particularly in rural and in lower socioeconomic areas, as families must wait for over a year to receive a formal diagnosis [3] and therefore treatment. Epidemiological estimates indicate that over 80% of U.S. counties do not have autism diagnostic resources [4]. Scalable and accessible tools would begin to address these inefficiencies in the healthcare system. Since autism consists of a largely behavioral phenotype, video data are a particularly powerful and rich means of capturing the range of social symptoms a child may exhibit in a fast and virtually cost-free manner. Accurate diagnoses and behavioral classifications have been inferred from categorical ordinal labels extracted by untrained humans from the short video clips [5–10], which are recorded by digital mobile and wearable interventions during use by the child or administering parent [11–22]. Such a process can be scaled through crowdsourcing platforms, which allow distributed workers from around the globe to perform short on-demand tasks.

Crowdsourcing offers a powerful mobilized telemedicine solution to providing a rapid and personalized diagnosis for and behavioral characterization of children at risk for developmental delays. Crowdsourcing is increasingly being used for sensitive work such as mental health tracking [23,24], body weight inference [25], prescription drug use and reactions [26,27], and investigating crime [28–30]. While at least partially automated diagnostics is an important goal for precision healthcare [31–34], the quantification and categorization of several social activities are beyond the scope of current machine learning methods [19], resulting in a major barrier in the field of precision medicine for behavioral conditions. While answers from a crowd worker on a variety of behavioral dimensions can provide a precision diagnosis for one individual, each label can be used as training data for a general-purpose machine learning model that can make precision medicine more automated and scalable. Achieving this goal, however, relies on high quality data from the crowd [35,36], necessitating careful characterization of worker performance and subsequent filtering of crowd workers.

Here, we evaluate the performance of individual workers within four independent pools of crowdsourced workers from Amazon Mechanical Turk (MTurk) [37,38], a popular paid crowdsourcing platform, and Microworkers [39,40], another paid crowdsourcing platform with a significantly larger international pool of workers compared to MTurk [41]. The workers watch unstructured videos of children with autism and neurotypical controls and fill out a series of multiple-choice questions about the child's behavior. The series of multiple-choice answers serve as a vector of categorical ordinal features used as input to a previously validated [42,43] logistic regression classifier distinguishing neurotypical children from autistic children. We assess the differences in classifier probabilities and final predictions across workers, finding that there are significant differences in worker performance despite identical video difficulty levels. These results suggest that crowd workers must be filtered before incorporation into clinical diagnostic practices.

2. Materials and Methods

Our methods consist of (1) first identifying a clinically representative video set, (2) choosing an appropriate classifier for evaluating worker responses, and (3) crowdsourcing a video rating task to a wide pool of global workers.

2.1. Clinically Representative Video Set

Clinically representative videos were downloaded from YouTube. We selected publicly available videos of both children with and without autism. Diagnosis was based on video title and description reported by the uploader. We only selected videos that matched all of the following criteria: (1) the child's hands and face are clearly visible, (2) there are opportunities for social engagement, and (3) there is at least one opportunity for using an object such as a toy or utensil. No further selection criteria were used.

All three rating groups on Microworkers received the same set of 24 videos with a mean duration of 47.75 s (SD = 30.71 s). Six videos contain a female child with autism, six videos contain a neurotypical female child, six videos contain a male child with autism, and six videos contain a neurotypical male child. The mean age of children in the video was 3.65 years (SD = 1.82 years).

We asked 4 licensed clinical experts (2 Child and Adolescent Psychiatrists, 1 Clinical Psychologist, and 1 Speech Language Pathologist) to watch each video of the 12 children with an autism diagnosis and to rate the severity of the child's autism symptoms according to the first question of the Clinical Global Impression (CGI) [44] scale measuring the "severity of illness" between 1 ("normal, not at all ill") to 7 ("among the most extremely ill patients"). We then recorded the mean rating rounded to the nearest whole number. There was one video with a mean rating of 2 ("borderline mentally ill"), four with a mean of 4 ("moderately ill"), five with a mean of 5 ("markedly ill"), and two with a mean of 6 ("severely ill"), validating that we posted a clinically representative set of videos on Microworkers.

We additionally conducted a post-hoc analysis of previously crowdsourced yet unpublished pilot test results from MTurk with the exact same rating tasks except using a separate set of 43 videos to rate with a mean duration of 43.85 s (SD = 26.06 s). Ten videos from this set contain a female child with autism, eleven videos contain a neurotypical female child, twelve videos contain a male child with autism, and ten videos contain a neurotypical male child. The mean age of children in the video set was 3.61 years (SD = 1.61 years). The 4 clinical experts rated the 22 children with autism in this set using the CGI. There were three videos with a mean rating of 2 ("borderline mentally ill"), five with a mean of 3 ("mildly ill"), three with a mean of 4 ("moderately ill"), six with a mean of 5 ("markedly ill"), and five with a mean of 6 ("severely ill"), validating that we posted a clinically representative set of videos on MTurk.

2.2. Video Observation Classifier

To evaluate the performance of crowd workers against a clinician gold standard, a previously validated binary logistic regression classifier [42,43] was trained on electronic health record data consisting of clinician filled Autism Diagnostic Observation Schedule (ADOS) [45] scoresheets for 1319 children with autism and 70 non-autism controls. We chose logistic regression over alternative classical machine learning techniques like support vector machines and alternating decision trees because of the previously published head-to-head comparison of these techniques by Tariq et al. [43], which found that logistic regression resulted in both the highest accuracy and highest unweighted average recall. We used the default *scikit-learn* parameters for logistic regression, except we evaluated both L1 and L2 regularization with an inverse regularization strength of 0.05, forcing strong regularization. We reported the metrics with the greatest accuracy of L1 or L2 regularization. Because our goal was to evaluate worker performance and not to maximize the performance of a classifier, we did not perform any further hyperparameter tuning.

Because logistic regression classifiers emit a probability for a binary outcome, we treat the probability as a confidence score of the crowdsourced workers' responses. Here, we exclusively analyze the probability of the correct class (referred to as PCC from here on out), which is p when the true class is autism and $1-p$ when the true class is neurotypical. When assessing classifier predictions, we use a threshold of 0.5. Throughout this paper, we refer to a worker's average PCC for videos the worker rated as a measure of the worker's video tagging capability. Similarly, we refer to a video's PCC as the difficulty level of the video.

2.3. Video Rating Tasks

We aimed to crowdsource workers from three culturally distinct countries where autism is prevalent yet access to resources is lacking. These are samples of areas where accessible, affordable, and scalable precision medicine solutions, such as instantiations of the technique described here, can enable access to care to underserved populations globally. In particular, we selected Bangladesh,

Kenya, and the Philippines, countries that collectively represent diverse areas containing problematic issues with autism prevalence and limited access to services [46–49].

In order to generalize our findings across these distinct groups of workers, we posted four sets of video rating tasks under the following hypotheses:

H1a. *There are workers on MTurk whose mean classifier PCC will exceed 75%.*

H1b. *There are "super recognizer" workers on MTurk whose mean classifier PCC will exceed 75% and whose mean will be over one standard deviation above 50%.*

H2a. *There are workers from Bangladesh on Microworkers whose mean classifier PCC will exceed 75%.*

H2b. *There are "super recognizer" workers from Bangladesh on Microworkers whose mean classifier PCC will exceed 75% and whose mean will be over one standard deviation above 50%.*

H3a. *There are workers from Kenya on Microworkers whose mean classifier PCC will exceed 75%.*

H3b. *There are "super recognizer" workers from Kenya on Microworkers whose mean classifier PCC will exceed 75% and whose mean will be over one standard deviation above 50%.*

H4a. *There are workers from the Philippines on Microworkers whose mean classifier PCC will exceed 75%.*

H4b. *There are "super recognizer" workers from the Philippines on Microworkers whose mean classifier PCC will exceed 75% and whose mean will be over one standard deviation above 50%.*

We evaluate the above hypotheses only for workers who rated at least ten videos and for videos that received at least ten sets of ratings from workers. Hypotheses H1a, H2a, H3a, and H4a verify that there exist workers whose mean classifier PCC is consistently higher than the classification decision boundary by a sizable margin (25%) that is consistent with the documented 75% agreement rate between qualified multidisciplinary team diagnosis [50] using the Autism Diagnostic Observation Schedule (ADOS) [45] and Gilliam Autism Rating Scale (GARS) [51] scales. Hypotheses H1b, H2b, H3b, and H4b are more stringent, requiring the worker to exhibit low enough variance in their answers such that one standard deviation below their mean PCC is still above the classifier decision boundary and therefore still yields the correct diagnostic prediction. This level of robustness to variability is reasonable given the measures of inter-rater reliability of ADOS scoresheets, with Cohen's kappa coefficients for individual ADOS items ranging between 0.24 and 0.94 [52].

The first set of tasks was posted on MTurk. The second, third, and fourth sets were posted to distinct groups of workers on Microworkers. The Microworkers crowdsourcing tasks were targeted to workers in Bangladesh, Kenya, and the Philippines in order to sample a sufficiently diverse global population of crowdworkers while comparing independent subsets of the crowd.

All four independent studies consisted of a series of 13 multiple choice questions which were fed as inputs into the video observation classifier (Figure 1). Although the videos did not necessarily contain evidence of all 13 behavioral features used as inputs, workers were asked to infer how the child would behave if placed in the situation in question.

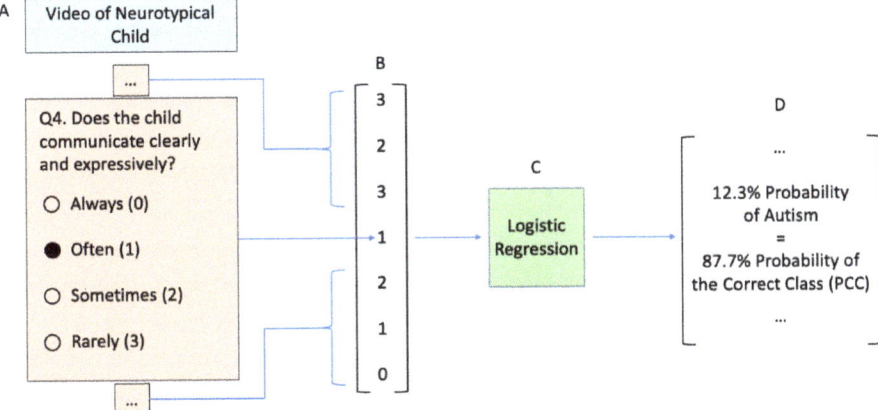

Figure 1. The process for calculating a probability score of autism from the categorical answers provided by crowdsourced workers. (**A**) Workers answer a series of multiple-choice questions per video that correspond to (**B**) categorical ordinal variables used in the input feature matrix to the (**C**) logistic regression classifier trained on electronic medical record data. This classifier emits a probability score for autism, which is the probability of the correct class when the true class is autism and 1 minus this probability when the true class is neurotypical (the latter case is depicted). (**D**) A vector of these probabilities is used to calculate mean worker and mean video probabilities of the correct class.

On MTurk, workers were only allowed to proceed with rating further videos if they passed a series of quality control metrics recording performance against the ADOS gold standard classifier (see section Materials and Methods: Video Observation Classifier) and the time spent working on the task. On Microworkers, worker filtering did not occur besides requiring a bare minimum of time rating each video (a minimum of 2 min per video was required to accept a worker's response).

3. Results

We analyze (1) the distribution of worker performance in different countries and crowd platforms, (2) the number of higher performing workers and "super recognizers" in each study group, and (3) the correlation between mean time spent on the task and mean worker performance for each study group.

3.1. Distribution of Worker Performance

For all four worker groups, there was major variation in the average probability score of the classifier per video (Figure 2) and per worker (Figure 3). The mean probability of the true class for the 43 videos with at least ten worker ratings on MTurk was 63.80% (SD = 13.78%), with a minimum of 16.90% and a maximum of 84.05%. On Microworkers, the mean PCC for videos with at least ten ratings were 63.15% (N = 24; SD = 10.42%; range = 33.73–79.03%) for Bangladesh, 67.75% (N = 24; SD = 14.68%; range = 32.71–88.91%) for Kenya, and 72.05% (N =2 4; SD = 13.05%; range = 47.84–90.80%) for the Philippines.

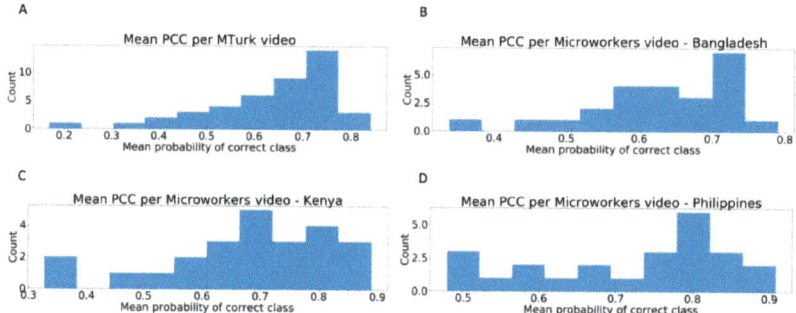

Figure 2. Distribution of average classifier probability of the correct class per video with at least ten ratings from (**A**) MTurk workers, (**B**) Bangladesh Microworkers, (**C**) Kenya Microworkers, and (**D**) Philippines Microworkers. There is wide variability in the difficulty level of rated videos.

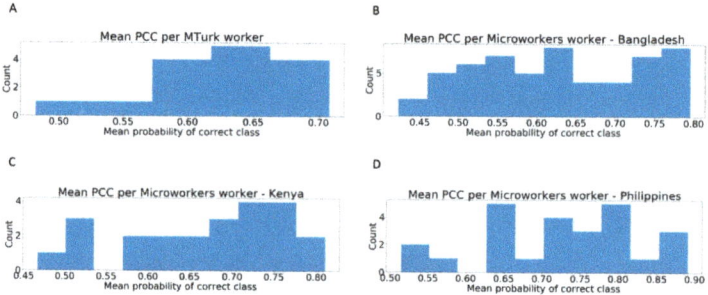

Figure 3. Distribution of average probability of the correct class per (**A**) MTurk worker, (**B**) Bangladesh Microworker, (**C**) Kenya Microworker, and (**D**) Philippines Microworker who provided at least ten ratings. There is wide variability in the ability of workers to provide accurate categorical labels.

The mean classifier PCC for the 15 workers with 10 or more videos rated on MTurk was 66.67% (SD = 5.98%), with a minimum of 48.16% and a maximum of 70.82%. On Microworkers, the mean worker classifier PCC for those who provided ten or more ratings were 62.53% (N = 56; SD = 10.43%; range = 42.21–79.53%) for Bangladesh, 66.67% (N = 23; SD = 9.75%; range = 46.62–81.03%) for Kenya, and 72.71% (N = 25; SD = 10.25%; range = 51.38–89.08%) for the Philippines.

Crucially, while there were individual differences in the subset of videos rated across workers, there was no significant difference in the difficulties of these videos across workers (Figure 4) for workers who rated at least ten videos and videos with at least ten ratings from workers. This confirms that the variability in worker performance in not attributable to the video difficulties. In all four groups, a Pearson correlation test between the mean video PCC and mean worker PCC yielded insignificant results ($r = 0.088$, $p = 0.07$ for MTurk; $r = 0.017$, $p = 0.62$ for Bangladesh Microworkers; $r = -0.018$, $p = 0.70$ for Kenya Microworkers; and $r = -0.030$, $p = 0.52$ for Philippines Microworkers).

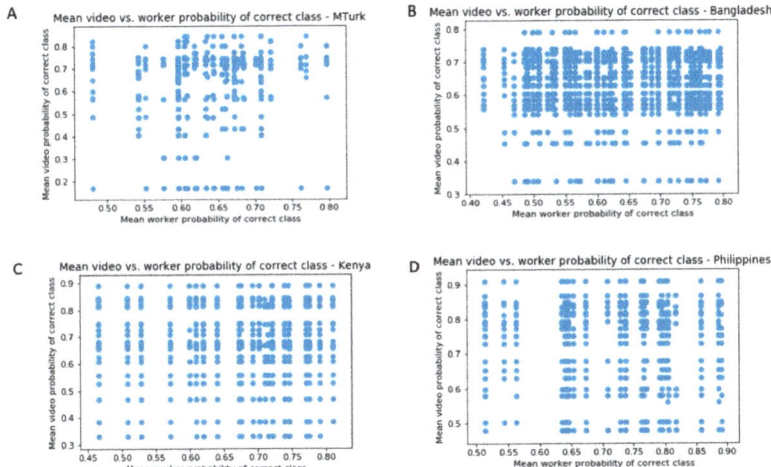

Figure 4. Mean classifier confidence per video vs. per worker for (**A**) MTurk workers, (**B**) Bangladesh Microworkers, (**C**) Kenya Microworkers, and (**D**) Philippines Microworkers for videos with at least 10 ratings and workers who provided at least ten ratings. Each vertical line of points contains the difficulty levels of videos rated for one worker, visually demonstrating that workers received similar distributions of video difficulties to rate despite displaying large variation in average diagnostic confidence.

3.2. Super Recognizers

Figures 3 and 4 reveal that hypotheses H1a, H2a, H3a, and H4a are confirmed: there were workers in all four study groups whose mean classifier PCC exceeded 75%. On MTurk, there was one worker whose mean was greater than one standard deviation above 50%, confirming hypothesis H1b. There were three Microworkers in the Bangladesh cohort, two Microworkers in the Kenya cohort and ten Microworkers in the Philippines cohort whose mean was greater than one standard deviation above 50%, confirming hypotheses H2b, H3b and H4b.

3.3. Effect of Time Spent Rating

Because of pervasive practices among MTurk workers of artificially inflating the time spent on the task out of fear of spending insufficient time on the task [53,54], we only analyzed timing information of Microworkers data. Several recorded times for MTurk tasks exceeded several hours, suggesting MTurk worker behavior of bloating task times.

There was no statistically significant Pearson correlation between mean time spent on the task and mean worker performance for the Kenya and Philippines Microworkers groups individually ($r = 0.191$, $p = 0.38$ for Kenya Microworkers; and $r = 0.193$, $p = 0.35$ for Philippines Microworkers). For Bangladesh Microworkers, there was a statistically significant correlation ($r = 0.326$, $p = 0.01$). When aggregating all Microworkers results, the correlation is slightly strengthened ($r = 0.358$, $p = 0.005$).

4. Discussion

We discuss (1) the overall implications of the worker variability in all study groups and the presence of "super recognizers," (2) the formalization of a crowd filtration process which can be leveraged for the identification of high performing crowd workers for a variety of precision medicine tasks, and (3) limitations of the present study and areas of potential future work.

4.1. General Implications

All four independent worker groups produced at least one worker who rated at least ten videos and whose mean classifier PCC exceeded 75%. There was one MTurk worker, three Microworkers in Bangladesh, two Microworkers in the Kenya cohort, and ten Microworkers in the Philippines cohort whose mean was greater than one standard deviation above 50%. It is unclear whether language barriers, differences in Microworker demographics across countries, or other factors are responsible for this inconsistency across countries.

We observe a high variation in worker performance in all four study groups. This variation in performance is distinct from other common crowdsourcing tasks such as image labeling, where worker responses are generally accepted to be high quality and therefore only simple quality control metrics (rather than filtering processes) are usually in place. These results suggest that there are innate differences between crowd workers' abilities to successfully and accurately label behavioral features from short unstructured videos of children. This variation in intrinsic ability to rate diagnostically rich features suggests that a filtering process must occur to curate a subset of the crowd who are skilled at inferring behavior patterns from videos. We term this skilled distributed workforce "super recognizers" as they appear consistently adept at recognizing and tagging core autism symptoms from unstructured video without prior training.

Further, we find that the time spent rating is weakly correlated with average performance, indicating that workers can be filtered for spending too little time on the tasks in aggregate. Although this trend was not observed in the Kenya and Philippines cohorts individually, this may likely be attributed to the smaller sample sizes of these groups. Including these data in the aggregate time correlation analysis bolstered the statistical significance of the correlation.

Gold standard classifiers trained on clinician-filled electronic health records are pertinent to scaling digital behavioral diagnostics. The source of training data is crucial, as behavioral instruments are not always consistent with categorizing diagnostic outcomes for the same individual [55]. The classifier used here was trained on ADOS records, but the children in the videos were not necessarily diagnosed via the ADOS, as there are several diagnostic instruments for autism [56–61] capturing overlapping yet distinct behaviors.

It is clear that different workers possess varying capabilities in behavioral video tagging, a nontrivial task. To realize economic crowdsourcing, several subsets of the crowd should be evaluated, with adept subgroups further pursued. Curating such a skilled crowd workforce in a developing country may lead to part time employment of "super recognizers" in telemedical practices in that country. This would eventually enable automated precision medicine through training machine learning classifiers using the labeled video data libraries accumulated through distributed behavioral video tagging.

4.2. Formalization of a Crowd Filtration Process

These results suggest that clinical workflows incorporating crowdsourced workers for pediatric diagnostics of complex behavioral conditions like autism should first filter down the crowd to a subset of workers who repeatedly and consistently perform well. Here, we propose a novel workflow for recruitment of crowdsourced workers to ensure high quality diagnostic evaluations of pediatric behavioral health conditions:

1. Train one or more machine learning classifiers using data accumulated by domain expert clinicians. These data may be actively acquired or mined from existing data sources. It is crucial that the gold standard data are representative of the target pediatric population.
2. Define a target performance metric for worker evaluation and a target number of workers to recruit.
3. Collect labels from a massive and distributed set of crowd workers (Figure 5).

4. Filter the crowd workers progressively and repeatedly until the target number of workers have reached or surpassed the target performance metric.
5. The final set of globally recruited "super recognizers" can be leveraged in precision health and precision medicine clinical workflows toward rating a worldwide pediatric population (Figure 5).

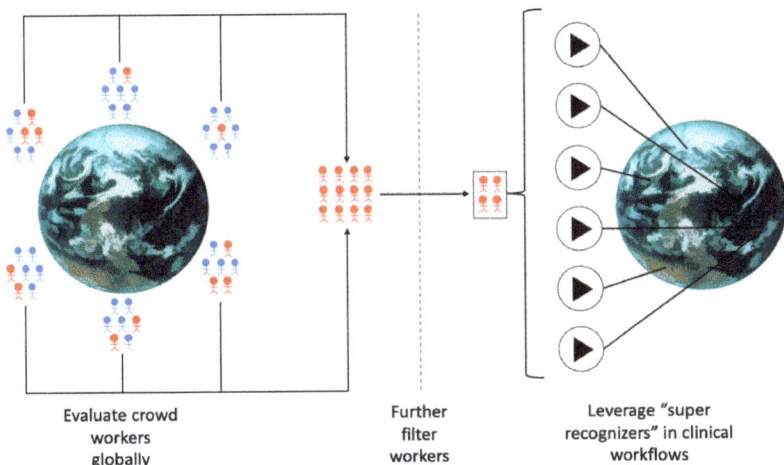

Figure 5. Crowd filtration pipeline. Crowdsourced workers are first evaluated globally. The highest performers from each location are further evaluated for one or more rounds until a final skilled workforce is curated. These "super recognizers" may then be repeatedly employed in global clinical workflows.

4.3. Limitations and Future Work

There are several limitations of the present study and fruitful avenues for future work. More structured videos, such as those collected in home smartphone autism interventions [15–19], may yield more consistent video difficulty levels due to the standardization of collected videos. Mobile therapeutics in conjunction with crowdsourcing may be leveraged toward longitudinal outcome tracking of symptoms [7]. Testing more subsets of the crowd, partitioned not only by location but by a wide array of demographic factors, will reveal economical subsets of the crowd for remote behavioral video tagging. To understand the reasons for differences in performance across subsets, videos of children that reflect the demographics of the population being targeted should be deployed and compared against a control set of videos. We welcome and call for replication crowdsourcing studies with separate video sets and crowd recruitment strategies. We also hope similar approaches to those tried here will be replicated for other behavioral conditions such as ADHD, speech delay, and OCD.

5. Conclusions

Crowdsourcing is a powerful yet understudied emerging tool for telemedical precision medicine and health. We have demonstrated that crowdsourced workers vary in their performance on behavioral tagging of clinically representative videos of autism and matched neurotypical controls, and we provide formalization of a crowd filtration process for curation of the most capable members of the crowd for repeated use in crowdsourcing-based clinical workflows. This process consists of training a classifier from records filled by domain experts, identifying quantitative metrics for evaluating workers, crowdsourcing a clinical task, filtering workers using the clinician-trained classifier, and repeating until the ideal workforce size has been reached.

As data from human crowd-powered telemedical precision medicine pipelines are recorded and stored in growing databases, computer vision classifiers of core autism symptoms such as hand stimming, eye contact, and emotion evocation can be trained using these labeled datasets. Curation of a workforce of "super recognizers" will allow clinicians to trust the diagnostic labels and allow engineers to use high quality features when training novel classifiers for precision medicine. This will enable an eventual increase in the automation, and therefore throughput, of precision medicine techniques for pediatric developmental delays such as autism.

Author Contributions: Conceptualization, P.W., E.L. and D.P.W.; data curation, P.W., K.D., A.K., K.P., and D.W.; formal analysis, P.W., E.L., and D.P.W.; funding acquisition, P.W., K.D., Y.P., A.K., and D.P.W.; investigation, N.H. and D.P.W.; methodology, P.W., E.L., K.D., Y.P., A.K., K.P., M.W.S., B.C., N.S., M.V., C.V., N.H., and D.P.W.; project administration, K.D., A.K., and D.P.W.; resources, K.D., Y.P., and D.P.W.; software, P.W. and D.P.W.; supervision, D.P.W.; validation, E.L., K.D., Y.P., A.K., K.P., M.W.S., B.C., N.S., M.V., C.V., N.H., and D.P.W.; visualization, P.W.; writing—original draft, P.W. and D.W.; writing—review and editing, E.L., K.D., Y.P., A.K., K.P., M.W.S., B.C., N.S., M.V., C.V., N.H. and D.P.W. All authors have read and agree to the published version of the manuscript.

Funding: These studies were supported by awards to DPW by the National Institutes of Health (1R21HD091500-01 and 1R01EB025025-01). Additionally, we acknowledge the support of grants to DPW from The Hartwell Foundation, the David and Lucile Packard Foundation Special Projects Grant, Beckman Center for Molecular and Genetic Medicine, Coulter Endowment Translational Research Grant, Berry Fellowship, Spectrum Pilot Program, Stanford's Precision Health and Integrated Diagnostics Center (PHIND), Wu Tsai Neurosciences Institute Neuroscience: Translate Program, Spark Program in Translational Research, Stanford's Institute of Human Centered Artificial Intelligence, the Weston Havens Foundation, as well as philanthropic support from Peter Sullivan. PW would like to acknowledge support from the Stanford Interdisciplinary Graduate Fellowship (SIGF).

Acknowledgments: We thank all crowd workers who participated in the study.

Conflicts of Interest: D.P.W. is the founder of Cognoa.com. This company is developing digital health solutions for pediatric care. C.V., N.H., and A.K. work as part-time consultant to Cognoa.com. All other authors declare no conflict of interests.

References

1. Fombonne, E. The rising prevalence of autism. *J. Child Psychol. Psychiatry* **2018**, *59*, 717–720. [CrossRef]
2. Matson, J.L.; Kozlowski, A.M. The increasing prevalence of autism spectrum disorders. *Res. Autism Spectr. Disord.* **2011**, *5*, 418–425. [CrossRef]
3. Gordon-Lipkin, E.; Jessica, F.; Georgina, P. Whittling down the wait time: Exploring models to minimize the delay from initial concern to diagnosis and treatment of autism spectrum disorder. *Pediatric Clin.* **2016**, *63*, 851–859.
4. Ning, M.; Daniels, J.; Schwartz, J.; Dunlap, K.; Washington, P.; Kalantarian, H.; Du, M.; Wall, D.P.; Cao, Y.; Antoniou, P. Identification and Quantification of Gaps in Access to Autism Resources in the United States: An Infodemiological Study. *J. Med. Internet Res.* **2019**, *21*, e13094. [CrossRef]
5. Tariq, Q.; Fleming, S.L.; Schwartz, J.; Dunlap, K.; Corbin, C.; Washington, P.; Kalantarian, H.; Khan, N.Z.; Darmstadt, G.L.; Wall, D.P.; et al. Detecting Developmental Delay and Autism Through Machine Learning Models Using Home Videos of Bangladeshi Children: Development and Validation Study. *J. Med. Internet Res.* **2019**, *21*, e13822. [CrossRef]
6. Washington, P.; Kalantarian, H.; Tariq, Q.; Schwartz, J.; Dunlap, K.; Chrisman, B.; Varma, M.; Ning, M.; Kline, A.; Stockham, N.; et al. Validity of Online Screening for Autism: Crowdsourcing Study Comparing Paid and Unpaid Diagnostic Tasks. *J. Med. Internet Res.* **2019**, *21*, e13668. [CrossRef]
7. Washington, P.; Park, N.; Srivastava, P.; Voss, C.; Kline, A.; Varma, M.; Tariq, Q.; Kalantarian, H.; Schwartz, J.; Patnaik, R.; et al. Data-Driven Diagnostics and the Potential of Mobile Artificial Intelligence for Digital Therapeutic Phenotyping in Computational Psychiatry. *Biol. Psychiatry Cogn. Neurosci. Neuroimaging* **2019**. [CrossRef]
8. Kosmicki, J.A.; Sochat, V.V.; Duda, M.; Wall, D.P. Searching for a minimal set of behaviors for autism detection through feature selection-based machine learning. *Transl. Psychiatry* **2015**, *5*, e514. [CrossRef]
9. Wall, D.P.; Kosmicki, J.; DeLuca, T.F.; Harstad, E.; Fusaro, V.A. Use of machine learning to shorten observation-based screening and diagnosis of autism. *Transl. Psychiatry* **2012**, *2*, e100. [CrossRef]
10. Abbas, H.; Garberson, F.; Liu-Mayo, S.; Glover, E.; Wall, D.P. Multi-modular Ai Approach to Streamline Autism Diagnosis in Young children. *Sci. Rep.* **2020**, *10*, 1–8. [CrossRef]

11. Voss, C.; Schwartz, J.; Daniels, J.; Kline, A.; Haber, N.; Washington, P.; Tariq, Q.; Robinson, T.N.; Desai, M.; Phillips, J.M.; et al. Effect of Wearable Digital Intervention for Improving Socialization in Children with Autism Spectrum Disorder: A Randomized Clinical Trial. *JAMA Pediatr.* **2019**, *173*, 446–454. [CrossRef]
12. Kline, A.; Voss, C.; Washington, P.; Haber, N.; Schwartz, H.; Tariq, Q.; Winograd, T.; Feinstein, C.; Wall, D.P. Superpower Glass. *GetMobile Mob. Comput. Commun.* **2019**, *23*, 35–38. [CrossRef]
13. Washington, P.; Catalin, V.; Aaron, K.; Nick, H.; Jena, D.; Azar, F.; Titas, D.; Carl, F.; Terry, W.; Dennis, W. Superpowerglass: A wearable aid for the at-home therapy of children with autism. *Proc. ACM Interact. Mob. Wearable Ubiquitous Technol.* **2017**, *1*, 112. [CrossRef]
14. Daniels, J.; Schwartz, J.N.; Voss, C.; Haber, N.; Fazel, A.; Kline, A.; Washington, P.; Feinstein, C.; Winograd, T.; Wall, D.P. Exploratory study examining the at-home feasibility of a wearable tool for social-affective learning in children with autism. *NPJ Digit. Med.* **2018**, *1*, 32. [CrossRef]
15. Kalantarian, H.; Jedoui, K.; Washington, P.; Tariq, Q.; Dunlap, K.; Schwartz, J.; Wall, D.P. Labeling images with facial emotion and the potential for pediatric healthcare. *Artif. Intell. Med.* **2019**, *98*, 77–86. [CrossRef]
16. Kalantarian, H.; Washington, P.; Schwartz, J.; Daniels, J.; Haber, N.; Wall, D. A Gamified Mobile System for Crowdsourcing Video for Autism Research. In Proceedings of the 2018 IEEE International Conference on Healthcare Informatics (ICHI), New York, NY, USA, 4–7 June 2018; pp. 350–352.
17. Kalantarian, H.; Washington, P.; Schwartz, J.; Daniels, J.; Haber, N.; Wall, D.P. Guess What? *J. Healthc. Informatics Res.* **2018**, *3*, 43–66. [CrossRef]
18. Kalantarian, H.; Jedoui, K.; Washington, P.; Wall, D.P. A Mobile Game for Automatic Emotion-Labeling of Images. *IEEE Trans. Games* **2018**, *1*. [CrossRef]
19. Kalantarian, H.; Jedoui, K.; Dunlap, K.; Schwartz, J.; Washington, P.; Husic, A.; Tariq, Q.; Ning, M.; et al. The Performance of Emotion Classifiers for Children with Parent-Reported Autism: Quantitative Feasibility Study. *JMIR Ment. Health* **2020**, *7*, e13174. [CrossRef]
20. Rudovic, O.; Lee, J.; Dai, M.; Schuller, B.W.; Picard, R.W. Personalized machine learning for robot perception of affect and engagement in autism therapy. *Sci. Robot.* **2018**, *3*, eaao6760. [CrossRef]
21. Egger, H.L.; Dawson, G.; Hashemi, J.; Carpenter, K.L.; Espinosa, S.; Campbell, K.; Brotkin, S.; Schaich-Borg, J.; Qiu, Q.; Tepper, M.; et al. Automatic emotion and attention analysis of young children at home: A ResearchKit autism feasibility study. *NPJ Digit. Med.* **2018**, *1*, 20. [CrossRef]
22. Kolakowska, A.; Landowska, A.; Anzulewicz, A.; Sobota, K. Automatic recognition of therapy progress among children with autism. *Sci. Rep.* **2017**, *7*, 13863. [CrossRef]
23. Chang, C.-H.; Saravia, E.; Chen, Y.-S. Subconscious Crowdsourcing: A feasible data collection mechanism for mental disorder detection on social media. In Proceedings of the 2016 IEEE/ACM International Conference on Advances in Social Networks Analysis and Mining (ASONAM), San Francisco, CA, USA, 18–21 August 2016; IEEE: Piscataway, NJ, USA, 2016; pp. 374–379.
24. Van Der Krieke, L.; Jeronimus, B.; Blaauw, F.J.; Wanders, R.B.; Emerencia, A.C.; Schenk, H.M.; De Vos, S.; Snippe, E.; Wichers, M.; Wigman, J.T.; et al. HowNutsAreTheDutch (HoeGekIsNL): A crowdsourcing study of mental symptoms and strengths. *Int. J. Methods Psychiatr. Res.* **2015**, *25*, 123–144. [CrossRef]
25. Weber, I.; Mejova, Y. Crowdsourcing health labels: Inferring body weight from profile pictures. In Proceedings of the 6th International Conference on Digital Health Conference, Montreal, QC, Canada, 11–13 April 2016; Association for Computing Machinery: New York, NY, USA, 2016; pp. 105–109.
26. Alvaro, N.; Conway, M.; Doan, S.; Lofi, C.; Overington, J.; Collier, N. Crowdsourcing Twitter annotations to identify first-hand experiences of prescription drug use. *J. Biomed. Informatics* **2015**, *58*, 280–287. [CrossRef]
27. Gottlieb, A.; Hoehndorf, R.; Dumontier, M.; Altman, R.B.; Johnson, K. Ranking Adverse Drug Reactions with Crowdsourcing. *J. Med. Internet Res.* **2015**, *17*, e80. [CrossRef]
28. Ariffin, I.; Solemon, B.; Abu Bakar, W.M.L.W. An evaluative study on mobile crowdsourcing applications for crime watch. In Proceedings of the 6th International Conference on Information Technology and Multimedia, Putrajaya, Malaysia, 18–20 November 2014; IEEE: Piscataway, NJ, USA, 2015; pp. 335–340.
29. Evans, M.B.; O'Hara, K.; Tiropanis, T.; Webber, C. Crime applications and social machines: Crowdsourcing sensitive data. In Proceedings of the 22nd International Conference on World Wide Web, Rio de Janeiro, Brazil, 13–17 May 2013; pp. 891–896.
30. Williams, C. Crowdsourcing Research: A Methodology for Investigating State Crime. *State Crime J.* **2013**, *2*, 30–51. [CrossRef]

31. Choy, G.; Khalilzadeh, O.; Michalski, M.; Synho, D.; Samir, A.E.; Pianykh, O.S.; Geis, J.R.; Pandharipande, P.V.; Brink, J.A.; Dreyer, K.J. Current Applications and Future Impact of Machine Learning in Radiology. *Radiology* **2018**, *288*, 318–328. [CrossRef]
32. Gargeya, R.; Leng, T. Automated Identification of Diabetic Retinopathy Using Deep Learning. *Ophthalmology* **2017**, *124*, 962–969. [CrossRef]
33. Iwabuchi, S.J.; Liddle, P.F.; Palaniyappan, L. Clinical Utility of Machine-Learning Approaches in Schizophrenia: Improving Diagnostic Confidence for Translational Neuroimaging. *Front. Psychol.* **2013**, *4*, 95. [CrossRef]
34. Yu, K.-H.; Beam, A.; Kohane, I.S. Artificial intelligence in healthcare. *Nat. Biomed. Eng.* **2018**, *2*, 719–731. [CrossRef]
35. Hsueh, P.-Y.; Melville, P.; Sindhwani, V. Data quality from crowdsourcing: A study of annotation selection criteria. In Proceedings of the NAACL HLT 2009 Workshop on Active Learning for Natural Language Processing, Yorktown Heights, NY, USA, 5 June 2009; pp. 27–35.
36. Welinder, P.; Perona, P. Online crowdsourcing: Rating annotators and obtaining cost-effective labels. In Proceedings of the 2010 IEEE Computer Society Conference on Computer Vision and Pattern Recognition-Workshops, San Francisco, CA, USA, 13–18 June 2010; IEEE: Piscataway, NJ, USA, 2010; pp. 25–32.
37. Kittur, A.; Chi, E.H.; Bongwon, S. Crowdsourcing user studies with Mechanical Turk. In Proceedings of the SIGCHI Conference on Human Factors in Computing Systems, New York, NY, USA, 5–10 April 2008; pp. 453–456.
38. Paolacci, G.; Jesse, C.; Panagiotis, G.I. Running experiments on amazon mechanical turk. *Judgm. Decis. Mak.* **2010**, *5*, 411–419.
39. Gardlo, B.; Ries, M.; Hossfeld, T.; Schatz, R. Microworkers vs. facebook: The impact of crowdsourcing platform choice on experimental results. In Proceedings of the 2012 Fourth International Workshop on Quality of Multimedia Experience, Yarra Valley, Australia, 5–7 July 2012; IEEE: Piscataway, NJ, USA, 2012; pp. 35–36.
40. Nguyen, N. Microworkers Crowdsourcing Approach, Challenges and Solutions. In Proceedings of the 2014 International ACM Workshop on Crowdsourcing for Multimedia, Orlando, FL, USA, 7 November 2014; p. 1.
41. Hirth, M.; Hossfeld, T.; Tran-Gia, P. Anatomy of a crowdsourcing platform-using the example of microworkers.com. In Proceedings of the 2011 Fifth International Conference on Innovative Mobile and Internet Services in Ubiquitous Computing, Korean Bible University, Seoul, Korea, 30 June–2 July 2011; IEEE: Piscataway, NJ, USA, 2011; pp. 322–329.
42. Levy, S.; Duda, M.; Haber, N.; Wall, D.P. Sparsifying machine learning models identify stable subsets of predictive features for behavioral detection of autism. *Mol. Autism* **2017**, *8*, 65. [CrossRef]
43. Tariq, Q.; Daniels, J.; Schwartz, J.; Washington, P.; Kalantarian, H.; Wall, D.P. Mobile detection of autism through machine learning on home video: A development and prospective validation study. *PLoS Med.* **2018**, *15*, e1002705. [CrossRef]
44. Guy, W. *ECDEU Assessment Manual for Psychopharmacology*; US Department of Health, Education, and Welfare, Public Health Service, Alcohol, Drug Abuse, and Mental Health Administration, National Institute of Mental Health, Psychopharmacology Research Branch, Division of Extramural Research Programs: Rockville, MD, USA, 1976.
45. Lord, C.; Rutter, M.; Goode, S.; Heemsbergen, J.; Jordan, H.; Mawhood, L.; Schopler, E. Austism diagnostic observation schedule: A standardized observation of communicative and social behavior. *J. Autism Dev. Disord.* **1989**, *19*, 185–212. [CrossRef]
46. Ahmed, N.; Raheem, E.; Rahman, N.; Khan, M.Z.R.; Al Mosabbir, A.; Hossain, M.S. Managing autism spectrum disorder in developing countries by utilizing existing resources: A perspective from Bangladesh. *Autism* **2018**, *23*, 801–803. [CrossRef]
47. Ehsan, U.; Sakib, N.; Haque, M.; Soron, T.; Saxena, D.; Ahamed, S.; Schwichtenberg, A.; Rabbani, G.; Akter, S.; Alam, F.; et al. Confronting Autism in Urban Bangladesh: Unpacking Infrastructural and Cultural Challenges. *EAI Endorsed Trans. Pervasive Health Technol.* **2018**, *4*. [CrossRef]
48. Gona, J.K.; Newton, C.R.; Rimba, K.K.; Mapenzi, R.; Kihara, M.; Van De Vijver, F.J.R.; Abubakar, A. Challenges and coping strategies of parents of children with autism on the Kenyan coast. *Rural. Remote Health* **2016**, *16*, 3517.

49. Ryan, C.M.M.; Diana, M.; Jumadiao, J.J.S.U.; Angel, J.J.Q.; Leonard, J.P.R.; Yoshiki, B.K. Awetism: A User Ergonomic Learning Management System Intended for Autism Diagnosed Students in the Philippines. In Proceedings of the International Conference on Industrial Engineering and Operations Management, Bandung, Indonesia, 6–8 March 2018.
50. Mazefsky, C.A.; Oswald, D. The discriminative ability and diagnostic utility of the ADOS-G, ADI-R, and GARS for children in a clinical setting. *Autism* **2006**, *10*, 533–549. [CrossRef]
51. James, E.G. *Gilliam Autism Rating Scale: Examiner's Manual*; Pro-Ed: Austin, TX, USA, 1995.
52. Zander, E.; Willfors, C.; Berggren, S.; Choque-Olsson, N.; Coco, C.; Elmund, A.; Moretti, Å.H.; Holm, A.; Jifält, I.; Kosieradzki, R.; et al. The objectivity of the Autism Diagnostic Observation Schedule (ADOS) in naturalistic clinical settings. *Eur. Child Adolesc. Psychiatry* **2015**, *25*, 769–780. [CrossRef]
53. Brawley, A.M.; Pury, C.L.S. Work experiences on MTurk: Job satisfaction, turnover, and information sharing. *Comput. Hum. Behav.* **2016**, *54*, 531–546. [CrossRef]
54. Necka, E.A.; Cacioppo, S.; Norman, G.J.; Cacioppo, J.T. Measuring the Prevalence of Problematic Respondent Behaviors among MTurk, Campus, and Community Participants. *PLoS ONE* **2016**, *11*, e0157732. [CrossRef]
55. Washington, P.; Paskov, K.M.; Kalantarian, H.; Stockham, N.; Voss, C.; Kline, A.; Patnaik, R.; Chrisman, B.; Varma, M.; Tariq, Q.; et al. Feature Selection and Dimension Reduction of Social Autism Data. *Pac. Symp. Biocomput.* **2020**, *25*, 707–718. [PubMed]
56. Lord, C.; Rutter, M.; Le Couteur, A. Autism Diagnostic Interview-Revised: A revised version of a diagnostic interview for caregivers of individuals with possible pervasive developmental disorders. *J. Autism Dev. Disord.* **1994**, *24*, 659–685. [CrossRef] [PubMed]
57. Rutter, M.; Bailey, A.; Lord, C.; Cianchetti, C.; Fancelli, G.S. *Social Communication Questionnaire*; Western Psychological Services: Los Angeles, CA, USA, 2003.
58. Sparrow, S.S.; Cicchetti, D.; Balla, D.A. *Vineland Adaptive Behavior Scales*, 2nd ed.; NCS Pearson Inc.: Minneapolis, MN, USA, 2005.
59. Carrow-Woolfolk, E. *Oral and Written Language Scales*; American Guidance Service: Circle Pines, MN, USA, 1995; Volume 93, pp. 947–964.
60. Phelps-Terasaki, D.; Phelps-Gunn, T. *Test of Pragmatic Language (TOPL-2)*; Pro-Ed: Austin, TX, USA, 2007.
61. Wechsler, D. *WISC-V: Technical and Interpretive Manual*; NCS Pearson, Incorporated: Bloomington, MN, USA, 2014.

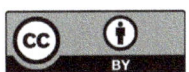

© 2020 by the authors. Licensee MDPI, Basel, Switzerland. This article is an open access article distributed under the terms and conditions of the Creative Commons Attribution (CC BY) license (http://creativecommons.org/licenses/by/4.0/).

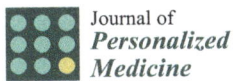 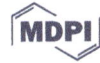

Article

The Autonomic Nervous System Differentiates between Levels of Motor Intent and End Effector

Jihye Ryu [1] and Elizabeth Torres [2],*

[1] Psychology Department, Rutgers University Center for Cognitive Science, Rutgers University, Piscataway, NJ 08854, USA; jr1102@psych.rutgers.edu
[2] Psychology Department, Rutgers University Center for Cognitive Science, Computational Biomedicine Imaging and Modeling Center at Computer Science Department, Rutgers University, Piscataway, NJ 08854, USA
* Correspondence: ebtorres@psych.rutgers.edu; Tel.: +1-732-208-3158

Received: 25 May 2020; Accepted: 28 July 2020; Published: 31 July 2020

Abstract: While attempting to bridge motor control and cognitive science, the nascent field of embodied cognition has primarily addressed intended, goal-oriented actions. Less explored, however, have been unintended motions. Such movements tend to occur largely beneath awareness, while contributing to the spontaneous control of redundant degrees of freedom across the body in motion. We posit that the consequences of such unintended actions implicitly contribute to our autonomous sense of action ownership and agency. We question whether biorhythmic activities from these motions are separable from those which intentionally occur. Here we find that fluctuations in the biorhythmic activities of the nervous systems can unambiguously differentiate across levels of intent. More important yet, this differentiation is remarkable when we examine the fluctuations in biorhythmic activity from the autonomic nervous systems. We find that when the action is intended, the heart signal leads the body kinematics signals; but when the action segment spontaneously occurs without instructions, the heart signal lags the bodily kinematics signals. We conclude that the autonomic nervous system can differentiate levels of intent. Our results are discussed while considering their potential translational value.

Keywords: embodied cognition; agency; action ownership; network analysis; graph theory; motor control; voluntary motion; precision medicine

1. Introduction

The field of embodied cognition (EC) has provided a powerful theoretical framework amenable to bridge the gap between research probing our mental states and research investigating our physical actions [1–3]. Indeed, within the framework of EC, the construct of agency conceived as a cognitive movement phenomenon [4–6] may provide a way to finally connect the disparate fields of cognitive science and motor control. An important component of agency is action ownership [6–8], i.e., the sense that sensory consequences of the actor's action are intrinsically part of the actor's inner sensations. When the actor owns the action, s/he has full control over those sensations that are internally self-generated and self-monitored by the actor's brain and yet extrinsically modulated by external sensory goals. A critical aspect of this internal–external loop is the identification of the level of actor's intent and its differential contribution to the action's intended and unintended sensory consequences.

In recent years, a body of knowledge has increased our understanding on the sensory consequences derived from intentional actions, as such action components deliver an overall sense of agency [9,10] through elements of body-ownership closely interrelated with motor control [11,12]. Less explored, however, have been parts of the action that are unintended or that transpire spontaneously and largely beneath awareness. Such actions' components exist at the involuntary (uncontrolled, random motions) and at the autonomic (pacemaker, periodic motions) levels of neuromotor control (Figure 1). They do not require explicit instructions or precisely defined external goals, yet they too contribute to the differentiation of levels of intent in our actions [13,14]. More importantly, at the cognitive level of decision making, these unintended movements contribute to the acquisition of decision accuracy within the context of the type of motor learning that is induced by different cognitive loads [15,16].

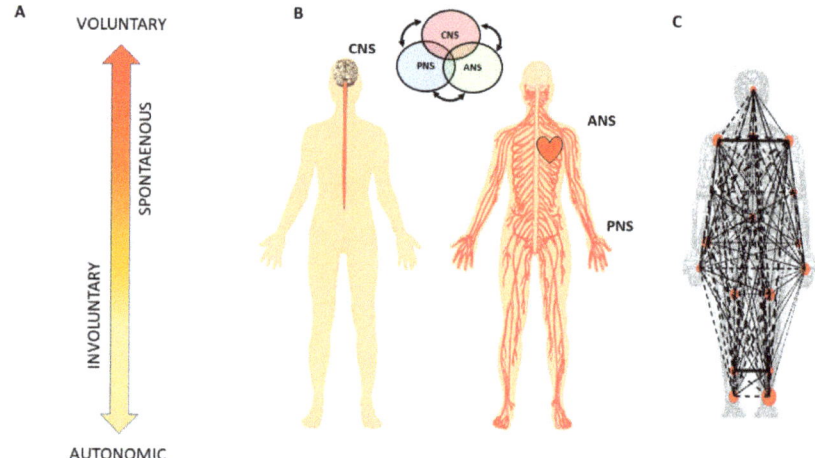

Figure 1. Defining quantitative aspects of agency for the study of embodied cognition. (**A**) A highly simplified schematics reflecting the phylogenetically orderly taxonomy of nervous system functions involving different levels of voluntary control (intent) ranging from deliberate to spontaneous movement segments, to involuntary motions and autonomic control. Levels correspond to three fundamental muscle types (skeletal for voluntary, smooth for involuntary, and cardiac for autonomic.) Multi-layered signals contributing from each of these layers are proposed to differentially contribute to the sense of action ownership and to the overall sense of agency via sensory consequences preceded by different levels of intent. (**B**) Contributions of the central and peripheral nervous systems (CNS and PNS, respectively), including the autonomic nervous system (ANS), can be tracked in a closed loop that helps the autonomous realization of intended thoughts into physical actions under volitional control. (**C**) Network connectivity analyses of kinematics and heart biorhythmic signals encompassing these levels of control enable the study of agency through objective quantitative methods.

At the motor control level, autonomous and spontaneous movements are important to develop a sense of action ownership in the face of motor redundancy [17]. Spontaneous motions can be covert, as those subtle motions occurring in a coma patient [18] or those occurring in a neonate [19]; or overt, as when they coexist with deliberate/staged ones, embedded in complex sports routines [13,14] and/or ballet choreographies [20]. Such complex overt movements require the coordination and control of many degrees of freedom (DoFs) across the body. Thus, as we produce fluid and timely goal-oriented actions, kinematic synergies self-emerge and dynamically recruit and release the bodily DoFs, according to task demands [21–23]. Conscious decisions generating movements that attain external goals take place as the brain interweaves deliberate and spontaneous movement segments. Such segments in our complex actions gracefully build an ebb and flow of actions intended to a goal, and sensory consequences from those actions [13]. Some of these sensations that voluntary movements give rise to [24] return to the brain as feedback from the intentional part of the movements, thought to contribute to our internal models of action dynamics [25,26]. This form of volitionally controlled kinesthetic reafference cumulatively helps us build accurate predictions of those intended sensory consequences [24], while other unintended movements return to the brain as spontaneous reafference in the precise sense that they do not follow from instructed acts. These spontaneous activities provide contextual cues that support motor learning, motor adaptation and action generalization across different situations [13], including pathologies of the nervous systems [27,28].

One informative aspect of this ebb and flow of intent and spontaneity in our actions is the fundamental differences that emerge in the geometric features of the positional trajectories that the moving body describes [29–31]. When the motions are intended, geometric measures related to path curvature and path length show invariance to changes in movement dynamics, i.e., these metrics remain robust to changes in speed, mass, etc. [21,31–34]. In contrast, trajectories from unintended motions produce different signatures of motor variability bound to return to the brain as *spontaneous feedback*. These internal sensations could help the brain differentiate contextual variations emerging from external environmental cues from sensory information that is internally self-generated by the nervous systems [13,14]. External information may include, for example, changes in visual and auditory inputs, such as shifts in lighting conditions, or modulations in sound and music [20,35].

The geometry of the uninstructed spontaneous movements' trajectories dramatically changes with fluctuations in the movements' dynamics. Changes in speed [21,30–32] or mass [14] affect their motor variability in fundamentally different ways (if we compare the signatures of variability derived from the spontaneous samples to those derived from deliberately staging the same movement trajectories [14,32].) More importantly, the fluctuations in the motor variability of these spontaneous motions can forecast symptoms of Parkinson's disease before the onset of high severity [27,36]. They have also aided in evoking the sense of action ownership and agency in young pre-verbal children [28]. For these reasons, here we posit that deliberate and spontaneous segments of complex covert actions ought to differentially contribute to our physical sense of action ownership and to our overall sense of agency. To examine this proposition, we follow a phylogenetically orderly taxonomy of the nervous systems' maturation (Figure 1B) and examine all levels of neuromotor control—from autonomic to deliberate—necessary to coordinate voluntary motions (Figure 1A).

More specifically, since autonomic systems are vital to our survival and wellbeing, they may remain impervious to subtle distinctions between deliberate and spontaneous motions that take place across the body, as the end effector completes goal-directed actions. Here we explore the interplay between autonomic signals and voluntary motor control in actions that integrate deliberate and spontaneous motions across the body. We use a new unifying statistical framework for individualized behavioral analyses and network connectivity analyses and offer a quantitative account of how these movement classes contribute to the overall embodied sense of agency.

2. Materials and Methods

2.1. Experimental Design

2.1.1. Participants

Nine undergraduate students (2 males and 7 females) between the ages of 18 and 22 years were recruited from the Rutgers human subject pool system. Two were left-handed and seven were right-handed, and all had normal or corrected-to-normal vision. All participants received credit for their participation, and provided informed consent, which was approved by the Rutgers University Institutional Review Board. The study took place at the Sensory Motor Integration Lab at Rutgers University.

During the experiment, movement kinematics and heart signals were recorded from each participant. However, one participant's recording had too much noise (i.e., inaccurate sensor position with error larger than 10 cm), so we excluded this participant's data in the analysis. For that reason, eight participants' motor and heart signals were analyzed.

2.1.2. Sensor Devices

Motion capture system (kinematics data): Fifteen electromagnetic sensors sampling at a frequency of 240 Hz (Polhemus Liberty, Colchester, VT, USA) were attached to the participant's upper body in the following locations: center of the forehead, thoracic vertebrate T7, right and left scapula, right and left upper arm, right and left forearm, performing hand, and the performing hand's index finger. These sensors were secured with sports bands to allow unrestricted movement during the recordings. Motor signals were recorded in real-time by Motion Monitor (Innovative Sports Training Inc., Chicago, IL, USA) software, where the participant's body was constructed by a biomechanical model, and movement data were preprocessed by an embedded filtering algorithm of the software, providing the position and kinematics of each sensor.

Electrocardiogram (heart data): Three sensors of electrocardiogram (ECG) from a wireless Nexus-10 device (Mind Media BV, Herten, The Netherlands) and Nexus 10 software Biotrace (Version 2015B) were used to record heart activity. At a sampling rate of 256 Hz, the sensors were placed across the chest according to a standardized lead II method.

2.1.3. Experimental Procedure

Participants sat at a desk facing an iPad tablet (Apple, Cupertino, CA, USA), which was used to display stimuli during the experiment, and participants responded by touching the tablet screen. The tablet display was controlled with an in-house developed MATLAB (Release 2015b, The MathWorks, Inc., Natick, MA, USA) program and TeamViewer application (Germany).

As shown in Figure 2, for each trial, the participant was presented with a circle on the tablet screen. This circle served as a prompt for the participant to touch the tablet screen within five seconds. After the touch, either 100 ms, 400 ms, or 700 ms elapsed, and the participant heard a tone at 1000 Hz for 100 ms. Then, on the tablet screen, the participant was presented with a sliding scale, ranging from 0 to 1 (second), to indicate how long he/she perceived the time elapsed between the touch and the tone. The response was to be made within five seconds upon the display of the sliding scale. The five second time-window was considered enough for the participant to provide a response, as it took approximately 1 s to touch the screen and retract the hand back to its original position. There was a total of three conditions, namely control, low cognitive load, and high cognitive load, and each condition consisted of 60 trials. In the control condition, the participant simply performed each trial with no additional task; under the low cognitive load condition, the participant performed each trial while repeatedly counting forward 1 through 5; under the high cognitive load condition, they counted backwards from 400 subtracting by 3 while they performed each trial. Participants counted forward and backward at their own comfortable pace, and they took breaks in between each condition. The experiment set up took about 30 min, and the recording took about 40 min.

2.2. Statistical Analysis Overview

2.2.1. Preprocessing

In this study, we extracted the kinematics (i.e., linear speed, angular acceleration) and heart data during time segments when the participant made a pointing motion towards the circle presented on the tablet screen, and we combined them across the three conditions. As a result, we analyzed the kinematics and heart data recorded while the participant made 180 pointing motions (less any trials that were deemed noisy; the most trials we excluded per participant due to instrumentation noise were 12 trials).

To analyze the ECG and kinematics data in tandem, we up-sampled the kinematics data from 240 Hz to 256 Hz using piecewise cubic spline interpolation. Note, the ECG signals were not synchronized with the kinematics data but were manually time stamped at the start and end of each experimental condition. For that matter, we expected the presence of a lag between the two modes of signals—kinematics and ECG—but the lag did not exceed 1 s.

To exclude effects of muscle motion from the ECG heart data, we bandpass filtered the data with Butterworth IIR for 5–30Hz at 2nd order. This filter was effective in identifying QRS complexes and extracting R-peaks in previous studies [16,37]. Here, the filter excluded the dominant frequency range where typical kinematics signals are present (see Appendix A Figure A1). We performed our analyses using both filtered and non-filtered EKG data and found similar trends and patterns. However, the paper only presents the results from using the filtered data, as it is a better reflection of the heart activity.

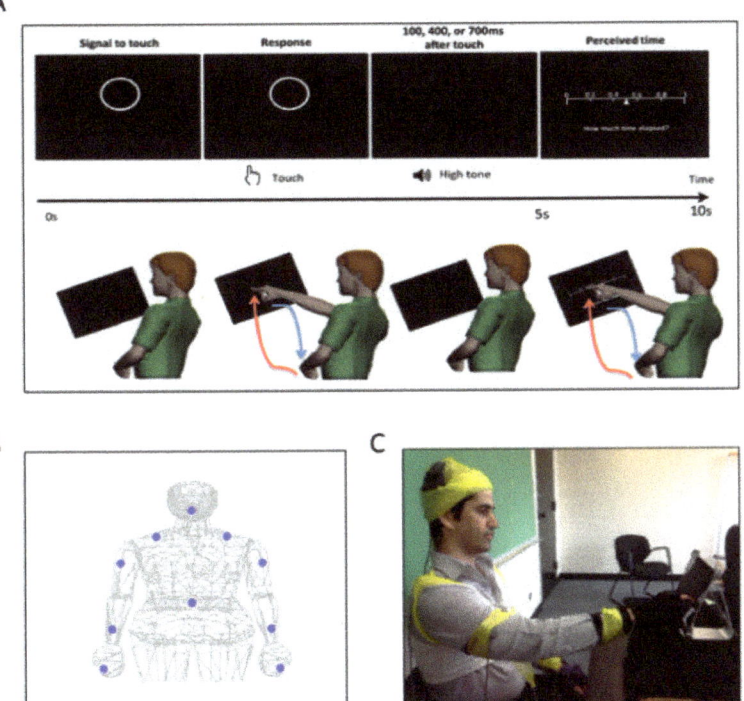

Figure 2. Experimental assay and instrumentation setup. (**A**) Experimental procedure. In a single trial, the participant was presented with a display screen, as shown on the top panel. During the first 5 s, the participant was presented with a circle as a prompt to touch the circle on the screen. After the touch, the participant heard a tone. The duration between the touch and the tone was randomly set to be 100 ms, 400 ms, or 700 ms. In the next 5 s, the participant was presented with a sliding scale, where s/he indicated how long the time was perceived to have elapsed between the touch and the tone, by touching the corresponding number on the scale. For each trial, the participant made two pointing gestures—one to touch the circle and another to indicate their time estimation on the sliding scale. Such pointing gesture was composed of a forward reaching segment (red) and a backward retracting segment (blue), as shown in the bottom panel. (**B**) Motion capture sensor positions. The sensors were attached on the following body parts: center of the forehead, thoracic vertebrate T7, right and left scapula, right and left upper arm, right and left forearm, non-performing hand, and the performing hand's index finger. (**C**) Snapshot of the experiment. During the experiment, the participant was seated in front of the tablet screen to perform the tasks, and wired sensors were secured with athletic tape.

2.2.2. Data Analysis Structure

We used the rationale in Figure 1 to structure our analyses, with a focus of two main axes denoting the level of motor intent and awareness that the brain may have during complex tasks (Figure 3A).

More precisely, one axis explored possible differentiations between time segments of the pointing movements that were deliberately aimed at an external target (forward/high motor intent) vs. segments that were consequential to the deliberate ones (backward/low motor intent). The latter may occur when the hand retracts back to rest, or when after touching the target the person transitions the hand in route to another goal-directed motion. These segments have been studied in our lab across very complex motions in sports (boxing, tennis) and in the performing arts (ballet, salsa dancing). We have coined them spontaneous movements and discovered that they have precise signatures that distinguish them from the deliberate ones. For this reason, we hypothesized here that these spontaneous motions would have different stochastic signatures or be differentially expressed in relation to the deliberate ones.

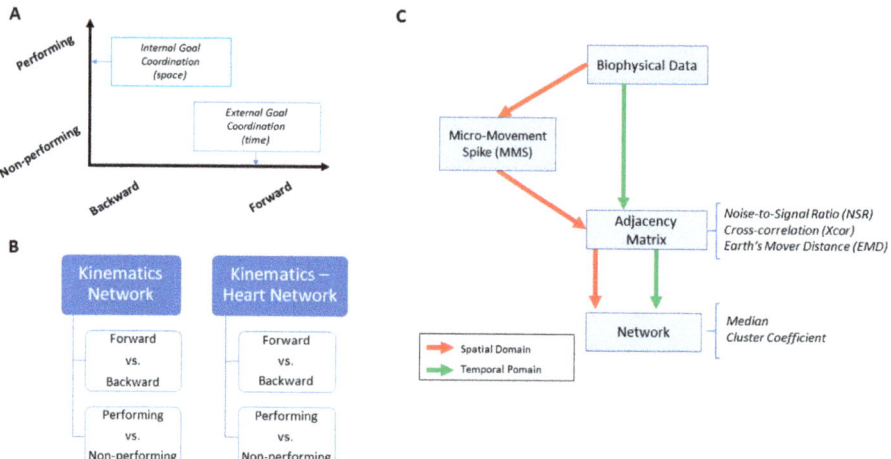

Figure 3. Overview of analytics pipeline. (**A**) Behavioral assay to quantify ranges of motor intent along two axes to highlight externally and internally defined goals. Along the former, motions are classified across time based on the end-effector's movement, ranging from backward–spontaneous (lower motor intent) to forward–deliberate (higher motor intent) motions. Along the other axis, motions are classified across locations of the body, based on the proximity to the end-effector, from non-performing side of the body parts (lower motor intent) to the performing side including the end-effector (higher motor intent). Note, the two axes are not necessarily orthogonal as the schematics imply. (**B**) Two types of network analyses were made. Within the kinematics network, kinematics data served to compare patterns of variability from movement segments of higher level of intent (deliberately aimed at the goal) and movement segments with lower level of intent (spontaneous retractions of the hand to rest, without instructions), including as well comparison of patterns from the performing and non-performing parts of the body. Within the kinematics-heart network, a similar comparison was made, with a layer of autonomic function added, using signals from the EKG sensors. (**C**) For the spatial domain of connectivity analysis, raw biophysical data (biorhythms) co-registered from multiple layers of the peripheral and autonomic nervous systems were converted to MMS and used to compute pairwise similarity/synchronicity metrics to build adjacency matrices to represent weighted/undirected graphs. For the temporal domain, the raw biophysical data were directly used to build adjacency matrices. For both domains, with the obtained adjacency matrices, network connectivity analyses combined with non-linear dynamical systems approaches were used to identify self-emerging kinematic synergies and various indexes to enable objective quantification of the embodied cognition phenomena.

The other axis explored possible contributions of body parts that were not directly related to the end effector (the performing hand) executing the pointing task. We reasoned that there may be higher motor intent devoted to the performing hand of the participant than to the non-performing side of the body. Furthermore, we explored how other body parts (also co-registered within the sensors' network) contributed to the overall performance of this task.

These two axes were explored at the voluntary level of motor control interleaving deliberate goal-directed (forward) actions and spontaneous (backward) segments of the full pointing loop. We also included in our analyses the autonomic level of control in the taxonomy of Figure 1A, and to that end, we co-registered the heart activity and incorporated it into the bodily kinematics activity (Figure 3B). We next explain how to overcome challenges in sensor data fusion from disparate systems along with new approaches to analyze these multi-modal data.

2.2.3. Challenges of Multilayered Data with Non-Linear Dynamics and Non-Normally Distributed Parameters

Disparate physical units: Different instruments to assess biorhythms from different layers of the nervous system (i.e., kinematics vs. EKG) output biosignals with different physical units (e.g., m/s from the kinematics speed, mV from the EKG). This poses a challenge to integrate these signals and examine their interrelations across these layers.

Allometric effects: Another issue is that when examining such data from different participants with different anatomical sizes, allometric effects may confound our results. This is so because, e.g., the speed ranges that a person attains depend on the length of the arm. Longer arms tend to broaden the ranges of speed and contribute to the distribution of speed values that the person attains in any given experiment. As such, we needed to account for these possible allometric effects.

Assumption of normality: Another related matter to the ranges of speed and their distributions is that they vary from person to person according to multiple factors (e.g., age, body mass, sex, fitness, etc.) [38]. These variations result in probability distributions with heavy tails, which are incompatible with common assumptions of normality in the literature. When the effects of the task, or the inherent motor noise in the system, are such that most values related to the speed distribute more densely toward the left of the frequency histogram (e.g., in autism exponentially distributed maximum speed amplitude is common [39]), assuming normality may incur spurious results. This is so because speed ranges from 0 to some limiting value for each person (the maximum speed that the person can reach before damaging the joints). As such, when one obtains the mean ± two standard deviation values to approximate standard error bars (which is very common in the motor control literature) while summarizing the statistical features of the data, the data may fall in the negative speed ranges (which is physically absurd).

Assessing similarity in probability space: Going beyond significant hypothesis testing models, one may need to assess the differences between probability distributions. To that end, one may need a proper similarity metric. Yet, when our data represent points in probability space, and the distributions are not symmetric, it is challenging to assess their similarity in a consistently proper way. Measures like the Fisher information metric are designed to compare symmetric distributions and the Kullback–Leibler divergence is computed asymmetrically between distributions (one-sided). We would like to have a proper (two-sided) distance metric to assess change and its rate when points are related to non-symmetric continuous probability density functions, or to their discrete approximations.

Degrees of freedom across intent levels of motor control: Multiple locations of the grid of sensors, co-registering biorhythms from different nervous systems, contribute differently to the overall behavior of the system. Some may be more directly related to action success, while others may provide support. Separating the bodily region within a kinematics-heart network can be challenging because of the non-linear dynamics of the interactive systems. Yet, most methods assume or impose local linearities to model such phenomena. Here we propose to approach this problem by treating the grid of sensors as a dynamically evolving weighted interconnected network, whereby we track self-emerging modules informing us of spontaneous synergies and connectivity patterns.

2.2.4. Some Solutions to the Challenges

New data type for disparate physical units: We created a data type called the micro-movement spikes (MMS), which is a unitless, standardized waveform derived from the moment to moment fluctuations in the raw data peaks' amplitude and/or timing. This data type extracts the fluctuations in amplitude and/or timing of any waveform with peaks and valleys (e.g., time series of speed values or kinematic related values derived from them). To that end, we obtained the empirically estimated moments from the peaks in the raw waveform. We then built a new waveform that can be normalized according to various criteria. This new waveform is then unitless and refers to a relative quantity (rather than to an absolute quantity).

Data standardization to account for allometric effects: The anthropology and paleontology literature has several solutions to address comparative data that may come from different bone sizes across, e.g., different humanoids [40,41]. Equation (1) provides an example of standardization to scale values derived from any waveform with peaks and valleys, which can be derived, e.g., from data series with different physical units, from effectors of different sizes.

$$StandardizedPeak = \frac{LocalPeak}{LocalPeak + Avrg_{min-to-min}} \quad (1)$$

The standardized quantities are in the real-valued [0,1] interval. They are coined MMS amplitudes and treated as a continuous random process. We characterized several complex behaviors from various layers of the nervous systems using the MMS and expressed them in two forms: (1) without preserving the original frames of the data, i.e., just focusing on the MMS amplitude fluctuations, and (2) conserving the original frames, in which case, we would 0-pad those that are not spikes or preserve their values as additional gross data contributing to the phenomena in question. Either way, these fluctuations ought not to be averaged out by assumptions of normality. Whereas in the extant literature these fluctuations are considered noise or superfluous, here we treated them as important signals.

Distribution-free approach to counter current assumption of normality: We did not assume normality in the data. Instead, we gathered enough data to empirically estimate the best family of probability distributions that fits the data. To that end, we here used maximum likelihood estimation (MLE) with 95% confidence intervals and sought the best continuous family that fit our data.

Distance metric to assess similarity in probability space: We here introduced the use of the earth mover's distance metric (EMD) [42–44] to approximate (using the frequency histograms of the MMS amplitudes) the stochastic shifts in probability space that occur for different movement types. This is an appropriate similarity metric that allowed us to examine the extent to which different levels of motor control change the stochastic patterns. We briefly describe it below:

The EMD, also known as the Kantarovich–Wasserstein distance [45], measures the distance between two discrete probability distributions. Given two discrete distributions P = {(p_1,w_{p1}), … (p_m,w_{pm})}, where pi is the cluster representative and w_{pi} is the weight of the cluster; and Q = {(p_1,w_{p1}), … (p_n,w_{pn})}, EMD computes how much mass is needed to transform one distribution into another. Defining D [d_{ij}] as the ground distance matrix, where d_{ij} is the ground distance between clusters p_i and q_j, and F = [f_{ij}] with f_{ij} as the flow between p_i and q_j; EMD is computed by minimizing the overall cost of such:

$$\text{Work } (P, Z, F) = \sum_{i=1}^{m} \sum_{j=1}^{n} d_{ij} f_{ij}$$

As there are infinite ways to do this, the following constraints are imposed to yield EMD values:

$$f_{ij} \geq 0 \; 1 \leq i \leq m, 1 \leq j \leq n$$

$$\sum_{j=1}^{n} f_{ij} \leq w_{p_i} \; 1 \leq i \leq m$$

$$\sum_{j=1}^{m} f_{ij} \leq w_{q_i} \ 1 \leq j \leq n$$

$$\sum_{i=1}^{m}\sum_{j=1}^{n} f_{ij} = \min\left(\sum_{i=1}^{m} w_{p_i}, \sum_{j=1}^{n} w_{q_j}\right)$$

$$\text{EMD}(P,Q) = \frac{\sum_{i=1}^{m}\sum_{j=1}^{n} d_{ij} f_{ij}}{\sum_{i=1}^{m}\sum_{j=1}^{n} f_{ij}}$$

<u>Network connectivity analyses to assess degrees of freedom recruitment across modalities of motor control</u>: We used graph theory to examine the inter-relations across the nodes of the multilayered kinematics-heart network. To that end, we derived an adjacency metric of pairwise quantities reflecting the cross-correlation between any pair of nodes in the grid. We then constructed weighted directed networks and borrowed connectivity metrics from brain-related research. We extended these methods to represent the peripheral network using the bodily biorhythms from multiple layers of the nervous systems' functioning, spanning from voluntary to autonomic (Figure 1A).

2.2.5. Choice of Kinematics Parameter

The recording of positions over time across 10 upper body parts allowed us to estimate two aspects of the biorhythmic data: spatial and temporal aspects, both of which are critical to characterize proper coordination and control. A parameter encompassing both aspects is the velocity. The derivative of position over time creates vector fields with direction and extent. Each point in the field (along the velocity trajectory) occurs in time and moves in space.

To assess spatial components, we used the scalar speed (distance traveled per unit time, where the unit time is taken constantly at the rate of 240 frames per second). We used the Euclidean norm to compute the length of the velocity vector at each unit time, thus quantifying the rate of change in position per unit time—the linear speed (m/s). Likewise, we used the orientation data from each sensor and obtained the angular velocity from the rotations of each body part. Using appropriately the quaternion representation of rotations and the Euclidean metric to quantify the magnitude of the angular velocity vector, we obtained the angular speed (deg/s). These waveforms derived from the first order change are useful, but at the time scale (~1/2 h) of our experimental assay, they provided fewer peaks per trial than waveforms derived from the second order change (i.e., linear acceleration (m/s^2) or angular acceleration (deg/s^2)).

As we needed many spikes for our distribution-fitting and stochastic analyses, we used the angular acceleration kinematics data. Note, it was possible to have had participants perform more trials to obtain a larger number of spikes using the linear speed; however, this would have fatigued the participants as the length of the experiment was around 70 min (inclusive of 40 min for set up). For that reason, within this amount of time, it was ideal to use the angular acceleration as our kinematic parameter of interest. This choice of parameter to analyze the stochastic patterns of the moment by moment fluctuations in signal amplitude (i.e., the spatial component of our analysis) provided a tighter confidence interval in the empirical estimation of the best probability distribution family fitting the data.

We also examined temporal components of the data. To that end, we used the linear speed patterns and the cross-correlation function. We extended our analyses to different kinematics parameters, and while they all showed similar patterns and trends, we found the linear speed to best characterize the differing patterns of motor intent. For that reason, we presented the results of the temporal analyses involving cross-correlation based network connectivity patterns using the linear speed as our waveform of choice (Figure 3C).

2.3. Data Analysis on Kinematics Network Connectivity

As a first step, we separated the kinematics data obtained from all 10 body parts, using the start and end time of the performing hand making a forward–deliberate motion, and the hand making a backward–spontaneous motion (Figure 4A). This was possible to do (automatically) because (1) the speed was near 0 at the onset of the motion towards the target; (2) the distance to the target monotonically decreased and once again the hand paused at the target at near 0 speed. As the deliberate (forward) segment was completed, the speed rose again away from 0, and the distance to the target increased as the hand followed the backward segment of the full pointing loop. The two segments could be automatically differentiated also because the deliberate (forward) one was less variable than the spontaneous (backward) one [14].

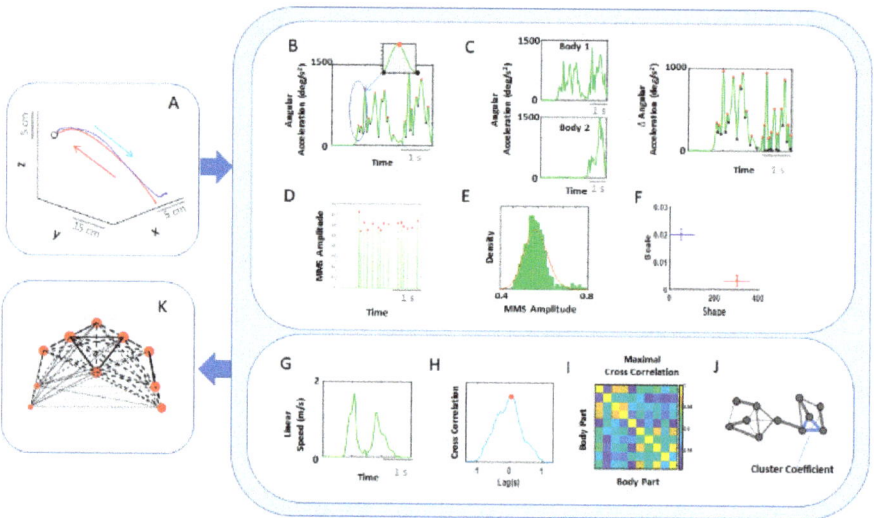

Figure 4. Analytical pipeline and visualization methods for the kinematics network. (**A**) Representative movement trajectory of the performing hand during a pointing motion to a target (denoted by a small open circle). Each trial was comprised of a forward–deliberate (red) and backward–spontaneous (blue) segment. These could be automatically separated by the speed and distance criteria (see Figure A2). (**B**) Time series of angular acceleration of the performing hand's index finger during a typical pointing task. To examine kinematics-based connectivity, we used the angular acceleration time series, focusing on the moment by moment fluctuations in waveform amplitude. Here, peaks (maxima) and valleys (minima) are shown in red and black dots, respectively. The inset shows a zoomed-in picture of a single angular acceleration segment (i.e., two local minima and a single peak in between, used for standardization described in Equation (1). (**C**) Pairwise absolute difference in waveform was obtained and standardized using Equation (1). The resulting waveform provided the input to obtain MMS. (**D**) MMS train scaling the waveform amplitude for a typical pointing task. All standardized spike amplitude values from (**B**) and (**C**) were maintained, while all non-spike values were set to 0. (**E**) Frequency histogram of MMS amplitudes fitted to a Gamma probability distribution function (PDF) using maximum likelihood estimation (MLE). (**F**) The empirically estimated Gamma parameters (shape and scale) were obtained and plotted on a Gamma parameter plane, with marker lines representing the 95% confidence interval. Noise-to-signal ratio (NSR) (i.e., fitted Gamma scale parameter) were later used for comparison between motor segments and different performing side. (**G**) Representative time series of linear speed of the performing hand's index finger in one trial. (**H**) Pairwise cross-correlation between two body parts. (**I**) Adjacency matrix obtained from all pairwise maximal cross-correlation across all body parts under consideration, to represent a weighted undirected graph. (**J**) Connectivity

metrics (e.g., clustering coefficient) were used to quantify patterns of temporal dynamics. (**K**) Network connectivity analyses to unveil self-emerging clusters, where nodes correspond to each body part. For the spatial domain, NSR derived from MMS amplitudes of angular accelerations were visualized as node size, and NSR derived from MMS amplitudes of pairwise absolute difference in angular acceleration as edge thickness. For the temporal domain, cluster coefficients were visualized as node size, and median cross-correlations as edge thickness.

For the connectivity analysis centered on spatial aspects of the signal amplitude, we pooled the angular acceleration data from each body part and extracted the MMS amplitudes (referred to as MMS from here on). We then built frequency histograms of the MMS and explored several families of PDFs using MLE. The continuous family of Gamma PDFs yielded the best fit (Figure A2) and served to provide the noise-to-signal ratio (NSR; computed to equal the Gamma scale parameter) for each body part (Figure 4B,D–F). These were then visualized as node size in the schematics of the network in Figure 4K across different motor intent levels.

To characterize the connectivity of 2 body parts, we took the pairwise absolute difference between angular acceleration and based on the obtained absolute difference time series, computed the corresponding MMS. We then fitted the Gamma scale parameters (i.e., NSR) (Figure 4C–F), which were visualized as edges in the schematics of the network in Figure 4K. The intuition behind taking the absolute difference in angular acceleration time series from two body parts is that this reflects the change in positional distance between those two body parts and thus represents the connectivity (physical distance) between those two. The NSR values were then compared between different movement segments (i.e., forward vs. backward) and different sides (i.e., performing vs. non-performing arm/hand), to understand the noise level during different levels of motor intent. Note, for each type of motor segment (i.e., forward vs. backward), and for each side (i.e., performing vs. non-performing), more than 2500 spike amplitude data were extracted. These spike amplitude data were then plotted on a frequency histogram using Freedman–Diaconis binning rule [46]. They were used for empirical estimation of the best PDF in an MLE sense. The results yielded the Gamma probability distribution function (PDF) (see Figure A2B).

Connectivity analyses on temporal aspects of coordination involved the linear speed from each pair of body parts. We computed pairwise cross-correlations to derive an adjacency matrix that would represent a weighted undirected graph. Here, the ij-link's weight is the maximum cross-correlation value between nodes i and j (that is, the corresponding two body parts). From these matrices, we computed clustering coefficients, which are measures that characterize the local connectivity (i.e., functional segregation). They would represent self-emerging kinematic synergies. Specifically, the degree of a node in the network (number of links at a node) between a set of nodes form triangles, and the fraction of triangle numbers formed around each node is known as the clustering coefficient (Figure 4G–J). This measure essentially reflects the proportion of the node's neighbors (i.e., nodes that are one degree away from the node of interest) that are also neighbors of each other [47]. Here, we computed the average intensity (geometric mean) of all triangles associated with each node, where the triangles reflect the degree strength, and is computed as shown below (using an algorithm by [48]; Equation (2)).

$$C_i = \sum_{i \in N} \frac{t_i}{k_i(k_i-1)} \qquad (2)$$

N: set of all nodes (composed of 10 body parts)
C_i: cluster coefficient for node i ($i \in N$)
t_i: geometric mean of triangles links formed around node i ($i \in N$)
k_i: number of degrees (links) formed around node i ($i \in N$)

To visualize the network, we represented the median pair-wise cross-correlation values as the edge thickness and median cluster coefficient values as the node size (Figure 4K). The median cross-correlation and cluster coefficient values were then compared between different movement segments (i.e., forward vs. backward) and different sides (i.e., performing vs. non-performing arm/hand) to understand how linear correlations differed across varying levels of motor control.

2.4. Data Analysis on Kinematics-Heart Network Connectivity

As with the kinematics connectivity analysis, we segmented the data of the filtered EKG data along with the kinematics data by the time intervals when the performing hand was making a deliberate forward motion and a spontaneous backward motion (Figure 5A).

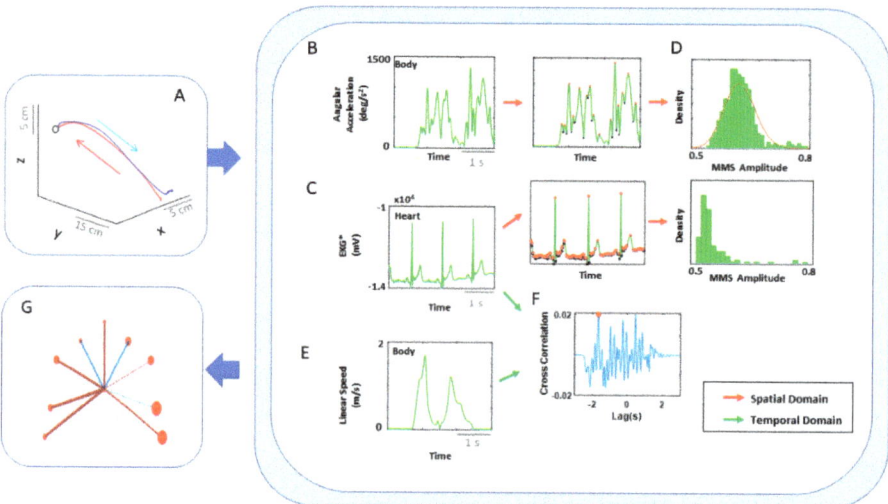

Figure 5. Analytical pipeline and visualization methods for the kinematics-heart network. (**A**) Typical movement trajectory of the performing hand position, while performing a single pointing action towards a target. Each trajectory was separated into forward–deliberate (red) and backward–spontaneous segments (blue) according to hand–target updated distance and near-zero-speed value (see Figure A2 for details). (**B**) Angular acceleration time series of the hand during a typical pointing task. MMS amplitudes from the angular acceleration time series were extracted for each body part. (**C**) Filtered EKG time series during a pointing task. MMS amplitudes from the filtered EKG time series were extracted. (**D**) Histograms of compiled MMS amplitudes. For spatial analysis, pairwise EMD was computed between histograms from each body part and heart activity. (**E**) Linear speed time series of the performing hand. For temporal analysis, linear speed kinematics time series was used. (**F**) Cross-correlation between a single body part's linear speed and filtered EKG signal. For each trial, cross-correlation was computed between a pair of filtered EKG and a single body part's linear speed time series, and the maximal value (red dot) and its corresponding lag values were extracted. (**G**) Visualization of connectivity. Network connectivity was visualized, where node size represented the EMD between the corresponding pair of body part and heart signals (i.e., spatial metric), and edge thickness represented the median cross-correlation values between the signal pairs (i.e., temporal metric). The edge colors were visualized, such that red would indicate EKG signals temporally leading linear speed signals, and blue would indicate linear speed leading EKG signals.

For the spatial domain of connectivity, we took the segmented data of angular acceleration and EKG data, extracted MMS from both signals, and plotted a histogram of the MMS. Because the MMS of EKG signals did not follow a Gamma distribution, in order to assess the connectivity between the two, we computed the earth mover's distance (EMD) between the histogram from a single body part and from the EKG data (Figure 5A–D).

For the temporal domain, we computed pairwise cross-correlations, along with lag, between the EKG filtered time series and each body part's linear velocity time series. In fact, in our analysis, we found an interesting pattern in directionality (i.e., lag) of correlation and deemed it informative to present them in the network graph. For that reason, edge thickness was represented by the median cross-correlation values, and color of the edges were visualized, where red indicated EKG signals leading linear velocity signals, and blue indicated linear velocity leading EKG signals (Figure 5G).

For all these metrics, we compared the medians between different movement segments (i.e., forward vs. backward) and different sides (i.e., performing vs. non-performing arm/hand), to understand how stochasticity and temporal dynamics changed across varying levels of motor intent between the heart (from ANS) and kinematics (from PNS/CNS).

3. Results

3.1. Higher Motor Intent Results in Higher NSR in Spatial Parameters

Motor intent in the context of our experimental assay specifically refers to the level of deliberateness (or spontaneity) of the movement segment in route to an external target (away from it). An instructed pointing action to touch the target is a goal-directed reach with high level of intent. In contrast, the uninstructed spontaneous retraction away from the target carries lower motor intent than the goal-directed one.

As a first set of analysis, the MMS extracted from the angular acceleration data from each body part were aggregated across all trials and conditions and arranged by different movement segments (forward–deliberate vs. backward–spontaneous) and different sides (performing vs. non-performing). The same was also done on the MMS extracted from the absolute difference in angular acceleration from all pairs of body parts. The NSR was found to be significantly higher when the motions were deliberate and on the performing side (Figure 6).

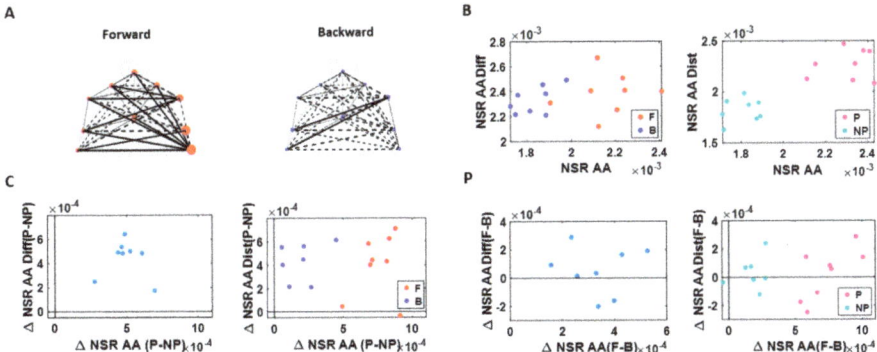

Figure 6. NSR signatures during pointing can differentiate the levels of intent. Comparison includes forward–deliberate vs. backward–spontaneous segments and performing vs. non-performing effector. (**A**) Network visualization of a right-handed representative participant. Node size is represented by the NSR derived from the corresponding body part's kinematics time series, and edge thickness is represented by the NSR of the absolute difference in kinematics between the corresponding pairs of body parts. Node size and edge thickness are graphed in the same scale across different movement segments (i.e., forward and backward segments). (**B**) NSR for different movement segment and sides. Each dot is the median NSR values for each participant's different movement segments (left) and different sides (right) from the unitless MMS derived from the angular acceleration (AA) fluctuations in amplitude. The x-axis denotes the NSR from individual body part's kinematics (NSR AA), and y-axis denotes the NSR from the MMS derived from the absolute pairwise body parts' difference (NSR AA Diff). Generally, for the former (NSR AA) measure, NSR is higher during a forward segment (F; red)

than during a backward segment (B; blue), and on the performing side (P; pink) than on the non-performing side (NP; cyan). (**C**) NSR difference between performing vs. non-performing side. Left panel shows the NSR median difference between the performing and non-performing side for each participant, denoted as a single marker. Right panel shows the NSR median difference between the performing and non-performing side for the forward motion (F; red) and backward motion (B; blue). When the difference between the performing and non-performing side is examined separately for each motion segment, the NSR AA difference is wider during forward motion segments (F; red) than during backward motion segments (B; blue). (**D**) NSR difference between forward vs. backward movement segment. Left panel shows the NSR median difference between the forward and backward motion segments for each participant, denoted as a single marker. Color scheme as in (**B**).

Specifically, NSRs of the kinematics time series from each body part shown was highest when an individual exerted higher motor control under higher level of motor intent, such as on the performing side of the body and during a forward–deliberate motion. Conversely, when an individual did not deliberately intend to move the arm, as exhibited on the non-performing side of the body and during a backward–spontaneous motion, the NSR was at its lowest. The NSRs for all pairs of body parts' absolute difference in angular acceleration (i.e., change in distance between the pairs of body parts), on the other hand, was higher on the performing side (vs. non-performing side) but did not show such a consistent pattern when comparing between the two motion segments (forward vs. backward). Details of the 95% confidence interval of the fitted Gamma scale parameter (i.e., the NSR) for all participants, all body parts (Figure A3), and all pairs of body parts (Figure A4) can be found in the Appendix A.

3.2. Higher Motor Intent Results in Higher Cross-Correlations and Clustering of Temporal Parameters

We used the MATLAB Network Connectivity toolbox [49] and examined the adjacency matrix derived from the pairwise maximal cross-correlation coefficient based on the time series of linear speed values. The clustering coefficient (CC) was obtained for each body part as a metric of functional segregation. For analysis, we examined the median cross-correlation values as a function of the CC values. Here we found that higher level of motor intent (i.e., during forward–deliberate motion performed with the performing hand) resulted in a tendency of increased CC and increased median cross-correlation values (Figure 7).

When we compared between different motion segments, median cross-correlations were higher for forward motions than for backward ones for all but two participants. When we compared between different sides, all participants showed higher correlation on the performing side than the non-performing one. The median CC was higher for forward motions than for backward segments for all participants and higher for the performing side than the non-performing side for all but two participants. For all participants, both measures showed statistical significance in their difference (see Table A1 of Appendix A for detailed statistical results).

The distinctions that we observed from these findings, on how different levels of motor intent had separable network connectivity patterns based on temporal aspects of the kinematics data, are consistent with the patterns uncovered using spatial aspects of the kinematics data. Specifically, when we exerted higher intent on our body, regardless of the physical trajectory of the motion, there was a stronger connectivity across our body parts. However, we noted that this pattern was not as uniform across all participants as we had found in the spatial aspect of the network analysis.

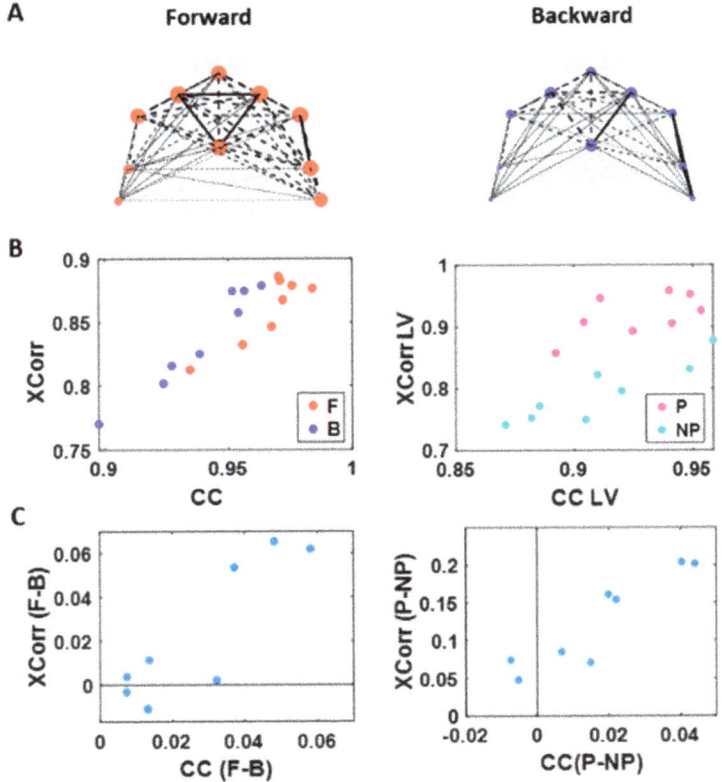

Figure 7. Network connectivity metric (cluster coefficient) and median cross-correlation differentiates between levels of intent. (**A**) Network visualization of a representative right-handed participant. Cross-correlation is represented by the line weight and cluster coefficient (CC) by the node size, during the forward (left) and backward movement segments (right). (**B**) Median cross-correlation (y-axis; Xcorr) and CC (x-axis) of linear speed for each participant's movement segment (left) and different sides (right). Forward motions (red) and performing side (pink) exhibits higher cross-correlation and CC values than backward segments (blue) and non-performing side (cyan). (**C**) Median cross-correlation and CC difference for different movement segments (left) and different sides (right). Each participant's data is denoted as a single marker. Higher motor intent tends to show higher cross-correlation and CC values.

3.3. Kinematics and EKG (Heart) Signals Show Larger Stochastic Differences for Higher Motor Intent and Control

To assess patterns of connectivity between biophysical signals derived from voluntary and autonomic levels of motor control we examined the kinematics (generated by the CNS–PNS) and the heart activity (generated by the ANS). The patterns of MMS stochasticity and temporal correlation across these systems distinguished levels of motor intent and control.

The analyses involving EKG and kinematics revealed larger stochastic differences in MMS data when higher motor intent and control were exerted. More precisely, the pairwise EMD showed higher differentiation between these two signals in all but one participant when forward motion was made, but only on the performing side of the body. Furthermore, all but two participants showed higher EMD on the performing side of the body, but only during forward motions. On the other hand, however, when backward motion was made, we found an opposite pattern, where all participants showed higher EMD on the non-performing side. We inferred that there may have been a modulating factor that underlied the stochastic relation between kinematics and heart signals.

When we examined the temporal relations between the two signals, by computing pair-wise cross-correlations, we saw higher cross-correlations when there was lower motor intent across all participants, that is, during backward motions and on the non-performing side. Here, we noted the low range of the correlation coefficient values of around 0.1. However, we saw a similar trend when this was based on the non-filtered raw EKG data, with a higher range around 0.6.

3.4. EKG Leads Kinematics under Higher Motor Intent, but Opposite Pattern Emerges in Spontaneous Motions Requiring Less Motor Intent

We also examined the lag values to assess which signal leads the other. We found that with motions under higher motor intent (i.e., during forward–deliberate motions performed with the performing side of the arm), EKG signals tended to lead the kinematics signal. On the other hand, in movements performed under lower intent (i.e., during backward–spontaneous motion, and on the non-performing side of the arm), kinematics signals tended to lead the EKG signals. This is depicted in Figure 8.

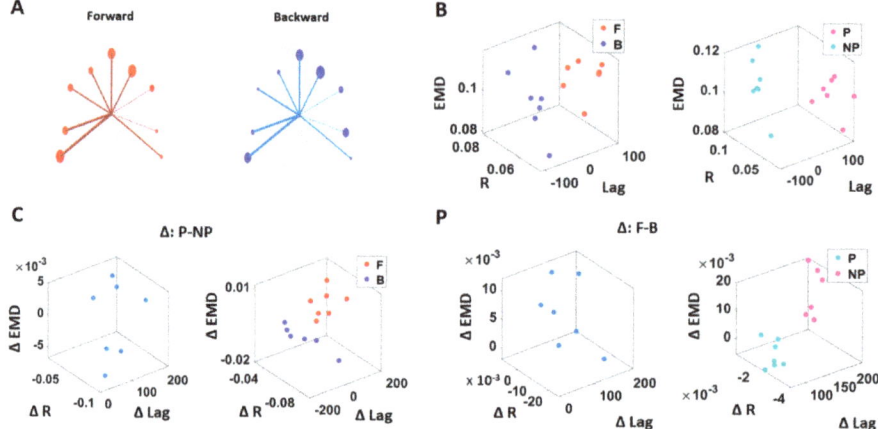

Figure 8. Differentiation of spatial and temporal connectivity within the kinematics-heart network according to levels of motor intent. (**A**) Network visualization of a right-handed representative participant. 1/EMD is represented by the node size, and median correlation is represented by the line weight. The color of edges indicates the temporal directionality between signals, where red indicates that heart leads the body linear speed and blue indicates that body linear speed leads the heart signals. (**B**) Median EMD (z-axis) and correlation (x-axis) and lag (y-axis) for each participant's movement segment (left) and different sides (right). There is an overall pattern where higher motor intent (denoted by red for forward motions, and pink for performing side) is exhibited by lower correlations and EKG leading the kinematics signal (i.e., lag is positive value). (**C**) Median EMD, correlation, and lag difference for different sides (left), and this difference separated by movement segment (right). We find a pattern where pairwise EMD show higher differentiation under higher motor intent on the performing side, but only when forward motion was made. (**D**) Median EMD, correlation, and lag difference for different movement segments (left), and this difference separated by sides (right). We find a pattern where pairwise EMD show higher differentiation under lower motor intent on the non-performing side, but only when the backward motion was made.

We caveat that because the EKG device and motion capture system were not exactly synchronized, the absolute lag value may not be as meaningful. Nevertheless, as we analyzed these data in terms of the difference (i.e., the delta lag values between forward and backward motions, and between performing and non-performing sides), it was indeed meaningful to find such patterns uniformly across all participants.

Table 1 summarizes the results that we showed in the sections above. We emphasize that although we examined a small number (eight) of participants, each individual's data were composed of a significant amount of data points with unique non-Gaussian stochastic characteristics. For that reason, instead of presenting the results with NHST (null hypothesis significant tests), we presented the results by comparing the median difference between data points, from different levels of intent, for each individual.

Table 1. Summary of the connectivity results, where symbols [1] are shown to indicate which category shows higher values.

		Kinematics (AA) Network			
		Forward	Backward	Performing	Non-Performing
Spatial	NSR AA	o		o	
	NSR AA Diff			o	
Temporal	Cross-Correlation	Δ		o	
	Cluster Coefficient	o			Δ
		Kinematics (LS)-Heart Network			
		Forward	Backward	Performing	Non-Performing
Spatial	EMD	Δ (P) [2]	-	Δ (F) [3]	o (B) [4]
Temporal	Cross-Correlation		Δ		o
	Lead *,[5]	EKG	LS	EKG	LS

[1] o indicates that it is higher for every participant; Δ indicates that it is higher for most participants.
[2] Forward–deliberate motions have higher EMD only on the performing (P) side. [3] Performing side has higher EMD only during forward–deliberate (F) motions. [4] Non-performing side has higher EMD only during backward–spontaneous (B) motions. [5] Lead* shows which signal leads between the 2 signals.

4. Discussion

This paper examined elements of the construct of agency from the embodied cognition framework and dissected several layers of neuromotor control contributing to the sense of action ownership. These layers, defined along a phylogenetically orderly taxonomy of maturation, follow a higher-to-lower gradient of intent, from voluntary, to involuntary, to autonomic signals. At the voluntary level, we followed the instructed–deliberate and the uninstructed–spontaneous segments of the target-directed pointing act, positing that they could differentiate between levels of intent and as such, delineate (from the fluctuations in their biorhythmic activity) when a given movement segment was deliberately performed with intent vs. when the segment happened spontaneously without instruction. This differentiation is important to distinguish the sensory consequences of voluntary acts from those of acts that are not intended or that occur autonomically. The sensory consequences of the latter have not been currently studied, yet they seem important to complement von Holst's and Mittelstaedt's principle of reafference as we know it today [24].

Our initial thought was that autonomic systems contributing to our brain's autonomy over the body and to our overall embodied sense of agency would remain impervious to stochastic shifts at the voluntary levels. We reasoned that given the vital role of these systems for survival, their robust signal would not reflect subtle changes in levels of intent, motor awareness, and voluntary control. As such, our guess was that if during voluntary movements, there were stochastic differences between instructed–deliberate and uninstructed–spontaneous segments of the reach, or between performing and non-performing sides of the body, such shifts in patterns of variability would not be appreciable in the heart signals' fluctuations. Our guess was altogether wrong. Not only were the heart signal differences quantifiable at the level of micro fluctuations in signal amplitude, these differences were appreciable as well in the inter-dynamics of the kinematics and cardiac signals.

4.1. The Autonomic Nervous System Differentiates across Levels of Motor Intent: Implications for Computational Models and Basic Cognitive Neuroscience

We found that when movements are intended and deliberately performed to attain the goal defined by an external (visual) target, the heart signal leads the movement kinematics signal. Yet, when these overt movements are spontaneous in nature, i.e., uninstructed and not pursuing the completion of a specific externally defined task goal, the heart signal lags the movement kinematics signal. Across spatial and temporal parameters, we found consistent trends and confirmed the trends through different parameters. Indeed, deliberate motions, executed with the performing effector, carry higher levels of NSR, denoting higher fluctuations away from the empirically estimated mean.

We interpret these findings considering the principle of reafference, treating micro-movements as a form of re-entrant sensory feedback [24]. Furthermore, we discuss the possible contributions of these self-generated signals to the self-emergence of cognitive agency from motor agency, namely the sense that one can physically realize what one mentally intends to do, confirm the consequences (both intended and unintended), and, as such, mentally own the physical action.

Von Holst and Mittelstaedt studied the complexities of reafference across the nervous systems in the 1950s. They tried to capture the inherent recursiveness that relates movements and their sensations as they flow within closed feedback loops between the external and the internal environments of the organism. They wrote, "Voluntary movements show themselves to be dependent on the returning stream of afference which they themselves cause." Undeniably, feedback from voluntary movements currently play an important role in theoretical motor control, particularly within the framework of internal models for action [25,26] and more recent models of stochastic feedback control [50]. Central to all these conceptualizations of the motor control problem has been the notion of anticipating the sensory consequences of impending intended actions. Nevertheless, nothing has been said about the consequences of action segments that bear a lower level of intent, which occur spontaneously, or that are altogether occurring autonomously.

The implications of our results are manifold: Modelers and experimenters in motor control do not seem to be aware of self-emergent, uninstructed, spontaneous motions. These motions are rather assumed to be far removed from cognitive processes, perhaps because they transpire largely beneath awareness (although see [13,51] more recently). Yet, unintended consequences from the uninstructed–spontaneous segments of the voluntary action seem as important as those sensory consequences that result from the instructed–deliberate segments. They may serve to inform learning new tasks, adapting to new environmental conditions or situations, and more generally, they may play a role as a surprise factor to aid propel curiosity and/or to stimulate creative, exploratory thinking. They may help make our "invisible" automatic movements visible to the conscious brain planning and controlling them, and/or to the external observer tracking our behaviors.

Neither these models, nor Von Holst's work considered the contributions of unintended consequences from spontaneous acts quantifiable at different anatomical and physiological layers of the nervous systems, while trying to model the basic problem that the organism faces, i.e., the paradox of understanding the "self", which entails parsing out external from internal reafference. Without a unifying framework to quantify these multilayered interactions and their contributions to the emergence of the notion of self, it becomes rather challenging to bridge the cognitive sense of agency, and more basically of action ownership, "I can do this!; It's me who's doing this!", with the type of autonomous motor control that enables successful self-initiation and completion of the intended act. We argue that inclusion of the unintended consequences from overt spontaneous motions and autonomic signals in our models of motor control will help define embodied agency and provide a new framework to objectively quantify it.

The present work provides empirical evidence that (1) different levels of cognitive intent, awareness, and control are indeed embodied and quantifiable in natural, unconstrained movements, and (2) there are important contributions to central cognitive control quantifiable at the periphery in spontaneous segments of our motions *and their consequences*, but also in motions from supporting (non-performing) body parts. Importantly, such differentiating contributions are also present in patterns from signals generated by the autonomic nervous systems. Recent work from our lab has examined cognitive load in relation to autonomic signals and found systematic changes bound to impact the type of feedback that these signals mediated by cardiac muscles generate within the nervous systems [16,52]. These aspects of the motor control problem are not considered at present in any of the mathematical and computational frameworks used to model the human brain, despite a body of empirical data differentiating classes of movements that are less sensitive to changes in dynamics [14,21,30–34] from those which are dynamic dependent [14].

Our work augments Von Holst's and Mittelstaedt's principle of reafference nontrivially by including reafferent contributions from other layers of the nervous systems (Figure 1A) and highlighting the need to update our conceptualization of internal models for action. In the past, the literature has focused on voluntary control and goal-directed behavior to define and to characterize agency [5,6,8,11]. However, if new generations of AI models aim to attain artificial autonomous agents with real agency, it may be necessary to reformulate our models and reconceptualize our experiments in embodied cognition to encompass these multiple layers of intent, awareness, and motor function. These results provide a way to distinguish levels of intent in the stochastic feedback from a robust (autonomic signal), as an important addition to prior work distinguishing levels in more variable speed and acceleration signals [14].

4.2. Distinguishing Performing vs. Non-Performing End Effector

Another aspect of this work explored the differentiation between the performing end effector and the non-performing one, within the context of connectivity network analyses and levels of NSR. There we found that the micro fluctuations in kinematics activity taken as a weighted directed graph representing an interconnected network of nodes (body parts), can automatically reveal which side of the body is performing the goal-directed task with intent vs. which side of the body is performing the uninstructed spontaneous segment. The importance of this result is several-fold: First, it demonstrates that we can gain information by considering arm movements within a broader context of bodily motions, treated as a fully interconnected network, rather than examining the end effector in isolation. The network connectivity analyses presented here adapt and extend similar methods used in brain analyses to full bodily motions. This is important to connect data from the CNS and the PNS within a full network (see here [52]) and infer the contributions of different bodily sides on the planning, execution, and coordination of the many DoFs of the body in motion. We need these empirical data to improve our multi-layered generative analytical models of neuromotor control involving different spaces of joints and end effectors [21,29,32,33]. Secondly, these results underscore the importance of not eliminating gross data through grand averaging methods that assume a priori a probability distribution and take theoretical means across all data. Here we personalize the analyses and for each participant, we examine the micro fluctuations (away from empirically estimated distribution moments) contributed by both the performing and the non-performing limbs. We do so within the context of full body macro- and micro-motions, thus considering the value of the NSR derived from the gross data that is often thrown away as superfluous noise. The importance of these new methods is that we can examine possible asymmetries in neurological disorders like Parkinson's disease, where, e.g., tremor may emerge at the performing hand and yet be forecasted in the NSR of activity recorded in the non-performing limbs. Differentiating performing from non-performing NSR in the context of voluntary motions is now possible using these new statistical methods and network connectivity analyses adapted to full body motions. This type of data is rarely examined in clinical work. Lastly, we offer new ways to examine kinematics synergies and possible patterns of co-articulation across the body, while examining the outcomes from the traditional pointing task now extended to also include the spontaneously retracting segments of the full pointing loop.

4.3. Implications of the Results for Translational Cognitive Science

An area where these results could be relevant is smart health and AI, connecting digital biomarkers with clinical observational criteria (e.g., [53]). In the clinical world, there are many problems that will require us to be mindful of this intended vs. unintended dichotomy, as there are phenomena that occur spontaneously and largely beneath awareness. It is difficult to model these phenomena within the voluntary reafference framework. The type of reafference that we need to model those problems belongs in the realm of self-emerging aspects of naturalistic behaviors. Among those which are disrupted due to pathologies of the nervous systems are sudden freezing of gait in Parkinson's disease, leading to the loss of balance and occasional falls; seizures across a broad range of disorders; heart attacks; a subset of repetitive behaviors and self-injurious or aggressive episodes in autism; among others. All these episodes have in common the element of surprise connected to their spontaneity. Several new emerging areas in basic research with a focus on the relationships between property and agency in neurological disorders can also be incorporated in new AI concepts for smart health [15,19,28,53–55].

No algorithm relying exclusively on intentional control signals can appropriately capture the essence of these phenomena. To properly characterize it, forecast it, and quickly detect it, we need veridical generative models that understand the differences between the consequences of something that was intended and under voluntary control, something that spontaneously happened, and something that happens autonomically, with high accuracy. We do not have autonomous robots with embodied agency yet, because their staged motions are mostly pre-programmed. These programs may only mimic the predictive consequences of voluntary actions. Self-correcting robotic systems, where such behaviors spontaneously self-emerge, are less common. It is perhaps self-emerging awareness derived from the consequences of spontaneous and autonomic phenomena that makes our embodied agency a special human trait contributing to intelligent control. This type of control, combining deliberate and spontaneous acts, may produce solutions that are capable of generalizing from a small set of specific situations; transfer the learning from one context to another (using contextual variations); and retain robustness to potential interference from new situations in unknown contexts. In future research, it will be important to understand how the type of differentiation that we discovered here, paired with externally vs. internally generated rewards, may contribute to the fast or slow acquisition of memories from transient acts vs. memories from systematic, periodic repetitions of those acts.

Here we offer a unifying framework with a taxonomy of function and differentiable levels of intent, awareness, and control paired with a new statistical platform for personalized analyses of natural behaviors. This new model aims to capture and characterize the micro-fluctuations in the gross data of our biorhythms that traditional approaches throw away as noise through grand averaging and *"one size fits all"* methods. Our approach allows integration of multilayered hierarchical signals and provides the means to differentiate re-entrant contributions from multilayered exo- and endo-afference. This can help our self-realization of embodied agency as the spontaneous transformation of mental intent into physical volition. We invite the reader to consider this new model for embodied cognition and offer novel avenues to bridge the currently disconnected fields of motor control and cognitive phenomena.

Author Contributions: Conceptualization, J.R. and E.T.; methodology, J.R. and E.T.; formal analysis, J.R. and E.T.; investigation, J.R. and E.T.; writing—original draft preparation, J.R. and E.T.; writing—review and editing, J.R. and E.T.; visualization, J.R. and E.T.; supervision, E.T.; funding acquisition, E.T. All authors have read and agreed to the published version of the manuscript.

Funding: This research was funded by the New Jersey Governor's Council for the Medical Research and Treatments of Autism CAUT17BSP024 and by the Nancy Lurie Marks Family Foundation to E.B.T. Career Development Award.

Conflicts of Interest: The authors declare no conflict of interest.

Appendix A

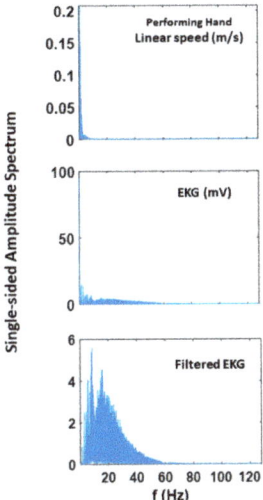

Figure A1. Fourier power spectrum of linear speed and EKG and filtered EKG signals extracted from 60 trials of pointing motion (i.e., 300 s).

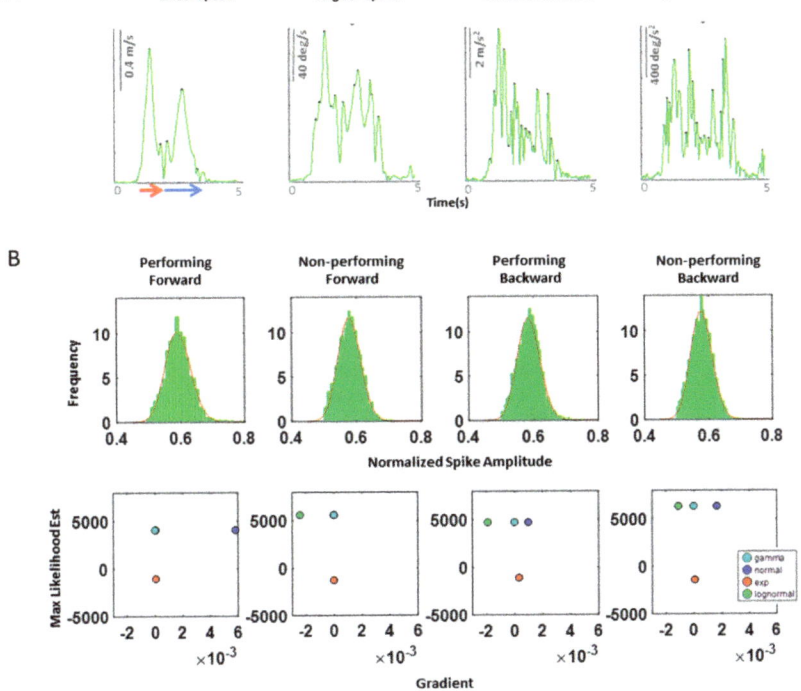

Figure A2. (**A**) Speed profile of a typical pointing motion. During a single pointing motion, a typical speed profile of linear speed, angular speed, linear acceleration, and angular acceleration are exhibited as such. Because angular acceleration is shown to have the largest number of peaks during a single pointing motion, we decided to examine this kinematic waveform, as this would provide the highest statistical power for the MLE process. Note, linear speed data was used to extract the timing that would separate the start and end time of a forward–deliberate motion (shown in red) and of a backward–spontaneous motion (shown in blue arrow). This was done by finding the timepoint when instantaneous zero linear speed occurs, since this indicates the moment the index finger reaches the target. (**B**) Maximum likelihood estimated values for the corresponding histogram on top of each graph. The horizontal axis contains the value of the gradient at the end of the optimization process, and the vertical axis contains the maximum likelihood estimation (MLE) value for the Gamma, normal, exponential, and lognormal distributions. Overall, we found that the Gamma and lognormal distributions have a good fit to these kinematics data. However, because Gamma distributions have been shown to be a better fit to the kinematics data from individuals with neurological disorders than lognormal distributions, for consistency, we chose to use the Gamma probability distribution for fitting purpose.

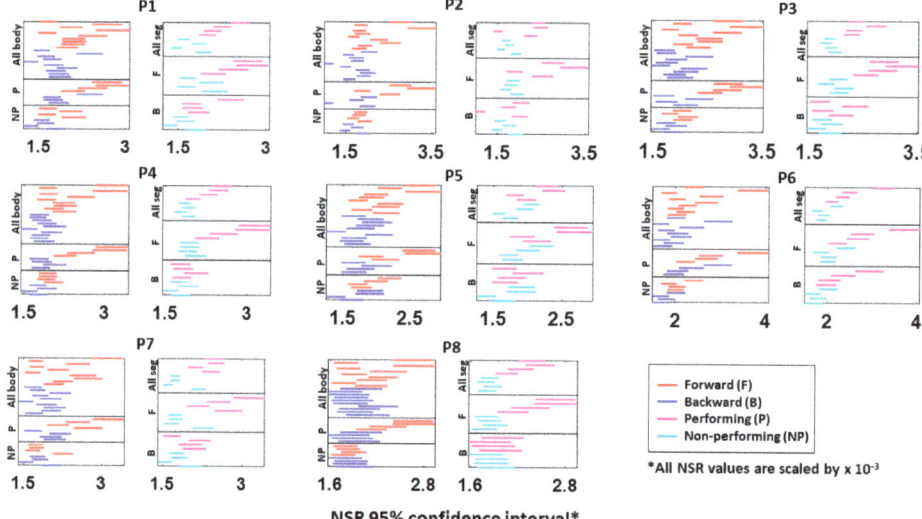

Figure A3. Fitted Gamma scale parameter (i.e., NSR) 95% confidence interval for a single body part's kinematics data. The 95% confidence interval is plotted for all eight participants (P1 to P8). Each row represents a single body part: under the "All body" category shows all 10 body parts during forward (red) and backward (blue) motions; under the "P (performing)" category shows the 4 body parts from the performing side of the arm; under the "NP (non-performing)" category shows the 4 body parts from the non-performing side of the arm; under the "All seg (all segment)" category shows the 4 body parts on the performing (pink) and non-performing (cyan) side during the entire pointing motion; under the "F (forward)" category shows the 4 body parts on both P and NP side during forward motion; and under the "B (backward)" category shows the 4 body parts on both P and NP side during backward motion.

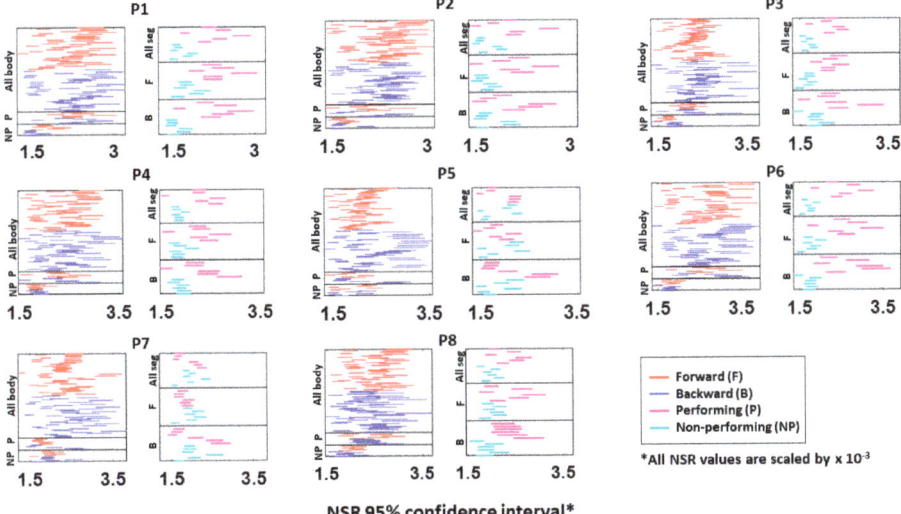

Figure A4. Fitted Gamma scale parameter (i.e., NSR) 95% confidence interval from the absolute difference in kinematics between pairs of body parts. The 95% confidence interval is plotted for all eight participants (P1 to P8). Each row represents a pair of body part: under the "All body" category shows all 45 body part ($_{10}C_2$) pairs during forward (red) and backward (blue) motions; under the "P (performing)" category shows the 6 body part pairs ($_4C_2$) from the performing side of the arm; under the "NP (non-performing)" category shows the 6 body parts pairs ($_4C_2$) from the non-performing side of the arm; under the "All seg (all segment)" category shows the 6 body parts pairs ($_4C_2$) on the performing (pink) and non-performing (cyan) side during the entire pointing motion; under the "F (forward)" category shows the 6 body parts pairs ($_4C_2$) on both P and NP side during forward motion; and under the "B (backward)" category shows the 4 body parts on both P and NP side during backward motion.

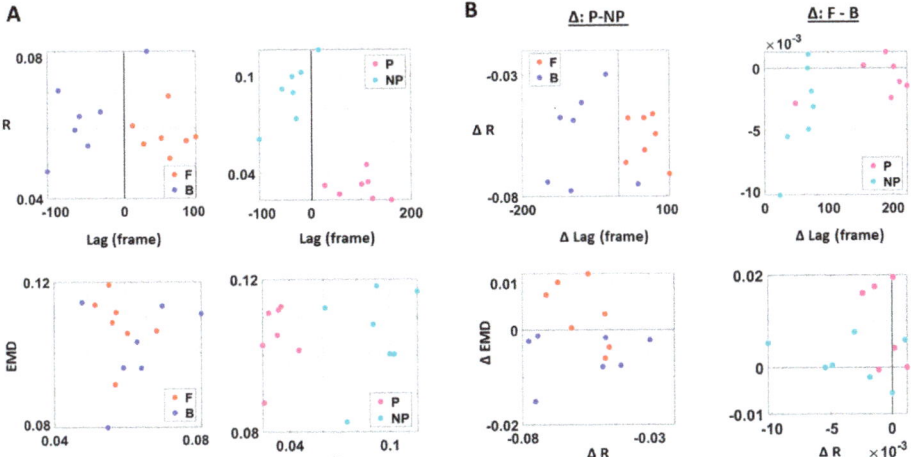

Figure A5. Different viewpoints of the 3D graphs in Figure 8. (**A**) Different viewpoint of graphs in Figure 8B. (**B**) Different viewpoints of graphs in Figure 8C (left) and Figure 8D (right).

Table A1. Kolmogorov–Smirnov test statistics (KS-stat) and their *p*-values (p) on cluster coefficients comparison (left) and cross-correlation (right) between different movement segments (forward (F) vs. backward (B)) and different sides (performing (P) vs. non-performing (NP)) [1].

Subject ID	Cluster Coefficient				Subject ID	Cross-Correlation			
	F vs. B		P vs. NP			F vs. B		P vs. NP	
	KS-stat	p	KS-stat	p		KS-stat	p	KS-stat	p
P01	0.29	<0.01 **	0.16	<0.01 **	P01	0.14	<0.01 **	0.40	<0.01 **
P02	0.55	<0.01 **	0.57	<0.01 **	P02	0.55	<0.01 **	0.57	<0.01 **
P03	0.38	<0.01 **	0.16	<0.01 **	P03	0.38	<0.01 **	0.16	<0.01 **
P04	0.09	<0.01 **	0.09	<0.01 **	P04	0.09	<0.01 **	0.09	<0.01 **
P05	0.14	<0.01 **	0.26	<0.01 **	P05	0.14	<0.01 **	0.26	<0.01 **
P06	0.17	<0.01 **	0.28	<0.01 **	P06	0.17	<0.01 **	0.28	<0.01 **
P07	0.35	<0.01 **	0.41	<0.01 **	P07	0.35	<0.01 **	0.41	<0.01 **
P08	0.13	<0.01 **	0.35	<0.01 **	P08	0.13	<0.01 **	0.35	<0.01 **

** *p*-value is less than 0.05. [1] Note, the Kolmogorov–Smirnov test was used, as this test is appropriate for data that do not follow a Gaussian distribution and has a large sample size ($n > 1000$) that may yield low statistical power.

References

1. Abrahamson, D.; Sánchez-García, R. Learning Is Moving in New Ways: The Ecological Dynamics of Mathematics Education. *J. Learn. Sci.* **2016**, *25*, 203–239. [CrossRef]
2. Maturana, H.R.; Varela, F.J. *Autopoiesis and Cognition: The Realization of the Living*; Boston studies in the philosophy of science; D. Reidel Publishing Company: Boston, MA, USA, 1980; p. 141.
3. Newen, A. The Embodied Self, the Pattern Theory of Self, and the Predictive Mind. *Front. Psychol.* **2018**, *9*, 2270. [CrossRef] [PubMed]
4. David, N.; Newen, A.; Vogeley, K. The "sense of agency" and its underlying cognitive and neural mechanisms. *Conscious. Cogn.* **2008**, *17*, 523–534. [CrossRef] [PubMed]
5. Frith, C.D. Action, agency and responsibility. *Neuropsychologia* **2014**, *55*, 137–142. [CrossRef]
6. Synofzik, M.; Vosgerau, G.; Newen, A. I move, therefore I am: A new theoretical framework to investigate agency and ownership. *Conscious Cogn.* **2008**, *17*, 411–424. [CrossRef]
7. Tsakiris, M.; Hesse, M.D.; Boy, C.; Haggard, P.; Fink, G.R. Neural Signatures of Body Ownership: A Sensory Network for Bodily Self-Consciousness. *Cereb. Cortex* **2007**, *17*, 2235–2244. [CrossRef]
8. Tsakiris, M.; Prabhu, G.; Haggard, P. Having a body versus moving your body: How agency structures body-ownership. *Conscious. Cogn.* **2006**, *15*, 423–432. [CrossRef]
9. Haggard, P.; Wing, A. On the Hand Transport Component of Prehensile Movements. *J. Mot. Behav.* **1997**, *29*, 282–287. [CrossRef]
10. Toni, I.; Thoenissen, D.; Zilles, K. Movement Preparation and Motor Intention. *NeuroImage* **2001**, *14*, S110–S117. [CrossRef]
11. Burin, D.; Livelli, A.; Garbarini, F.; Fossataro, C.; Folegatti, A.; Gindri, P.; Pia, L. Are Movements Necessary for the Sense of Body Ownership? Evidence from the Rubber Hand Illusion in Pure Hemiplegic Patients. *PLoS ONE* **2015**, *10*, e0117155. [CrossRef]
12. Della Gatta, F.; Garbarini, F.; Puglisi, G.; Leonetti, A.; Berti, A.; Borroni, P.A. Decreased motor cortex excitability mirrors own hand disembodiment during the rubber hand illusion. *eLife* **2016**, *5*, e14972. [CrossRef] [PubMed]
13. Torres, E.B. Two classes of movements in motor control. *Exp. Brain Res.* **2011**, *215*, 269–283. [CrossRef] [PubMed]
14. Torres, E.B. Signatures of movement variability anticipate hand speed according to levels of intent. *Behav. Brain Funct.* **2013**, *9*, 10. [CrossRef]
15. Torres, E.B.; Brincker, M.; Isenhower, R.W.I.; Yanovich, P.; Stigler, K.A.; Nurnberger, J.I.J.; Metaxas, D.N.; José, J.V. Autism: The micro-movement perspective. *Front. Integr. Neurosci.* **2013**, *7*, 32. [CrossRef] [PubMed]
16. Ryu, J.; Torres, E.B. Characterization of Sensory-Motor Behavior Under Cognitive Load Using a New Statistical Platform for Studies of Embodied Cognition. *Front. Hum. Neurosci.* **2018**, *12*, 1–19. [CrossRef]
17. Bernstein, N.A. *The Coordination and Regulation of Movements*; Pergamon Press: London, UK, 1967.

18. Torres, E.B.; Lande, B. Objective and personalized longitudinal assessment of a pregnant patient with post severe brain trauma. *Front. Hum. Neurosci.* **2015**, *9*, 128. [CrossRef]
19. Torres, E.B.; Smith, B.; Mistry, S.; Brincker, M.; Whyatt, C. Neonatal Diagnostics: Toward Dynamic Growth Charts of Neuromotor Control. *Front. Pediatr.* **2016**, *4*, 121. [CrossRef]
20. Kalampratsidou, V.; Torres, E.B. Peripheral Network Connectivity Analyses for the Real-Time Tracking of Coupled Bodies in Motion. *Sensors* **2018**, *18*, 3117. [CrossRef]
21. Torres, E.B.; Zipser, D. Reaching to Grasp with a Multi-Jointed Arm. I. Computational Model. *J. Neurophysiol.* **2002**, *88*, 1–13. [CrossRef]
22. Scholz, J.P.; Schöner, G. The uncontrolled manifold concept: Identifying control variables for a functional task. *Exp. Brain Res.* **1999**, *126*, 289–306. [CrossRef]
23. Latash, M.L.; Scholz, J.P.; Schöner, G. Motor Control Strategies Revealed in the Structure of Motor Variability. *Exerc. Sport Sci. Rev.* **2002**, *30*, 26–31. [CrossRef] [PubMed]
24. Von Holst, E.; Mittelstaedt, H. The principle of reafference: Interactions between the central nervous system and the peripheral organs. In *Perceptual Processing: Stimulus Equivalence and Pattern Recognition*; Dodwell, P.C., Ed.; Appleton-Century-Crofts: New York, NY, USA, 1950; pp. 41–72.
25. Kawato, M.; Wolpert, D. Internal models for motor control. *Novartis Found. Symp.* **1998**, *218*, 291–304.
26. Wolpert, D.M.; Miall, R.C.; Kawato, M. Internal models in the cerebellum. *Trends Cogn. Sci.* **1998**, *2*, 338–347. [CrossRef]
27. Torres, E.B.; Heilman, K.M.; Poizner, H. Impaired endogenously evoked automated reaching in Parkinson's disease. *J. Neurosci.* **2011**, *31*, 17848–17863. [CrossRef]
28. Torres, E.B.; Yanovich, P.; Metaxas, D.N. Give spontaneity and self-discovery a chance in ASD: Spontaneous peripheral limb variability as a proxy to evoke centrally driven intentional acts. *Front. Integr. Neurosci.* **2013**, *7*, 46. [CrossRef]
29. Torres, E.B. Theoretical Framework for the Study of Sensori-motor Integration. Ph.D. Thesis, University of California, San Diego, CA, USA, 2001; p. 115.
30. Atkeson, C.G.; Hollerbach, J.M. Kinematics Features of unrestrained vertical arm movements. *J. Neurosci.* **1985**, *5*, 2318–2330. [CrossRef]
31. Nishikawa, K.C.; Murray, S.T.; Flanders, M. Do arm postures vary with the speed of reaching? *J. Neurophysiol.* **1999**, *81*, 2582–2586. [CrossRef]
32. Torres, E.B.; Zipser, D. Simultaneous control of hand displacements and rotations in orientation-matching experiments. *J. Appl. Physiol.* **2004**, *96*, 1978–1987. [CrossRef]
33. Torres, E.; Andersen, R. Space-time separation during obstacle-avoidance learning in monkeys. *J. Neurophysiol.* **2006**, *96*, 2613–2932. [CrossRef]
34. Torres, E.B. New symmetry of intended curved reaches. *Behav. Brain Funct.* **2010**, *6*, 21. [CrossRef]
35. Kalampratsidou, V.; Torres, E.B. Sonification of heart rate variability can entrain bodies in motion. In Proceedings of the 7th International Symposium on Movement and Computing, Jersey City, NJ, USA, 15–17 July 2020; ACM: New York, NY, USA, 2020. [CrossRef]
36. Yanovich, P.; Isenhower, R.W.; Sage, J.; Torres, E.B. Spatial-Orientation Priming Impedes Rather than Facilitates the Spontaneous Control of Hand-Retraction Speeds in Patients with Parkinson's Disease. *PLoS ONE* **2013**, *8*, e66757. [CrossRef] [PubMed]
37. Kathirvel, P.; Sabarimalai Manikandan, M.; Prasanna, S.R.M.; Soman, K.P. An efficient R-peak detection based on new nonlinear transformation and first-order Gaussian differentiator. *Cardiovasc. Eng. Technol.* **2011**, *2*, 408–425. [CrossRef]
38. Torres, E.B.; Isenhower, R.W.; Nguyen, J.; Whyatt, C.; Nurnberger, J.I.; José, J.V.; Silverstein, S.M.; Papathomas, T.V.; Sage, J.; Cole, J. Toward Precision Psychiatry: Statistical Platform for the Personalized Characterization of Natural Behaviors. *Front. Neurol.* **2016**, *7*, 8. [CrossRef] [PubMed]
39. Torres, E.B. Atypical signatures of motor variability found in an individual with ASD. *Neurocase* **2013**, *19*, 150–165. [CrossRef]
40. Mosimann, J.E. Size allometry: Size and shape variables with characterizations of the lognormal and generalized gamma distributions. *J. Am. Stat. Assoc.* **1970**, *65*, 930–945. [CrossRef]
41. Lleonart, J.; Salat, J.; Torres, G.J. Removing allometric effects of body size in morphological analysis. *J. Theor. Biol.* **2000**, *205*, 85–93. [CrossRef]

42. Monge, G. Memoire sur la theorie des deblais et des remblais. In *Histoire de l' Academie Royale des Science*; Avec les Memoired de Mathematique et de Physique; De L'imprimerie Royale: Paris, France, 1781.
43. Arjovsky, M.; Chintala, S.; Bottou, L. Wasserstein Generative Adversarial Networks. In Proceedings of the 34th International Conference on Machine Learning, Sydney, Australia, 6–11 August 2017.
44. Rubner, Y.; Tomasi, C.; Guibas, L.J. A Metric for Distributions with Applications to Image Databases. In Proceedings of the Sixth International Conference on Computer Vision, Bombay, India, 7 January 1998; p. 59.
45. McClelland, J.; Koslicki, D. EMDUniFrac: Exact linear time computation of the UniFrac metric and identification of differentially abundant organisms. *J. Math. Boil.* **2018**, *77*, 935–949. [CrossRef]
46. Freedman, D.; Diaconis, P. On the histogram as a density estimator: L_2 theory. *Z. Wahrscheinlichkeitstheorie verw Geb.* **1981**, *57*, 453–476. [CrossRef]
47. Watts, D.J.; Strogatz, S.H. Collective dynamics of 'small-world' networks. *Nature* **1998**, *393*, 440. [CrossRef]
48. Onnela, J.P.; Saramäki, J.; Kertész, J.; Kaski, K. Intensity and coherence of motifs in weighted complex networks. *Phys. Rev. E* **2005**, *71*, 065103. [CrossRef]
49. Rubinov, M.; Sporns, O. Complex network measures of brain connectivity: Uses and interpretations. *Neuroimage* **2010**, *52*, 1059–1069. [CrossRef] [PubMed]
50. Todorov, E. Stochastic optimal control and estimation methods adapted to the noise characteristics of the sensorimotor system. *Neural Comput.* **2005**, *17*, 1084–1088. [CrossRef]
51. Torres, E.B. Objective Biometric Methods for the Diagnosis and Treatment of Nervous System Disorder. *Elsevier* **2018**, 580.
52. Ryu, J.; Vero, J.; Torres, E.B. Methods for Tracking Dynamically Coupled Brain-Body Activities during Natural Movement. In Proceedings of the MOCO '17 4th International Conference on Movement Computing, London, UK, 28–30 June 2017; ACM: New York, NY, USA, 2017.
53. Ryu, J.; Vero, J.; Dobkin, R.D.; Torres, E.B. Dynamic Digital Biomarkers of Motor and Cognitive Function in Parkinson's Disease. *J. Vis. Exp.* **2019**, *149*, e59827. [CrossRef] [PubMed]
54. Nguyen, J.; Majmudar, U.; Papathomas, T.V.; Silverstein, S.M.; Torres, E.B. Schizophrenia: The micro-movements perspective. *Neuropsychologia* **2016**, *85*, 310–326. [CrossRef]
55. Wu, D.; José, J.V.; Nurnberger, J.I.; Torres, E.B. A Biomarker Characterizing Neurodevelopment with applications in Autism. *Sci. Rep.* **2018**, *8*, 614. [CrossRef]

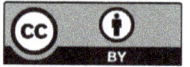

© 2020 by the authors. Licensee MDPI, Basel, Switzerland. This article is an open access article distributed under the terms and conditions of the Creative Commons Attribution (CC BY) license (http://creativecommons.org/licenses/by/4.0/).

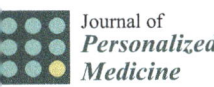

Review

A Systematic Literature Review on the Application of Machine-Learning Models in Behavioral Assessment of Autism Spectrum Disorder

Nadire Cavus [1,2], Abdulmalik A. Lawan [1,3,*], Zurki Ibrahim [4], Abdullahi Dahiru [5], Sadiya Tahir [6], Usama Ishaq Abdulrazak [7] and Adamu Hussaini [3,8]

1. Department of Computer Information Systems, Near East University, Nicosia 99138, Cyprus; nadire.cavus@neu.edu.tr
2. Computer Information Systems Research and Technology Centre, Near East University, Nicosia 99138, Cyprus
3. Department of Computer Science, Kano University of Science and Technology, Wudil 713281, Nigeria; adamu.hussaini2510@gmail.com
4. Department of Medical Genetics, Near East University, Nicosia 99138, Cyprus; zurkiibrahim@yahoo.com
5. College of Nursing and Midwifery, School of Nursing, Kano 700233, Nigeria; abdullahidahiru84@gmail.com
6. Department of Pediatrics, Murtala Muhammad Specialist Hospital, Kano 700251, Nigeria; taheersadiyah@gmail.com
7. Department of Emergency Medicine, Peterborough City Hospital, North West Anglia NHS Foundation Trust, Peterborough PE3 9GZ, UK; usamia12@gmail.com
8. Crestic Laboratory, Universite de Reims, 51100 Reims, France
* Correspondence: aalawan@kustwudil.edu.ng; Tel.: +23-4706-649-8622

Citation: Cavus, N.; Lawan, A.A.; Ibrahim, Z.; Dahiru, A.; Tahir, S.; Abdulrazak, U.I.; Hussaini, A. A Systematic Literature Review on the Application of Machine-Learning Models in Behavioral Assessment of Autism Spectrum Disorder. *J. Pers. Med.* 2021, *11*, 299. https://doi.org/10.3390/jpm11040299

Academic Editor: Elizabeth B. Torres

Received: 23 March 2021
Accepted: 12 April 2021
Published: 14 April 2021

Publisher's Note: MDPI stays neutral with regard to jurisdictional claims in published maps and institutional affiliations.

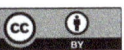

Copyright: © 2021 by the authors. Licensee MDPI, Basel, Switzerland. This article is an open access article distributed under the terms and conditions of the Creative Commons Attribution (CC BY) license (https://creativecommons.org/licenses/by/4.0/).

Abstract: Autism spectrum disorder (ASD) is associated with significant social, communication, and behavioral challenges. The insufficient number of trained clinicians coupled with limited accessibility to quick and accurate diagnostic tools resulted in overlooking early symptoms of ASD in children around the world. Several studies have utilized behavioral data in developing and evaluating the performance of machine learning (ML) models toward quick and intelligent ASD assessment systems. However, despite the good evaluation metrics achieved by the ML models, there is not enough evidence on the readiness of the models for clinical use. Specifically, none of the existing studies reported the real-life application of the ML-based models. This might be related to numerous challenges associated with the data-centric techniques utilized and their misalignment with the conceptual basis upon which professionals diagnose ASD. The present work systematically reviewed recent articles on the application of ML in the behavioral assessment of ASD, and highlighted common challenges in the studies, and proposed vital considerations for real-life implementation of ML-based ASD screening and diagnostic systems. This review will serve as a guide for researchers, neuropsychiatrists, psychologists, and relevant stakeholders on the advances in ASD screening and diagnosis using ML.

Keywords: autism spectrum disorder; screening; diagnosis; artificial intelligence; machine learning

1. Introduction

Autism spectrum disorder (ASD) is a lifelong neurodevelopmental disorder associated with communication impairment, restrictive and compulsive behavior. According to the fifth edition of the diagnostic and statistical manual of mental disorders (DSM-5), the primary indicators for diagnosing ASD are deficits in social communication and the manifestation of repetitive and restricted patterns of activities, behavior, or interests [1]. The rising prevalence of ASD necessitates the need for early and cost-effective diagnosis to set the path for efficient, and appropriate treatment [2,3]. Moreover, early diagnosis of ASD leads to improved outcomes in communication and social interaction and guides parents to the right interventions in school, home, and clinic [4–6]. However, apart from the cost-ineffectiveness of the current diagnostic instruments, studies have indicated the delay of the clinical processes of diagnosing ASD [7–10]. Addressing these challenges lead to several suggestions, including the so-called quick and accurate Machine Learning (ML)-enabled ASD assessment systems [11–14]. The promising results realized with ML algorithms across various research fields motivated these suggestions and made it a vital step toward quick and cost-effective assessment of ASD symptoms.

The gap in the existing literature is the absence of a definitive explanation on the sufficiency and readiness of the ML models toward real-life implementation. Recently, there is an increasing number of studies on the development of ML models for diagnosing ASD based on either genetic [15,16], brain imaging [17–19], physical biomarkers [20–24], or behavioral data. However, despite the high evaluation metrics reported in the ML-based behavioral studies, there is little evidence on the clinical use of the resulting ML models [11]. Generally, apart from improving the accuracy metrics of the ML models, previous studies focused on improving diagnostic speed by reducing the model parameters using various dimensionality reduction techniques. Worthy of note, both the ML algorithms and the dimensionality reduction techniques are data-centric; they are independent of the conceptual basis upon which professionals build and utilize ASD assessment instruments [25]. Thus, the clinical validity of the resulting ML models could be explained based on the alignment of the data-centric techniques with the conceptual basis of diagnosing ASD. Nonetheless, other factors that might limit the clinical validity and real-life implementation of the models include the reported discrepancies within the data repositories [26,27].

The present review explores the advances in the application of machine learning in the behavioral assessment of ASD. Accordingly, recent articles were systematically reviewed on the application of machine learning models toward quick and accurate assessment of ASD. Based on the reviewed literature, we sought the answer on whether the recent findings could sufficiently translate to real-life implementation of ML-based ASD screening and diagnostic models. Nonetheless, previous literature reviews assessed the performance of ML models in ASD screening and diagnosis based on the common evaluation metrics of sensitivity, specificity, and accuracy, among others [25,28]. However, none of the existing literature reviews systematically analyzed the subject area and provided enough evidence on the readiness and sufficiency of the models toward real-life implementation of the ML-based systems. For instance, Song et al. [28] reviewed 13 relevant studies that utilized varying data types and discussed the possibility of achieving effective classification of ASD based on the study findings. Similarly, Thabtah [25] identified some limitations within the commonly employed research methodologies and proposed intuitive stages toward appending the ML models into ASD screening apps. In this work, key challenges were highlighted alongside the commonly utilized assessment tools, datasets, and data intelligence techniques, and solutions were suggested toward valid implementations of real-life ML-based ASD screening and diagnostic systems.

2. Methodology
2.1. Search Strategy

The present review involved a systematic search, which is conducted in October 2020. To identify the most relevant studies, the authors ensured careful planning and allocation of tasks at every stage of the systematic literature review. The search strategy was tailored to the four most popular scientific databases of the study field, namely, Web of Science, PubMed, IEEEXplore, and Scopus. Furthermore, the search query utilized includes the following terms "Autism Spectrum Disorder" OR "Autistic Disorder" OR "Autism" AND "Screening" OR "Assessment" OR "Identification" OR "Test" OR "Detection" AND "Machine Learning" OR "Artificial Intelligence". The search filters covered a period of ten years from 2011 to 2020 and were limited to journal articles published in the English language. Beyond the above-mentioned databases, relevant publications were accessed from other databases on the advances in ASD assessment.

2.2. Selection Criteria

The article selection process was based on the PRISMA statement [29]. Relevant studies have utilized PRISMA in providing critical appraisal on the advances in the assessment of autism and other neuropsychiatric disorders [19,24,28,30–33]. The determining factor in the inclusion criteria involves any published full-text journal article on the use of ML in ASD screening or diagnosis. At the initial screening stage, after duplicates removal, the authors assessed the records against the inclusion criteria to decide on worthy articles for the systematic literature review. The decisions for inclusion/exclusion on the records were recorded in a separate column within the combined excel sheet imported from the databases. Thus, for records whose titles and corresponding abstracts aligned with the preset inclusion criteria, full-text articles of the studies were retrieved for the subsequent screening stage. In the next PRISMA screening stage, all the authors reviewed the downloaded papers, independently, to ascertain their relevance with the search query used, as well as the set research question. The authors utilized the WhatsApp discussion group in resolving disagreements in the selection process.

Specifically, three hundred and sixty-seven records were carefully assessed for eligibility. One hundred and eighty studies out of the 367 records were discarded, due to the following reasons: Book chapters (n = 17), conference papers (n = 138), editorial materials (n = 11), literature reviews (n = 15), not written in English (n = 9). The remaining one hundred and seventy-seven studies were further assessed; one hundred and forty-four records were eliminated because they are either based on brain imaging data (n = 57), genetic data (n = 35), or physical/metabolic biomarkers (n = 32), while others are intervention studies (n = 20). Consequently, thirty-three full-text articles were retrieved, read, and qualitatively assessed. Nonetheless, additional articles were excluded because ML is not the main method employed (n = 7), and ASD is not the main neuropsychiatric disorder assessed (n = 4). Finally, 22 studies met the inclusion criteria. The PRISMA flow diagram (Figure 1) summarized the above-mentioned systematic literature review process, and Table 1 itemized the key items of the inclusion and exclusion criteria of the study.

Table 1. Inclusion and exclusion criteria of the study.

Inclusion Criteria
Journal articles published in the English language
Documents published within the last ten years from 2011 to date
Full-text papers that are accessible and downloadable
Studies that utilized behavioral data
Studies that employed machine learning as the main technique
Studies that considered autism as the main disorder assessed
Exclusion criteria
Papers that are written in other languages
Duplicated papers
Full-text of the document is not accessible on the internet
The study aim is not clearly defined
Studies that are not relevant to the stated research question
Relevant studies, but machine learning is not the main method
Relevant studies, but autism is not the main disorder assessed
Conferences papers, editorial materials, and literature reviews
Studies that utilized data from either brain imaging, genetic, or physical/metabolic biomarkers.
Intervention studies

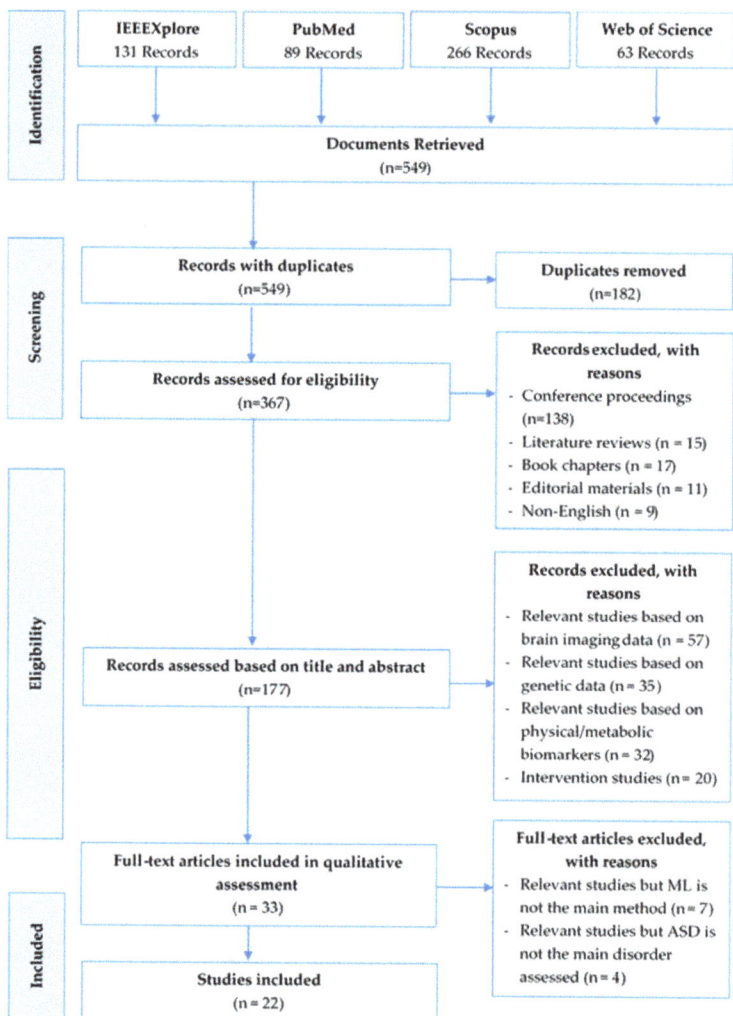

Figure 1. PRISMA flow diagram of the search results.

2.3. Quality Assessment

The authors carefully adhered to the planned, systematic literature review process to maintain the study's quality. Particularly, at every phase of the systematic literature review, the authors ensured careful planning and allocation of tasks. The first author created an online Mendeley repository and monitored the progress of the review based on preset milestones to ensure that all tasks complied with the scheduled deadlines. The Mendeley repository was also used in keeping track of the data extraction stages, noting essential observations and sharing vital contents related to the study. The authors further upheld peer-reviewing at each phase of the study to enhance the systematic literature review. Nevertheless, unbiased and constructive assessments on the systematic approach used in this study were sought from external professionals on ASD diagnostic procedures with expertise in systematic literature reviews.

2.4. Data Extraction

As the final stage of the study's PRISMA, the data extraction stage, 22 articles were appraised critically, and the following information was extracted from the studies:

- Author(s) (year),
- Number of citations,
- Source(s) of the research data,
- Data collection/assessment instrument,
- ML model(s)developed,
- Best performing model(s),
- The key finding(s).

3. Results

3.1. Descriptive Analysis on Trends and Status of the Study on ML in ASD Assessment

Based on the exported data, the trend of studies on the use of ML in the behavioral assessment of ASD showed the most cited references, the most cited journals, as well as citation and publication frequencies across the years.

With the increasing application of ML in healthcare studies, as shown in Figure 2, there are more publications on ML and ASD assessment. From 2012 to 2018, not so many studies cared about the application of ML in ASD assessment. However, with the recently increased patronage of ML techniques across various fields, there is an increasing demand for intelligent tools for accurate assessment of ASD. From Figure 3, most of the articles contributing to the area were published in Translational Psychiatry (n = 5), followed by the Health Informatics Journal (n = 3). The remaining fifteen journals depicted published one article, each.

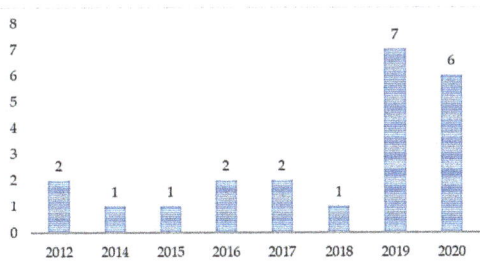

Figure 2. Article distribution over the years.

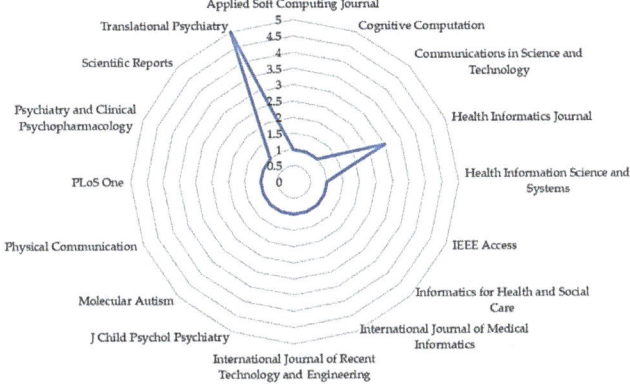

Figure 3. The number of articles published by journals.

Based on the citation data exported, as shown in Table 2, we can see that the most cited references are Wall et al. [34] (n = 160), Wall et al. [35] (n = 106), Duda et al. [36] (n = 89), Kosmicki et al. [37] (n = 84), and Bone et al. [38] (n = 77). Most of the significant references; with the highest number of citations, were published in Translational Psychiatry [34,36,37] (Figure 4, n = 408) in the years 2012 (Figure 5, n = 266), 2015 (Figure 5, n = 84), and 2016 (Figure 5, n = 166). Figure 4 highlighted the citation data of the eight most cited journals involved in the study; Translational Psychiatry (n = 408), PLoS One (n = 106), Journal of Children Psychological Psychiatry (n = 77), and so on.

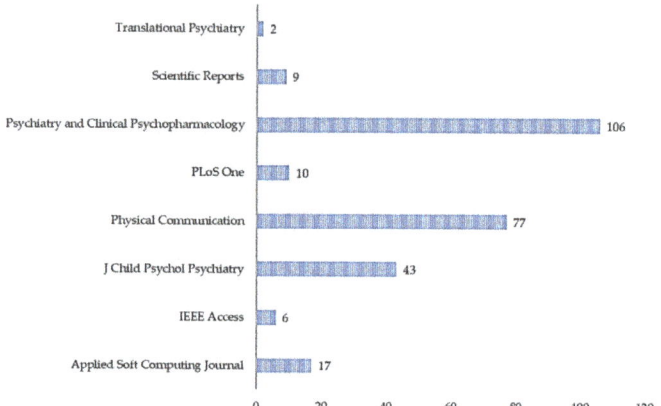

Figure 4. Sum of citations per journal.

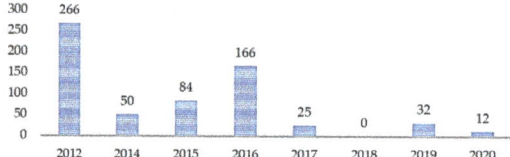

Figure 5. Number of citations across years.

3.2. Dimensionality Reduction Techniques

Most of the studies primarily aimed at streamlining the data collection instruments, followed by evaluating the performance of various ML algorithms on the streamlined datasets [35,37,39–41]. While various feature selection methods were applied in streamlining the most influential features of the data collection instruments from the datasets, other studies utilized various feature transformation techniques in reducing the input parameters. For instance, in the work of Puerto et al. [42], the inputs were fuzzified into membership values before applying the classification algorithms. Similarly, before implementing the classification models, Baadel et al. [43] and Akter et al. [44] transformed the inputs using clustering and feature transformation functions, respectively. Nonetheless, other studies employed a trial-error approach in selecting the most influential features. The trial-error approach involves repetitive evaluation of the ML models using a varying combination of the features; the most influential combination achieves superior results with fewer input parameters. Specifically, the studies utilized various feature selection techniques, including trial-error [13,34,35,39,45], Variable Analysis (Va) [46,47], information gain (IG) and chi-square testing (CHI) [48], sequential feature selection (SFS) [49], correlation-based feature selection (CFS) and minimum redundancy maximum relevance (mRMR) [12]. Additionally, ML-based feature selection techniques employed include recursive feature selection [40], sparsity/parsimony enforcing regularization techniques [50], stepwise backward feature selection [37], and forward feature selection [36].

3.3. Models Implementation

As shown in Table 2, the commonly implemented ML algorithms are Random Forest (RF) [12,43,47,51], Support Vector Machines (SVM) [37,38,40,49,50], Alternative Decision Tree (ADTree) [34,35,39,45], and Logistic Regression (LR) [13,37,48]. To achieve comparative results, most of the studies employed several algorithms, such as Adaboost, Artificial Neural Network (ANN), Linear Discriminant Analysis (LDA), Naïve Bayes, and K-Nearest Neighbor (KNN).

3.4. Data Collection/Assessment Instruments

The most utilized data collection instruments are AQ-10 [11,13,43,44,46–49,51,52], Q-CHAT-10 [11,44,46,52], ADOS [34,37,39,40,42,50], ADI-R [35,38,42], and Social Responsiveness Scale (SRS) [36,38,53]. Others include Autism Behavior Checklist, Aberrant Behavior Checklist, Clinical Global Impression [45], and MCHAT-based Pictorial Autism Assessment Schedule (PASS) [12]. Thus, the need for improving the reliability of these assessment instruments and ascertaining their relevance in ML modelling remains.

3.5. Sources of Data

The most prominent sources of data utilized in the studies include Boston Autism Consortium (AC), Autism Genetic Resource Exchange (AGRE), Simons Simplex Collection (SSC) [34–37,39,50,53], National Database for Autism Research (NDAR) [37,39], and Simons Variation In Individuals Project (SVIP) [37,39,50]. Other studies utilized data sets from ASDTest: Kaggle and UCI ML repository [11,13,43,44,46–49,51,52], Association of Parents and Friends for the Support and Defense of the rights of people with Autism (APADA) [42], PASS app [12], Ondokuz Mayis University Samsun [45], and ASD outpatient clinics in Germany [40]. To achieve standardized comparative results, there is a need for standardized ASD data repositories for machine learning studies [25].

3.6. Research Procedures

Apart from the common aim of streamlining the various data collection instruments followed by model evaluation, other studies focused on either optimizing the machine-learning algorithms [49,51], proposing input optimization techniques [43,44,46,47], or implementing ML-based screening apps [11,12]. For instance, Goel et al. [51] proposed Modified Grasshopper Optimization Algorithm (MGOA) for improved performance over common ML algorithms. The proposed MGOA (GOA with Random Forest classifier) outperformed other basic models and predicted ASD with approximate accuracy, specificity, and sensitivity of 100%. Similarly, Suresh et al. [49] proposed Differential Evaluation (DE) Algorithm to find the optimal solution of SVM parameters. The proposed DE tuned SVM achieved better performance over SVM, ANN and DE optimized ANN in classifying ASD. As stated earlier, apart from trial-error, studies employed either feature selection or transformation techniques for dimensionality reduction. For instance, Thabtah et al. [46] demonstrated the superiority of Va over IG, Correlation, CFS, and CHI in reducing AQ-10 items. Va derived fewer features, while maintaining competitive predictive accuracy, sensitivity, and specificity rates. A replicated study by Pratama et al. [47] produced a higher sensitivity of 87.89% in Adults AQ with RF and an increased specificity level of 86.33% in Adolescents AQ with SVM. Despite the good performance of the above-mentioned techniques in automating feature selection processes across various applications [54,55], none of the previous studies justified the conformity of the feature selection methods with the conceptual basis upon which professionals built and utilize ASD diagnostic instruments. Furthermore, unlike other medical diagnoses, the absence of definitive measures and medical tests for diagnosing ASD makes it difficult to numerical quantify the disorder based on few parameters. Notably, accurate assessment of ASD relied on the precise application of the commonly used behavioral scales built based on the knowledge and expertise of the professionals. Thus, applying human knowledge is imperative to reliable ASD diagnosis. Based on that, there is a need for quantifying the trade-offs of dimensionality reduction (ensuring fewer items for quick assessment) and validity (preservation of the human knowledge for correct diagnosis). Specifically, a machine-learning model built based on fewer behavioral features that do not sufficiently capture the human knowledge of the assessment instrument, will not be valid for clinical use. Thus, there is a need for applying dimensionality reduction techniques that professionals could track their ability to preserve the validity of the assessment instruments.

Nonetheless, various feature transformation techniques were equally utilized in the dimensionality reduction processes. For instance, Akter et al. [44] utilized three feature transformation techniques; Log, Z-score, and Sine functions, and evaluated the performance of nine different ML models on the transformed datasets. Log, Z-score, and Sine functions normalize data by converting excessively skewed entities into a normal distribution, converting features into −1 to 1 value range, and transforming instances to the Sine 0–2π value intervals, respectively. Akter et al. [44] recorded varying superior performances of the ML models, and the feature transformation approaches across the datasets. The feature transformations resulting in the best classifications were Z-score and Sine function on children, adolescents, and toddlers' datasets, respectively. However, despite the reported improved performances of the ML models on the transformed datasets and the theoretical understanding of the capabilities of the transformation functions, studies have demonstrated how these transformations compromise the relevance of the original data to the transformed data [56–59]. Researchers ought to be mindful of the limitations in using these transformations in terms of the relevance of the original to the transformed data during results interpretation. For instance, Feng [59] demonstrated such irrelevancies between the statistical findings of standard tests performed on original and log-transformed data. Similarly, several studies have highlighted some of the pitfalls and inconsistencies in the application of Z-scores and its concepts that overlooked the meaning of the original data, its standard deviations, and confusing applications [56–58].

Recent studies further demonstrated how ML-enable ASD screening and diagnostic models could be developed, evaluated, and implemented. Recently, Baadel et al. [43] proposed Clustering-based Autistic Trait Classification (CATC), which identifies ASD-based traits' similarity, unlike the commonly used scoring functions. CATC showed significant improvement in the ASD classification based on clustered inputs. Comparative evaluation of various classification algorithms showed better improvement with the Random Forest classifier. On the implementation of mobile apps for ASD screening, Wingfield et al. [12], and Shahamiri and Thabtah [11] embedded RF and CNN-based scoring models, respectively, while Thabtah [13] employed ML to validate ASDTest; a mobile screening app embedded with non-ML functions. In all the foregoing studies, the commonly used evaluation metrics are classification accuracy, sensitivity, and specificity. Specificity is the ratio of non-ASD cases that are correctly classified (i.e., true negatives rate) and sensitivity is the ratio of true ASD cases that are correctly classified (i.e., true positives rate), while classification accuracy is derived from sensitivity and specificity—as the measure of precisely classified cases from the total number of the cases.

Table 2. Information extracted from the articles.

Article/Citations	Aim	Tool	Data Source	FS/FT	FS/FT Method	Modeling Algorithms	Key Findings
Goel et al. [51] C = 10	Proposed Optimization Algorithm for improved performance over common ML	AQ-10 (child, adolescent, adult)	ASDTest	-	-	GOA, BACO, LR, NB, KNN, RF-CART + ID3, * MGOA	The proposed MGOA (GOA with Random Forest classifier) predicted ASD cases with approximate accuracy, specificity, and sensitivity of 100%.
Shahamiri and Thabtah [11] C = 0	Implementation and evaluation of CNN-based ASD scoring system	Q-CHAT-10, AQ-10	ASDTest	-	-	C4.5, Bayes Net, RIDOR, * CNN	The performance evaluation showed the superior performance of CNN over other algorithms; indicating the robustness of the implemented system.
Thabtah and Peebles [52] C = 28	Demonstrate the superiority of Rules-based ML over other models	Q-CHAT-10, AQ-10 (child, Adolescent, adult)	ASDTest	-	-	RIPPER, RIDOR, Nnge, Bagging, CART, C4.5, and PRISM, * RML	Empirically evaluated rule induction, Bagging, Boosting, and decision trees algorithms on different ASD datasets. The superiority of the RML model was reported in not only classifying ASD but also offer rules that can be utilized in understanding the reasons behind the classification.
Wall et al. [35] C = 106	Streamlining ADR-I and evaluate ML performance	ADI-R	AGRE, SSC, AC	FS	Trial-error	* ADTree, BFTree, ConjunctiveRule, DecisionStump, FilteredClassifier, J48, J48graft, JRip, LADTree, Nnge, OneR, OrdinalClassClassifier, PART, Ridor, and SimpleCart	The best model utilized 7 of the 93 items contained in the ADI-R in classifying ASD with 99.9% accuracy.
Duda et al. [39] C = 50	Streamlining ADOS and demonstrate the superior performance of ADTree over common hand-crafted methods	ADOS	AC, AGRE, SSC, NDAR, SVIP	FS	Trial-error	ADTree	72% reduction in the items from ADOS-G with >97% accuracy.
Küpper et al. [40] C = 2	Streamlining ADOS and demonstrate the performance of SVM	ADOS	ASD outpatient clinics in Germany	FS	Recursive Feature Selection	SVM	SVM achieved good sensitivity and specificity with fewer ADOS items pointing to 5 behavioral features.
Wall et al. [34] C = 160	Streamlining ADOS and evaluate ML performance	ADOS	AC, AGRE, SSC	FS	Trial-error	* ADTree, BFTree, Decision Stump, Functional Tree, J48, J48graft, Jrip, LADTree, LMT, Nnge, OneR, PART, Random Tree, REPTree, Ridor, Simple Cart	The ADTree model utilized 8 of the 29 items in Module 1 of the ADOS and classified ASD with 100% accuracy.
Levy et al. [50] C = 21	Streamlining ADOS and evaluate ML performance	ADOS	AC, AGRE, SSC, SVIP	FS	Sparsity/parsimony enforcing regularization techniques	LR, Lasso, Ridge, Elastic net, Relaxed Lasso, Nearest shrunken centroids, LDA, * LR, * SVM, ADTree, RF, Gradient boosting, AdaBoost	With at most 10 features from ADOS's Module 3 and Module 2, AUC of 0.95 and 0.93 was achieved, respectively.

Table 2. Cont.

Article/Citations	Aim	Tool	Data Source	FS/FT	FS/FT Method	Modeling Algorithms	Key Findings
Kosmicki et al. [37] C = 84	Streamlining ADOS and evaluate ML performance	ADOS	AC, AGRE, SSC, NDAR, SVIP	FS	Stepwise Backward Feature Selection	ADTree, * SVM, Logistic Model Tree, * LR, NB, NBTree, RF	The best performing models have utilized 9 of the 28 items from module 2, and 12 of the 28 items from module 3 in classifying ASD with 98.27% and 97.66% accuracy, respectively.
Thabtah [13] C = 31	Propose ASDTest; AQ-based mobile screening app, streamline AQ-10 items, and evaluate the performance of 2 ML models	AQ-10 (child, adolescent, adult)	ASDTest	FS	Trial-error	NB, * LR	Feature and predictive analyses demonstrate small groups of autistic traits improving the efficiency and accuracy of screening processes.
Thabtah et al. [46] C = 47	Demonstrate the superiority of Va over other FS methods based on the performance of ML models on the streamlined datasets	Q-CHAT-10, and AQ-10 (child, adolescent, adult)	ASDTest	FS	Va, IG, Correlation, CFS, and CHI	Repeated Incremental Pruning to Produce Error Reduction (RIPPER), C4.5 (Decision Tree)	Va derived fewer features from adults, adolescents, and child datasets with optimal model performance. Demonstrate the efficacy of Va over IG, Correlation, CFS, and CHI in reducing AQ-10 items
Thabtah et al. [48] C = 13	Streamlining AQ-10 and demonstrate the superior performance of LR over common hand-crafted methods	AQ-10 (adolescent, adult)	ASDTest	FS	IG, CHI	LR	LR showed acceptable performance in terms of sensitivity, specificity, and accuracy among others.
Suresh Kumar and Renugadevi [49] C = 0	Algorithm Optimization (improvement in accuracy compared to common ML)	AQ-10 (child, adolescent, adult)	ASDTest	FS	SFS	SVM, ANN, * DE SVM, DE ANN	DE optimized SVM outperformed ANN and DE optimized ANN in classifying ASD. DE is effective.
Pratama et al. [47] C = 0	Input Optimization using Va	AQ-10 (child, adolescent, adult)	ASDTest	FS	Va	SVM, * RF, ANN	RF succeeded in producing higher adult AQ sensitivity (87.89%), and a rise in the specificity level of AQ-Adolescents was better produced using SVM (86.33%).
Usta et al. [45] C = 9	ML Performance Evaluation	Autism Behavior Checklist, Aberrant Behavior Checklist, Clinical Global Impression	Ondokuz Mayis University Samsun	FS	Trial-error	NB, LR, * ADTree	The ML modeling revealed the significant influence of other demographic parameters in ASD classification.

Table 2. Cont.

Article/Citations	Aim	Tool	Data Source	FS/FT	FS/FT Method	Modeling Algorithms	Key Findings
Wingfield et al. [12] C = 3	Propose PASS; a culturally sensitive app embedded with ML model	PASS	VPASS app	FS	CFS, mRMR	* RF, NB, Adaboost, Multilayer Perceptron, J48, PART, SMO	PASS app overcomes the cultural variation in interpreting ASD symptoms, and the study demonstrated the possibility of removing feature redundancy.
Duda et al. [36] C = 89	ML Performance Evaluation in classifying ASD from ADHD	SRS	AC, AGRE, SSC	FS	Forward Feature Selection	ADTree, RF, SVM, LR, Categorical lasso, LDA	All the models could classify ASD from ADHD by utilizing 5 of the 65 items of SRS with high average accuracy (AUC = 0.965).
Duda et al. [53] C = 25	Improve models' reliability using expanded datasets for classifying ASD from ADHD	SRS	AC, AGRE, SSC, and crowdsourced data	FS	-	SVM, LR, * LDA	LDA model achieved an AUC of 0.89 with 15 items.
Bone et al. [38] C = 77	Demonstrate the improved accuracy of SVM over common hand-crafted rules	ADI-R, SRS	Balanced Independent Dataset	FT	Tuned parameters across multiple levels of cross-validation	SVM	The SVM model utilized five of the fused ADI-R and SRS items and classified ASD sufficiently with below (above) 89.2% (86.7%) sensitivity and 59.0% (53.4%) specificity.
Puerto et al. [42] C = 17	Propose MFCM-ASD and evaluate its performance against other ML models	ADOS, ADI-R	APADA	FT	Inputs fuzzification	* MFCM-ASD, SVM, Random forest, NB	The superior performance of MFCM characterized by its robustness makes it an effective ASD diagnostic technique.
Akter et al. [44] C = 6	Compare FT methods and evaluate the performance of ML models on the transformed datasets	Q-CHAT-10, and AQ-10 (child, adolescent, adult)	ASDTest	FT	Log, Z-score, and Sine FT	Adaboost, FDA, C5.0, LDA, MDA, PDA, SVM, and CART	Varying superior performances of the ML models and FT approaches were achieved across the datasets.
Baadel et al. [43] C = 2	Input Optimization using a clustering approach	AQ-10 (child, adolescent, adult)	ASDTest	FT	CATC	OMCOKE, RIPPER, PART, * RF, RT, ANN	CATC showed significant improvement in screening ASD based on traits' similarity as opposed to scoring functions. The improvement was more pronounced with RF classifier.

ASD, autism spectrum disorder; FS, feature selection; FT, feature transformation; ML, machine learning; ANN, artificial neural network; SVM, support vector machine; CNN, convolutional neural network; RF, random forest; LR, logistic regression; ADTree, alternative decision tree; LDA, linear discriminant analysis; MGOA, modified grasshopper optimization algorithm; BACO, binary ant colony optimization; NB, naïve Bayes; KNN, K-nearest neighbor; RIPPER, repeated incremental pruning to produce error reduction; ADOS, autism diagnostic observation schedule; ADI-R, autism diagnostic interview-revised; Q-CHAT, quantitative checklist for autism toddlers; AQ, autism quotient; SRS, social responsiveness scale; PASS, pictorial autism assessment schedule; AC, boston autism consortium; AGRE, autism genetic resource exchange; SSC, Simons Simplex Collection; NDAR, National Database for Autism Research; SVIP, Simons Variation In Individuals Project; APADA, Association of Parents and Friends for the Support and Defense of the Rights of People with Autism; MFCM, multilayer fuzzy cognitive maps; CATC, clustering-based autistic trait classification. * Best performing models.

4. Discussion

The search for cost-effective ASD assessment coupled with the global rise in ASD cases attracted the implementation of quick and accurate assessment measures based on data intelligence techniques, including machine-learning algorithms. Despite the various attempts in ML-based ASD assessment using functional magnetic resonance imaging (MRI), eye tracking, and genetic data, among others, the promising results based on behavioral data call for further research. For instance, Plitt et al. [60] found that ASD classification via behavioral measures consistently surpassed rs-fMRI classifiers. Accordingly, in line with the common research aim of the behavioral studies, various dimensionality reduction techniques were employed to improve the diagnostic speed of the resulting ML models. However, unlike the reduced dimensions, there is enough evidence on the good reliability, high internal consistency, and convergent validity between the common assessment instruments within large samples [61–65]. Furthermore, studies have ascertained the robustness of the common assessment instruments in the quantitative measurement of the various dimensions of communication, interpersonal behavior, and stereotypic/repetitive behavior associated with ASD. Therefore, it will be difficult to sufficiently measure the key dimensions of the instruments using the fewer items generated by the common dimensionality reduction techniques. For instance, while professionals interpret SRS scores based on the sum of its 65 items, Bone et al. [38], Duda et al. [36], and Duda et al. [53] implemented SRS-enabled machine-learning models with at most 5, 5, and 15 items, respectively. Specifically, Duda et al. [36] and Duda et al. [53] focused on classifying ASD from ADHD using the SRS data from AC, AGRE, SSC. Duda et al. [36] implemented ADTree, RF, SVM, LR, Categorical lasso, and LDA models and achieved the highest area under the curve (AUC) of 0.965 in classifying ASD from ADHD by utilizing five of the 65 items of SRS identified using forward feature selection. Duda et al. [53] validated the findings of Duda et al. [36] with crowdsourced data to improve the model's capability on 'real-world' data, and the findings revealed that LDA outperformed LR and SVM by achieving an AUC of 0.89 with 15 items. Despite the high metrics reported by the studies, based on the standard clinical procedures for ASD diagnosis, the ML models are neither clinically sufficient nor readily implementable for real-life use.

Similarly, Wall et al. [35] compared the performance of 15 different ML algorithms on AGRE, SSC, and AC datasets and found ADTree to outperformed other models by utilizing 7 of the 93 items contained in the ADI-R in classifying ASD with 99.9% accuracy. In a similar study by Wall et al. [34], ADTree outperformed 17 comparative models by achieving 100% accuracy with 8 of the 29 items in Module 1 of ADOS. Moreover, Duda et al. [39] demonstrated the superior performance of ADTree in achieving 97% classification accuracy with a 72% reduction in ADOS-G items. Nonetheless, Levy et al. [50] and Kosmicki et al. [37] reduced the items of ADOS using sparsity/parsimony enforcing regularization and stepwise backward feature selection techniques, respectively, and reported the superior performance of LR and SVM over other ML algorithms. Specifically, in the study by Levy et al. [50], with at most 10 features from ADOS's Module 3 and Module 2, AUC of 0.95 and 0.93 was achieved, respectively. While Kosmicki et al. [37] recorded an accuracy of 98.27% and 97.66% with 9 of the 28 items from module 2, and 12 of the 28 items from module 3, respectively. Recently, Küpper et al. [40] utilized ADOS data from a clinical sample of adolescents and adults with ASD and reported good performance of SVM on fewer items reduced using the recursive feature selection technique. The foregoing studies have demonstrated how ML-enable ASD screening and diagnostic models could be developed and evaluated. However, numerous challenges associated with the behavioral assessment instruments, data repositories, and applied data intelligence algorithms need to be understood and addressed.

Although ML-based approaches are data-centric and are expected to improve objectivity and automation [66], with the global rise in ASD cases, the capacity to quickly and accurately assess ASD requires a careful understanding of the conceptual basis of the assessment instruments, as well as their relevance to the logical concepts of the ML algorithms.

Nonetheless, discrepancies within the data repositories, such as data imbalance, limit the clinical relevance of the high evaluation metrics reported in the studies [26,27]. For instance, Torres et al. [67] studied the statistical properties of ADOS scores from 1324 records and identified various factors that could undermine the scientific viability of the scores. Particularly, the empirical distributions in the generated scores break the theoretical conditions of normality and homogeneous variance, which are critical for independence between bias and sensitivity. Thus, Torres et al. [67] suggested readjusting the scientific use of ADOS, due to the variation in the distribution of the scores, lack of appropriate metrics for characterizing changes, and the impact of both on sensitivity-bias codependencies and longitudinal tracking of ASD. In essence, the applied data intelligence algorithms, and the resulting models, missed the human knowledge upon which the assessment instruments were built and applied by the professionals [25]. Additionally, most of the studies overlooked the inherent limitations associated with the dimensionality reduction techniques, and the assessment instruments [7–9]. Thus, the need for ascertaining the clinical relevance of the data-centric approaches and readjusting the scientific use of the assessment instruments remains. Obviously, in the future, it can be said that the trend in the application of ML in the behavioral assessment of ASD will go on. On the other hand, the pressing demands for cost-effective assessment of ASD remain. Thus, future studies need to revisit the relevance of the data collection instruments to ML algorithms.

5. Conclusions and Recommendations

Machine learning has been broadly applied in the behavioral assessment of ASD based on a variety of data types as input to data-intelligence algorithms. Commonly utilized inputs include the items of screening tools, such as ADI-R and ADOS-G. Popular ML algorithms used are SVMs, variants of the decision trees, random forests, and neural networks. However, the multitudes of challenges in accurate ASD assessments are yet to be addressed by the suggested machine learning approaches. Specifically, the high metrics achieved with the data-intelligence techniques have not guaranteed the clinical relevance of the ML models. Additionally, the commonly used evaluation measures of classification accuracy, specificity, and sensitivity, among others cannot sufficiently reflect the human knowledge applied by professionals in assessing behavioral symptoms of ASD. Consequently, understanding the clinical basis of the assessment tools and the logical concepts of the data-intelligence techniques will lead to promising studies on the real-life implementation of cost-effective ASD assessment systems. The novelty in the present review is that while previous literature reviews focused on the performance of various data intelligent techniques on different data sets, this work systematically reviewed the literature and provide a definitive explanation on the relevance of the reported findings toward the real-life implementation of the ML-based assessment systems. The authors hope that the findings of this systematic literature review will guide researchers, caregivers, and relevant stakeholders on the advances in ASD assessment with ML.

Nonetheless, a few of the limitations associated with the present work include overlooking other non-English documents. Thus, possible excellent studies reported in other languages might have been missed. Secondly, the search filters spanned ten years and were limited to the four scientific databases mentioned. Furthermore, the records retrieved relied on the few search terms utilized in the search query. Therefore, relaxing the search filters across additional databases could yield additional relevant studies. Lastly, the present review considered only full-text online journal articles. Consequently, the findings are limited to the studies included. The future research agenda will be based on relaxing the search criteria to incorporate other scholastic databases for further comparative results. In addition, future studies could relax the search filters to include books, conference papers, and so on. Noteworthy, to build on or replicate the reviewed studies, future research should explore data-intelligence techniques that will achieve not only excellent evaluation metrics, but also adhere to the conceptual basis upon which professionals diagnose ASD.

Author Contributions: Conceptualization, A.A.L., N.C. and Z.I.; methodology, A.A.L., N.C., Z.I., S.T., U.I.A., A.D. and A.H.; resources, A.A.L., N.C., Z.I. and A.D.; data curation, A.A.L.; writing—original draft preparation, A.A.L. and N.C.; writing—review and editing, A.A.L., N.C., A.D., S.T., U.I.A., A.H. and Z.I.; visualization, A.A.L.; supervision, N.C., S.T., U.I.A. and A.D. All authors have read and agreed to the published version of the manuscript.

Funding: This research received no external funding.

Institutional Review Board Statement: Not applicable.

Informed Consent Statement: Not applicable.

Data Availability Statement: Data sharing is not applicable to this article.

Conflicts of Interest: The authors declare no conflict of interest.

References

1. American Psychiatric Association. *Diagnostic and Statistical Manual of Mental Disorders (DSM-5)*, 5th ed.; American Psychiatric Publishing: Philadelphia, PA, USA, 2013.
2. Chauhan, A.; Sahu, J.; Jaiswal, N.; Kumar, K.; Agarwal, A.; Kaur, J.; Singh, S.; Singh, M. Prevalence of autism spectrum disorder in Indian children: A systematic review and meta-analysis. *Neurol. India* **2019**, *67*, 100. [CrossRef] [PubMed]
3. Baio, J.; Wiggins, L.; Christensen, D.L.; Maenner, M.J.; Daniels, J.; Warren, Z.; Kurzius-Spencer, M.; Zahorodny, W.; Rosenberg, C.R.; White, T.; et al. Prevalence of Autism Spectrum Disorder Among Children Aged 8 Years—Autism and Developmental Disabilities Monitoring Network, 11 Sites, United States, 2014. *MMWR Surveill. Summ.* **2018**, *67*, 1–23. [CrossRef] [PubMed]
4. Durkin, M.S.; Elsabbagh, M.; Barbaro, J.; Gladstone, M.; Happe, F.; Hoekstra, R.A.; Lee, L.C.; Rattazzi, A.; Stapel-Wax, J.; Stone, W.L.; et al. Autism screening and diagnosis in low resource settings: Challenges and opportunities to enhance research and services worldwide. *Autism Res.* **2015**, *8*, 473–476. [CrossRef] [PubMed]
5. Matson, J.L.; Konst, M.J. Early intervention for autism: Who provides treatment and in what settings. *Res. Autism Spectr. Disord.* **2014**, *8*, 1585–1590. [CrossRef]
6. Case-Smith, J.; Weaver, L.L.; Fristad, M.A. A systematic review of sensory processing interventions for children with autism spectrum disorders. *Autism* **2015**, *19*, 133–148. [CrossRef] [PubMed]
7. Guthrie, W.; Wallis, K.; Bennett, A.; Brooks, E.; Dudley, J.; Gerdes, M.; Pandey, J.; Levy, S.E.; Schultz, R.T.; Miller, J.S. Accuracy of autism screening in a large pediatric network. *Pediatrics* **2019**, *144*, e20183963. [CrossRef]
8. Øien, R.A.; Candpsych, S.S.; Volkmar, F.R.; Shic, F.; Cicchetti, D.V.; Nordahl-Hansen, A.; Stenberg, N.; Hornig, M.; Havdahl, A.; Øyen, A.S.; et al. Clinical features of children with autism who passed 18-month screening. *Pediatrics* **2018**, *141*, e20173596. [CrossRef]
9. Surén, P.; Saasen-Havdahl, A.; Bresnahan, M.; Hirtz, D.; Hornig, M.; Lord, C.; Reichborn-Kjennerud, T.; Schjølberg, S.; Øyen, A.-S.; Magnus, P.; et al. Sensitivity and specificity of early screening for autism. *BJPsych Open* **2019**, *5*, 1–8. [CrossRef]
10. Yuen, T.; Carter, M.T.; Szatmari, P.; Ungar, W.J. Cost-Effectiveness of Universal or High-Risk Screening Compared to Surveillance Monitoring in Autism Spectrum Disorder. *J. Autism Dev. Disord.* **2018**, *48*, 2968–2979. [CrossRef]
11. Shahamiri, S.R.; Thabtah, F. Autism AI: A New Autism Screening System Based on Artificial Intelligence. *Cognit. Comput.* **2020**, *12*, 766–777. [CrossRef]
12. Wingfield, B.; Miller, S.; Yogarajah, P.; Kerr, D.; Gardiner, B.; Seneviratne, S.; Samarasinghe, P.; Coleman, S. A predictive model for paediatric autism screening. *Health Inform. J.* **2020**, *26*, 2538–2553. [CrossRef]
13. Thabtah, F. An accessible and efficient autism screening method for behavioural data and predictive analyses. *Health Inform. J.* **2019**, *25*, 1739–1755. [CrossRef]
14. Campbell, K.; Carpenter, K.L.H.; Espinosa, S.; Hashemi, J.; Qiu, Q.; Tepper, M.; Calderbank, R.; Sapiro, G.; Egger, H.L.; Baker, J.P.; et al. Use of a Digital Modified Checklist for Autism in Toddlers–Revised with Follow-up to Improve Quality of Screening for Autism. *J. Pediatr.* **2017**, *183*, 133–139.e1. [CrossRef]
15. Ghafouri-Fard, S.; Taheri, M.; Omrani, M.D.; Daaee, A.; Mohammad-Rahimi, H.; Kazazi, H. Application of Single-Nucleotide Polymorphisms in the Diagnosis of Autism Spectrum Disorders: A Preliminary Study with Artificial Neural Networks. *J. Mol. Neurosci.* **2019**, *68*, 515–521. [CrossRef] [PubMed]
16. Sekaran, K.; Sudha, M. Predicting autism spectrum disorder from associative genetic markers of phenotypic groups using machine learning. *J. Ambient Intell. Humaniz. Comput.* **2020**, *12*, 1–14. [CrossRef]
17. Jack, A. Neuroimaging in neurodevelopmental disorders: Focus on resting-state fMRI analysis of intrinsic functional brain connectivity. *Curr. Opin. Neurol.* **2018**, *31*, 140–148. [CrossRef]
18. Fu, C.H.Y.; Costafreda, S.G. Neuroimaging-based biomarkers in psychiatry: Clinical opportunities of a paradigm shift. *Can. J. Psychiatry* **2013**, *58*, 499–508. [CrossRef]
19. Moon, S.J.; Hwang, J.; Kana, R.; Torous, J.; Kim, J.W. Accuracy of machine learning algorithms for the diagnosis of autism spectrum disorder: Systematic review and meta-analysis of brain magnetic resonance imaging studies. *J. Med. Internet Res.* **2019**, *6*, e14108. [CrossRef]

20. Sarabadani, S.; Schudlo, L.C.; Samadani, A.A.; Kushski, A. Physiological Detection of Affective States in Children with Autism Spectrum Disorder. *IEEE Trans. Affect. Comput.* **2020**, *11*, 588–600. [CrossRef]
21. Liu, W.; Li, M.; Yi, L. Identifying children with autism spectrum disorder based on their face processing abnormality: A machine learning framework. *Autism Res.* **2016**, *9*, 888–898. [CrossRef] [PubMed]
22. Alcañiz Raya, M.; Chicchi Giglioli, I.A.; Marín-Morales, J.; Higuera-Trujillo, J.L.; Olmos, E.; Minissi, M.E.; Teruel Garcia, G.; Sirera, M.; Abad, L. Application of Supervised Machine Learning for Behavioral Biomarkers of Autism Spectrum Disorder Based on Electrodermal Activity and Virtual Reality. *Front. Hum. Neurosci.* **2020**, *14*, 90. [CrossRef] [PubMed]
23. Hashemi, J.; Dawson, G.; Carpenter, K.L.H.; Campbell, K.; Qiu, Q.; Espinosa, S.; Marsan, S.; Baker, J.P.; Egger, H.L.; Sapiro, G. Computer Vision Analysis for Quantification of Autism Risk Behaviors. *IEEE Trans. Affect. Comput.* **2018**, *3045*, 1–12. [CrossRef]
24. Dahiya, A.V.; McDonnell, C.; DeLucia, E.; Scarpa, A. A systematic review of remote telehealth assessments for early signs of autism spectrum disorder: Video and mobile applications. *Pract. Innov.* **2020**, *5*, 150–164. [CrossRef]
25. Thabtab, F. Machine learning in autistic spectrum disorder behavioral research: A review and ways forward. *Inform. Health Soc. Care* **2019**, *44*, 278–297. [CrossRef]
26. Alahmari, F. A Comparison of Resampling Techniques for Medical Data Using Machine Learning. *J. Inf. Knowl. Manag.* **2020**, *19*, 1–13. [CrossRef]
27. Abdelhamid, N.; Padmavathy, A.; Peebles, D.; Thabtah, F.; Goulder-Horobin, D. Data Imbalance in Autism Pre-Diagnosis Classification Systems: An Experimental Study. *J. Inf. Knowl. Manag.* **2020**, *19*, 1–16. [CrossRef]
28. Song, D.-Y.; Kim, S.Y.; Bong, G.; Kim, J.M.; Yoo, H.J. The Use of Artificial Intelligence in Screening and Diagnosis of Autism Spectrum Disorder: A Literature Review. *J. Korean Acad. Child Adolesc. Psychiatry* **2019**, *30*, 145–152. [CrossRef]
29. Moher, D.; Liberati, A.; Tetzlaff, J.; Altman, D.G.; Group, T.P. Preferred Reporting Items for Systematic Reviews and Meta-Analyses: The PRISMA Statement. *PLoS Med.* **2009**, *6*, e1000097. [CrossRef]
30. Low, D.M.; Bentley, K.H.; Ghosh, S.S. Automated assessment of psychiatric disorders using speech: A systematic review. *Laryngoscope Investig. Otolaryngol.* **2020**, *5*, 96–116. [CrossRef]
31. Lebersfeld, J.B.; Swanson, M.; Clesi, C.D.; Kelley, S.E.O. Systematic Review and Meta-Analysis of the Clinical Utility of the ADOS-2 and the ADI-R in Diagnosing Autism Spectrum Disorders in Children. *J. Autism Dev. Disord.* **2021**, *51*, 1–14. [CrossRef]
32. Kulage, K.M.; Goldberg, J.; Usseglio, J.; Romero, D.; Bain, J.M.; Smaldone, A.M. How has DSM-5 Affected Autism Diagnosis? A 5-Year Follow-Up Systematic Literature Review and Meta-analysis. *J. Autism Dev. Disord.* **2020**, *50*, 2102–2127. [CrossRef]
33. Smith, I.C.; Reichow, B.; Volkmar, F.R. The Effects of DSM-5 Criteria on Number of Individuals Diagnosed with Autism Spectrum Disorder: A Systematic Review. *J. Autism Dev. Disord.* **2015**, *45*, 2541–2552. [CrossRef]
34. Wall, D.; Kosmicki, J.; Deluca, T.; Harstad, E.; Fusaro, V. Use of machine learning to shorten observation-based screening and diagnosis of autism. *Transl. Psychiatry* **2012**, *2*, e100-8. [CrossRef]
35. Wall, D.; Dally, R.; Luyster, R.; Jung, J.Y.; DeLuca, T. Use of artificial intelligence to shorten the behavioral diagnosis of autism. *PLoS ONE* **2012**, *7*, e43855. [CrossRef]
36. Duda, M.; Ma, R.; Haber, N.; Wall, D. Use of machine learning for behavioral distinction of autism and ADHD. *Transl. Psychiatry* **2016**, *6*, 1–5. [CrossRef]
37. Kosmicki, J.; Sochat, V.; Duda, M.; Wall, D. Searching for a minimal set of behaviors for autism detection through feature selection-based machine learning. *Transl. Psychiatry* **2015**, *5*, 1–7. [CrossRef]
38. Bone, D.; Bishop, S.L.; Black, M.P.; Goodwin, M.S.; Lord, C.; Narayanan, S.S. Use of machine learning to improve autism screening and diagnostic instruments: Effectiveness, efficiency, and multi-instrument fusion. *J. Child Psychol. Psychiatry Allied Discip.* **2016**, *57*, 927–937. [CrossRef]
39. Duda, M.; Kosmicki, J.; Wall, D. Testing the accuracy of an observation-based classifier for rapid detection of autism risk. *Transl. Psychiatry* **2015**, *5*, e556. [CrossRef]
40. Küpper, C.; Stroth, S.; Wolff, N.; Hauck, F.; Kliewer, N.; Schad-Hansjosten, T.; Kamp-Becker, I.; Poustka, L.; Roessner, V.; Schultebraucks, K.; et al. Identifying predictive features of autism spectrum disorders in a clinical sample of adolescents and adults using machine learning. *Sci. Rep.* **2020**, *10*, 1–11. [CrossRef]
41. Bellesheim, K.R.; Cole, L.; Coury, D.L.; Yin, L.; Levy, S.E.; Guinnee, M.A.; Klatka, K.; Malow, B.A.; Katz, T.; Taylor, J.; et al. Family-driven goals to improve care for children with autism spectrum disorder. *Pediatrics* **2018**, *142*, e20173225. [CrossRef]
42. Puerto, E.; Aguilar, J.; López, C.; Chávez, D. Using Multilayer Fuzzy Cognitive Maps to diagnose Autism Spectrum Disorder. *Appl. Soft Comput. J.* **2019**, *75*, 58–71. [CrossRef]
43. Baadel, S.; Thabtah, F.; Lu, J. A clustering approach for autistic trait classification. *Inform. Health Soc. Care* **2020**, *45*, 309–326. [CrossRef]
44. Akter, T.; Shahriare Satu, M.; Khan, M.I.; Ali, M.H.; Uddin, S.; Lio, P.; Quinn, J.M.W.; Moni, M.A. Machine Learning-Based Models for Early Stage Detection of Autism Spectrum Disorders. *IEEE Access* **2019**, *7*, 166509–166527. [CrossRef]
45. Usta, M.B.; Karabekiroglu, K.; Sahin, B.; Aydin, M.; Bozkurt, A.; Karaosman, T.; Aral, A.; Cobanoglu, C.; Kurt, A.D.; Kesim, N.; et al. Use of machine learning methods in prediction of short-term outcome in autism spectrum disorders. *Psychiatry Clin. Psychopharmacol.* **2019**, *29*, 320–325. [CrossRef]
46. Thabtah, F.; Kamalov, F.; Rajab, K. A new computational intelligence approach to detect autistic features for autism screening. *Int. J. Med. Inform.* **2018**, *117*, 112–124. [CrossRef]

47. Pratama, T.G.; Hartanto, R.; Setiawan, N.A. Machine learning algorithm for improving performance on 3 AQ-screening classification. *Commun. Sci. Technol.* **2019**, *4*, 44–49. [CrossRef]
48. Thabtah, F.; Abdelhamid, N.; Peebles, D. A machine learning autism classification based on logistic regression analysis. *Health Inf. Sci. Syst.* **2019**, *7*, 1–11. [CrossRef]
49. Suresh Kumar, R.; Renugadevi, M. Differential evolution tuned support vector machine for autistic spectrum disorder diagnosis. *Int. J. Recent Technol. Eng.* **2019**, *8*, 3861–3870. [CrossRef]
50. Levy, S.; Duda, M.; Haber, N.; Wall, D. Sparsifying machine learning models identify stable subsets of predictive features for behavioral detection of autism. *Mol. Autism* **2017**, *8*, 1–17. [CrossRef]
51. Goel, N.; Grover, B.; Gupta, D.; Khanna, A.; Sharma, M. Modified Grasshopper Optimization Algorithm for detection of Autism Spectrum Disorder. *Phys. Commun.* **2020**, *41*, 101115. [CrossRef]
52. Thabtah, F.; Peebles, D. A new machine learning model based on induction of rules for autism detection. *Health Inform. J.* **2020**, *26*, 264–286. [CrossRef]
53. Duda, M.; Haber, N.; Daniels, J.; Wall, D. Crowdsourced validation of a machine-learning classification system for autism and ADHD. *Transl. Psychiatry* **2017**, *7*, 2–8. [CrossRef] [PubMed]
54. Alhaj, T.A.; Siraj, M.M.; Zainal, A.; Elshoush, H.T.; Elhaj, F. Feature Selection Using Information Gain for Improved Structural-Based Alert Correlation. *PLoS ONE* **2016**, *11*, e0166017. [CrossRef] [PubMed]
55. Roobaert, D.; Karakoulas, G.; Chawla, N.V. Information Gain, Correlation and Support Vector Machines. In *Feature Extraction*; Springer: Berlin/Heidelberg, Germany, 2006; Volume 207, pp. 463–470.
56. Wiesen, J. Benefits, Drawbacks, and Pitfalls of z-Score Weighting. In Proceedings of the 30th Annual IPMAAC Conference, Las Vegas, NV, USA, 27 June 2006; pp. 1–41.
57. Lapteacru, I. On the Consistency of the Z-Score to Measure the Bank Risk. *SSRN Electron. J.* **2016**, *4*, 1–33. [CrossRef]
58. Curtis, A.; Smith, T.; Ziganshin, B.; Elefteriades, J. The Mystery of the Z-Score. *AORTA* **2016**, *4*, 124–130. [CrossRef] [PubMed]
59. Feng, C.; Wang, H.; Lu, N.; Chen, T.; He, H.; Lu, Y.; Tu, X.M. Log-transformation and its implications for data analysis. *Shanghai Arch. Psychiatry* **2014**, *26*, 105–109. [CrossRef] [PubMed]
60. Plitt, M.; Barnes, K.A.; Martin, A. Functional connectivity classification of autism identifies highly predictive brain features but falls short of biomarker standards. *NeuroImage Clin.* **2015**, *7*, 359–366. [CrossRef]
61. Chan, W.; Smith, L.E.; Hong, J.; Greenberg, J.S.; Mailick, M.R. Validating the social responsiveness scale for adults with autism. *Autism Res.* **2017**, *10*, 1663–1671. [CrossRef]
62. Becker, M.M.; Wagner, M.B.; Bosa, C.A.; Schmidt, C.; Longo, D.; Papaleo, C.; Riesgo, R.S. Translation and validation of Autism Diagnostic Interview-Revised (ADI-R) for autism diagnosis in Brazil. *Arq. Neuropsiquiatr.* **2012**, *70*, 185–190. [CrossRef]
63. Falkmer, T.; Anderson, K.; Falkmer, M.; Horlin, C. Diagnostic procedures in autism spectrum disorders: A systematic literature review. *Eur. Child Adolesc. Psychiatry* **2013**, *22*, 329–340. [CrossRef]
64. Medda, J.E.; Cholemkery, H.; Freitag, C.M. Sensitivity and Specificity of the ADOS-2 Algorithm in a Large German Sample. *J. Autism Dev. Disord.* **2019**, *49*, 750–761. [CrossRef]
65. Chojnicka, I.; Pisula, E. Adaptation and Validation of the ADOS-2, Polish Version. *Front. Psychol.* **2017**, *8*, 1–14. [CrossRef]
66. Achenie, L.E.K.; Scarpa, A.; Factor, R.S.; Wang, T.; Robins, D.L.; McCrickard, D.S. A Machine Learning Strategy for Autism Screening in Toddlers. *J. Dev. Behav. Pediatr.* **2019**, *40*, 369–376. [CrossRef]
67. Torres, E.B.; Rai, R.; Mistry, S.; Gupta, B. Hidden aspects of the research ADOS are bound to affect autism science. *Neural Comput.* **2020**, *32*, 515–561. [CrossRef]

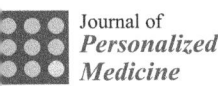

Review

Autism Spectrum Disorder from the Womb to Adulthood: Suggestions for a Paradigm Shift

Cristina Panisi [1,2,*], Franca Rosa Guerini [3,*], Provvidenza Maria Abruzzo [4], Federico Balzola [5], Pier Mario Biava [6], Alessandra Bolotta [4], Marco Brunero [7], Ernesto Burgio [8], Alberto Chiara [9], Mario Clerici [3,10], Luigi Croce [11], Carla Ferreri [12], Niccolò Giovannini [13], Alessandro Ghezzo [4], Enzo Grossi [14], Roberto Keller [15], Andrea Manzotti [16], Marina Marini [4,*], Lucia Migliore [17], Lucio Moderato [1], Davide Moscone [18], Michele Mussap [19], Antonia Parmeggiani [20], Valentina Pasin [21], Monica Perotti [22], Cristina Piras [23], Marina Saresella [3], Andrea Stoccoro [17], Tiziana Toso [24], Rosa Anna Vacca [25], David Vagni [26], Salvatore Vendemmia [27], Laura Villa [28], Pierluigi Politi [2] and Vassilios Fanos [19,29]

1. Fondazione Istituto Sacra Famiglia ONLUS, Cesano Boscone, 20090 Milan, Italy; lmoderato@sacrafamiglia.org
2. Department of Brain and Behavioral Sciences, University of Pavia, 27100 Pavia, Italy; pierluigi.politi@unipv.it
3. IRCCS Fondazione Don Carlo Gnocchi, ONLUS, 20148 Milan, Italy; mario.clerici@unimi.it (M.C.); msaresella@dongnocchi.it (M.S.)
4. DIMES, School of Medicine, University of Bologna, 40126 Bologna, Italy; provvidenza.abruzzo2@unibo.it (P.M.A.); alessandra.bolotta3@unibo.it (A.B.); a.ghezzo@fondazionedanelli.org (A.G.)
5. Division of Gastroenterology, Azienda Ospedaliero-Universitaria Città della Salute e della Scienza di Torino, University of Turin, 10126 Turin, Italy; federico.balzola@usa.net
6. Scientific Institute of Research and Care Multimedica, 20138 Milan, Italy; piermario.biava@gmail.com
7. Department of Pediatric Surgery, Fondazione IRCCS Policlinico San Matteo, 27100 Pavia, Italy; marcobrunero@hotmail.it
8. ECERI—European Cancer and Environment Research Institute, Square de Meeus 38-40, 1000 Bruxelles, Belgium; eburg@libero.it
9. Dipartimento Materno Infantile ASST, 27100 Pavia, Italy; alberto_chiara@asst-pavia.it
10. Department of Pathophysiology and Transplantation, University of Milan, 20122 Milan, Italy
11. Centro Domino per l'Autismo, Universita' Cattolica Brescia, 20139 Milan, Italy; luigi.croce@unicatt.it
12. National Research Council of Italy, Institute of Organic Synthesis and Photoreactivity (ISOF), 40129 Bologna, Italy; carla.ferreri@isof.cnr.it
13. Department of Obstetrics and Gynecology, Fondazione IRCCS Ca' Granda Ospedale Maggiore Policlinico, 20122 Milan, Italy; niccologiovannini@hotmail.com
14. Autism Research Unit, Villa Santa Maria Foundation, 22038 Tavernerio, Italy; enzo.grossi51@gmail.com
15. Adult Autism Centre DSM ASL Città di Torino, 10138 Turin, Italy; rokel2003@libero.it
16. RAISE Lab, Foundation COME Collaboration, 65121 Pescara, Italy; manzotti.andrea68@gmail.com
17. Medical Genetics Laboratories, Department of Translational Research and of New Surgical and Medical Technologies, University of Pisa, 56126 Pisa, Italy; lucia.migliore@unipi.it (L.M.); andrea.stoccoro@unipi.it (A.S.)
18. Associazione Spazio Asperger ONLUS, Centro Clinico CuoreMenteLab, 00141 Rome, Italy; davide.moscone@cuorementelab.it
19. Neonatal Intensive Care Unit, Department of Surgical Sciences, Puericulture Institute and Neonatal Section, Azienda Ospedaliera Universitaria, 09100 Cagliari, Italy; mumike153@gmail.com (M.M.); vafanos@tin.it (V.F.)
20. Child Neurology and Psychiatry Unit, IRCCS ISNB, S. Orsola-Malpighi Hospital, Department of Medical and Surgical Sciences, University of Bologna, 40138 Bologna, Italy; antonia.parmeggiani@unibo.it
21. Milan Institute for health Care and Advanced Learning, 20124 Milano, Italy; dott.pasinvalentina@gmail.com
22. Università Telematica Pegaso, 80134 Napoli, Italy; monicaperotti@virgilio.it
23. Department of Biomedical Sciences, University of Cagliari, 09042 Cagliari, Italy; cristina.piras@unica.it
24. Unione Italiana Lotta alla Distrofia Muscolare UILDM, 35100 Padova, Italy; dr.tizianatoso@gmail.com
25. Institute of Biomembranes, Bioenergetics and Molecular Biotechnologies (IBIOM), National Research Council of Italy, 70126 Bari, Italy; r.vacca@ibiom.cnr.it
26. Institute for Biomedical Research and Innovation (IRIB), National Research Council of Italy, 98164 Messina, Italy; david.vagni@irib.cnr.it
27. Department of Pediatric, Moscati Hospital, 81031 Aversa, Italy; dotvendemmia@libero.it
28. Scientific Institute, IRCCS Eugenio Medea, Via Don Luigi Monza 20, 23842 Bosisio Parini, Italy; laura.villa@lanostrafamiglia.it
29. Neonatal Intensive Care Unit, Azienda Ospedaliera Universitaria, 09042 Cagliari, Italy

Citation: Panisi, C.; Guerini, F.R.; Abruzzo, P.M.; Balzola, F.; Biava, P.M.; Bolotta, A.; Brunero, M.; Burgio, E.; Chiara, A.; Clerici, M.; et al. Autism Spectrum Disorder from the Womb to Adulthood: Suggestions for a Paradigm Shift. *J. Pers. Med.* **2021**, *11*, 70. https://doi.org/10.3390/jpm11020070

Academic Editor: Elizabeth B. Torres
Received: 5 December 2020
Accepted: 19 January 2021
Published: 25 January 2021

Publisher's Note: MDPI stays neutral with regard to jurisdictional claims in published maps and institutional affiliations.

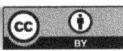

Copyright: © 2021 by the authors. Licensee MDPI, Basel, Switzerland. This article is an open access article distributed under the terms and conditions of the Creative Commons Attribution (CC BY) license (https://creativecommons.org/licenses/by/4.0/).

* Correspondence: cristina.panisi01@universitadipavia.it (C.P.); fguerini@dongnocchi.it (F.R.G.); marina.marini@unibo.it (M.M.); Tel.: +39-333-4616502(C.P.)

Abstract: The wide spectrum of unique needs and strengths of Autism Spectrum Disorders (ASD) is a challenge for the worldwide healthcare system. With the plethora of information from research, a common thread is required to conceptualize an exhaustive pathogenetic paradigm. The epidemiological and clinical findings in ASD cannot be explained by the traditional linear genetic model, hence the need to move towards a more fluid conception, integrating genetics, environment, and epigenetics as a whole. The embryo-fetal period and the first two years of life (the so-called 'First 1000 Days') are the crucial time window for neurodevelopment. In particular, the interplay and the vicious loop between immune activation, gut dysbiosis, and mitochondrial impairment/oxidative stress significantly affects neurodevelopment during pregnancy and undermines the health of ASD people throughout life. Consequently, the most effective intervention in ASD is expected by primary prevention aimed at pregnancy and at early control of the main effector molecular pathways. We will reason here on a comprehensive and exhaustive pathogenetic paradigm in ASD, viewed not just as a theoretical issue, but as a tool to provide suggestions for effective preventive strategies and personalized, dynamic (from womb to adulthood), systemic, and interdisciplinary healthcare approach.

Keywords: Autism Spectrum Disorder (ASD); pathogenesis; prevention; epigenetics; immune activation; gut dysbiosis; mitochondrial impairment; oxidative stress; metabolomics; machine learning

1. Introduction

Autism spectrum disorder (ASD) is currently diagnosed on the basis of the clinical assessment of behavioral features [1], and is characterized by a wide spectrum of presentation and frequent association with medical comorbidities [2]. People with ASD show an increasing endophenotypic complexity suggesting a systemic disorder with multilevel health needs. The manifold phenotype and the dramatic increase in prevalence in the last decades—currently 1:54 in the USA [3]—require the conceptualization of a pathogenic paradigm able to explain both the clinical and the epidemiological findings.

In research, there is a need to take stock of the situation in two main issues. First, effective strategies aimed at reversing the course of prevalence are urgently required. Secondly, evidence concerning the biological complexity of ASD requests a coherent translation into the healthcare model and the clinical practice.

Fetal neural programming, occurring during the ontogenesis, and early live neuroplasticity are crucial events in neurodevelopment and identify the time window of maximum brain opportunity in the embryo-fetal period and in the first two years of life (the so-called 'First 1000 Days') [4].

In this period, exogenous insults and changes in the maternal milieu are expected to have the maximum disturbing effect and lifelong consequences on health. The dynamic molecular machinery involved in the ontogenesis transforms early life inputs into long-term programmatic outcomes, influencing the enzymatic and immuno-neuroendocrine pathways, which define the basis of the homeostasis during intrauterine and postnatal life [5].

Several biological abnormalities are involved in the etiopathogenesis of ASD. Our study reviews the main topics addressed in biological research—genetics, epigenetics, environmental issues, immunogenetics, immunology, microbiology, and metabolic and electrophysiological impairments—with particular reference to their synergistic interactions and their links with the clinical phenotype. Therefore, a dynamic (from the womb to adulthood) perspective and the concept of multisystem disorder seems to be the most plausible framework for the study of neurodevelopmental disorders.

Machine learning will also be proposed as the most suitable method consistent with the biological complexity of ASD.

The healthcare model currently aimed at supporting autistic people is quite fragmented, and often fails to integrate psychoeducational and biological interventions. Drawing a 'fil rouge'—from the genome to the effector biochemical pathways, and from them to the multifaceted clinical phenotype in ASD—seems to be the premise for the long looked-for breakthrough in clinical practice.

The conceptualization of the pathogenetic paradigm is proposed as the premise for necessary changes in clinical practice, highlighting a common thread, from primary prevention in pregnancy, to the healthcare model addressed, to the complex lifelong needs of people with ASD.

According to a dynamic and systemic perspective, neurodevelopmental disorders seem to be better depicted by a trajectory of possible and, at least partially, modifiable frailty rather than by a static picture resulting from a fixed and inevitable brain damage.

Consequently, this paradigm encourages the best efforts for effective primary prevention strategies addressed to the 'First 1000 Days', in order to turn this time window into the best chance for human health. At the same time, evidence concerning numerous biologic abnormalities in ASD provide suggestions for some already feasible adaptations of the healthcare model addressed to autistic people.

1.1. Clinical Features of People with ASD: Not Only a Behavioral Disorder

Autism is an early onset—and in most cases, lifelong—neurodevelopmental disorder, currently diagnosed through standardized behavioral testing between the ages of 2 and 4 years. The broad range of presentation accounts for the standard definition of Autism Spectrum Disorder (ASD) as an alteration in social communication and interaction across multiple contexts, in conjunction with repetitive behaviors, a restricted pattern of interests, and sensory abnormalities [1]. In the most common early onset pattern, atypical features in vocal–verbal language and socio-communicative development are detected in the first 12 months, and failure in acquiring skills is reported. However, some children initially show a period of apparently typical development, followed by a loss of previously established skills. The phenomenon is termed 'regression' and typically occurs between 15 and 30 months of age, with a mean of 21 months [6]. There is no consensus regarding the prevalence of regression within autism and other ASD diagnoses [6]. The phenomenon certainly needs to be better understood as well as defined by symptoms, including regressive events that may occur later in life. A wide range of different combinations of behavioral characteristics, beside numerous emotional and cognitive features, contribute to the wide variability of the clinical picture and to the varied impact on major life areas [7] and quality of life [8]. The presence and severity of intellectual impairment is the most relevant characteristic influencing the outcome [9]. The wide range of combinations within the spectrum poses the difficult challenge in responding to this variegated group of people, endowed with unique needs and unique strengths, in a personalized manner.

The striking increase in prevalence in the last decades [3] demands deep reflection and evaluation. Increased awareness of the disorder and evolving diagnostic criteria have undoubtedly contributed to this result. On the other hand, a broad scientific consensus converges on the concept that change in diagnostic criteria is not enough to explain such a significant rise in the occurrence of ASD [10], and environmental factors are supposed to fill the gap.

Currently, many areas are engaged in research on ASD, including genetics, epigenetics, immunogenetics, immunology, microbiology, and biochemistry—the last, in particular, with regard to mitochondrial impairment and oxidative stress. As the submerged part of an iceberg, the biological complexity underlying behavioral abnormalities accounts for a systemic disorder, not limited to the brain, but involving other organs and systems as well. This is consistent with the frequent occurrence of comorbidities [2]—in particular, immunologic [11] and GI abnormalities [12]. They are not just ancillary characteristics, but rather the result of a systemic disorder, impacting on the health of people with ASD and requiring to be properly faced.

1.2. Genetics, Epigenetics, and Environment: Who's to Blame?

Quantitative genetic studies, including twin studies, have suggested a role of genetics in ASD [13–15].

The genetic architecture in ASD is complex: Hundreds of gene variants, identified using genome-wide association studies (GWAS) [16] and copy number variants (CNVs) [17,18], as well as de novo mutations in non-coding regions, affecting transcriptional and posttranscriptional regulation [19], have been found associated with ASD. None of the individual genes identified to date account for more than 1% of ASD cases. Though many candidate gene-disease associations were suggested, molecular investigations have yet to identify a consistent association of ASD with biological markers [20]. This also reflects the complexity of the ASD phenotype, which overlaps with several neurodevelopmental/psychiatric disorders [21,22] and involves numerous non-neurological comorbidities [23]. ASD susceptibility evaluation using family-based genetic studies is now accompanied by population-based epidemiologic studies, which pointed to the role of environmental factors [24] in explaining the rate of non-genetic variance [25,26].

Altogether, the genetic data suggest the need to depart from a linear genetic model. The striking increase in prevalence in ASD makes implausible the hypothesis of an increasing number of monogenic diseases, and for this reason an epigenetic model has been suggested. Epigenetics refers to changes in gene regulatory mechanisms that are independent from alteration of the underlying DNA coding sequences [27]. Epigenetics tunes gene expression based on changes in the cellular environment, in an adaptive and predictive sense, predisposing cellular molecular equipment aimed at homeostasis [28].

DNA methylation, histone tails modifications, and non-coding RNAs (i.e., microRNAs) are the most commonly studied epigenetic effectors [29]. They influence the establishment of gene transcription patterns through multiple mechanisms, regulating the accessibility of genomic loci to a large number of regulatory factors (i.e., transcription factors, enhancers, silencers) as well as the expression/stability of mRNAs. Changes in epigenetic signatures during the developmental stage finely tune the differentiation of precursor cells into their specific mature state [30]. Therefore, epigenetic markers display a relatively high level of plasticity during periods of cellular differentiation, including neurodevelopment [31]. Since the embryo-fetal period and the first two years of life represent the temporal window of maximum neuroplasticity, environmental exposure occurring during pregnancy is expected to lead to long-term modifications in epigenetic patterns and to have maximum impact on neurodevelopment [32].

Synaptic plasticity and chromatin binding are the most important biological functions emerged from the analysis of hundreds of genes associated with ASD [33,34]. The enrichment of chromatin binding genes associated with ASD suggests their potential role in the etiology of this disorder. Rett syndrome is a well-known example of a genetic neurodevelopmental condition that includes autistic behavior, and whose etiology is directly related to epigenetic regulation. Rett syndrome is caused by mutations in MECP2 gene, which encodes for the methylated DNA binding protein MeCP2 [35], causing either the activation or the inhibition of gene transcription, depending on the genomic context [36]. Interestingly, beside Rett syndrome, also Fragile X syndrome, Angelman syndrome, and Beckwith-Wiedemann syndrome, are all caused by epigenetic dysregulation, and each one shares a phenotypic overlap with ASD [37,38].

Many epigenetic markers are differentially expressed in ASD. A recent systematic review by Dall'Aglio et al. [39] analyzed studies on epigenetic modifications found in ASD and other neurodevelopmental disorders, focusing on global and gene-specific methylation, as well as on epigenome-wide DNA methylation (EWAS) in brain and blood tissues, and on histone modifications in the brain tissue. A number of shared biological pathways of relevance to neurodevelopment, were reported by independent EWAS, including synaptic and neuronal processes, immune response processes, brain development, and cellular differentiation [39]. In candidate genes studies, the identification of differential DNA methylation in the proximity of three genes—PRRT1, C11orf21/TSPAN32, and OR2L13—

was confirmed in multiple independent analyses. The function of these genes is still little known, anyway, they are probably involved in neurological disorders. Analogously, histone modifications (methylation and acetylation) in association with ASD were consistently found in the gene coding for H3K27 in the cerebellum and cortex of autistic patients [39].

Moreover, several studies evidenced that short non-coding RNAs, such as microRNAs, are differentially expressed in brain tissue [40] as well as in the periphery (i.e., serum/plasma, saliva) [41,42] of ASD patients compared to typically developing controls.

Therefore, moving from a traditional paradigm focusing exclusively on a linear genetic model, epidemiological and clinical findings in ASD suggest the conceptualization of a model integrating genetics (hardware), environment (information), and epigenetics (software). Thus, the focus is shifted from the highly phylogenetically conserved human DNA sequence to the misleading way by which the stored instructions are read. The following paragraph explains in detail the epigenetic paradigm.

1.3. Widening the Gaze: From ASD to the Epidemiological Transition of NCDs

The plausibility of the epigenetic paradigm regarding ASD is supported by a wider phenomenon involving numerous non-communicable diseases and disorders (NCDs), which showed a striking increase in prevalence in the last decades, in parallel with neurodevelopmental disorders [43,44].

We are witnessing a profound epidemiological transformation, which concerns immuno-allergic, inflammatory, metabolic, chronic-degenerative, neurodevelopmental, neuropsychiatric, neurodegenerative, and neoplastic diseases [45]. The phenomenon as a whole suggests a common pathogenetic model. As the time frame is too short for genetic changes to have had an appreciable impact on the prevalence of the abovementioned diseases, it is more plausible that the increase reflects changes in gene programming (epigenetics) induced by a growing number of environmental stressors during critical time windows in development [46,47]. This interpretation is the basis of the theory of the epigenetic/embryo-fetal origin of diseases (DOHaD—Developmental Origin of Health and Diseases) [48]. The DOHaD theory suggests a systemic perspective, in order to explain the reasons of the profound transformation of human health and disease. The theory takes into account the impact of environmental stressors on reactive–adaptive and predictive epigenetic modifications (fetal programming) in cell and tissue differentiation, with long-term consequences on individual development and transgenerational impact. Imperfect correspondence between embryo-fetal programming and postnatal environment (that is, mismatch between the prenatal prediction and the actual postnatal environment) might also contribute to the onset of NCDs [45].

Beyond the definition, in the essence, epigenetics means a new systemic genome model which places the DNA sequence in the center of a dynamic, fluid, unitary, and interactive molecular network, involving the inner and the outside environment [28]. The genome is proposed as a fluid system, made up of the DNA sequence, the responsive histone structure, and information from the surrounding environment, in the broader sense of the term. The epigenome—as a software switching genes on and off [28]—tunes the matching between information coming from outside (environment) and information codified by millions of years in the DNA (that is the hardware). Through mechanisms modulating the programming, transcription, and translation of the message, the epigenome orchestrates the "natural genetic engineering" for the structural and functional changes of cells and tissues, contributing to the evolving phenotype, both in physiological and pathological situations [49].

During pregnancy, the placenta "translates" the external environment to the fetus through epigenetic molecular adaptations, in particular by modifying the methylation of imprinted genes, which act as key controllers for fetal development. A wide range of maternal inputs (i.e., over and under-nutrition, smoking, drug and alcohol intake, environmental toxicants, infections, and stress) can induce changes in placental physiology, ranging from alterations in placental morphology and weight, to the more subtle changes in placental gene expression, involving important signals directed towards the fetus [50]. Imprinted genes display a variety of cellular roles, such as cell cycle control, ion channels, protein synthesis/degradation, and nutrient transport. They are maximally expressed during the prenatal and/or postnatal period, and predominate in tissues governing resource allocation (brain, placenta, adipose tissue, and pancreatic beta cells). Consistently with these findings, a substantial number of imprinted genes are critical for placental function and normal fetal growth and development [51].

Epigenetic programming is highly sensitive to changes in the cellular environment. Indeed, epigenetic regulation is a widely utilized adaptive mechanism, allowing cells to maintain a favorable metabolic status under different conditions, including exposure to physiological substances (e.g., hormones, neurotransmitters, or growth-regulation factors), xenobiotics (e.g., pollutants, toxic chemicals), or even infectious agents (e.g., bacteria or viruses, fungi or parasites) [52]. Epigenetic regulation may facilitate adaptation to changes in the cellular environment through stable alterations of cellular phenotype, potentially resulting in progressive differentiation and maturation during fetal and possibly postnatal development [53].

During the ontogenesis, epigenetic software is programmed in an adaptive and predictive sense, driving cellular differentiation and setting up the metabolic, immunologic, and endocrine pathways for lifelong homeostasis. As far as neurodevelopment is concerned, the 'First 1000 Days' are the period in which neuroplasticity is most lively, for neuronal proliferation, differentiation, migration, synaptogenesis, and pruning. In other words, this is the most vulnerable time window for the wiring of individual connectome [54,55]. For the same reasons, the 'First 1000 Days' offer a unique opportunity to provide the best setting for the best lifelong trajectory in neurodevelopment [4].

1.4. Maternal Immune Response in Neurodevelopmental Disorders

Mounting evidence suggests the existence of a link between immune function and neurodevelopmental disorders [56,57]. The immune system plays a fundamental role in brain development, both in the physiological and in the pathological trajectories. Immune response impacts on neuronal migration, synaptogenesis, white matter organization, and remodeling (pruning), that is, on some of the crucial steps of neural network development [58–61]. Therefore, it is not surprising that an abnormal immune response might influence neurodevelopment [57].

Maternal infections and autoimmune diseases provided the first demonstration of the possible impact of immune response on brain development during pregnancy.

In the period following the Rubella outbreak of the 1960s, ASD was diagnosed in 5–10% of children born to mothers that were infected by the Rubella virus [62,63]. The prevalence of ASD and schizophrenia was found to be significantly higher in children exposed to infection than in those not exposed [64]. Afterwards, similar correlations were found with influenza, measles, mumps, varicella, and polio epidemics [65]. Several prospective studies confirmed the association between maternal viral infections and the onset of neuropsychiatric disorders in children, and over the years the list lengthened with the inclusion of bacterial infections (tonsillitis, sinusitis, pneumonia) and parasites (Toxoplasma gondii) [64,66]. A Swedish research found a 30% increase in ASD when the mothers were hospitalized for viral infections during pregnancy, and a significant association was found between viral infections and ASD in offspring [67].

The recent outbreak of the Zika virus raises concerns about the increased risk of ASD, given the high number of babies born with microcephaly, structural brain abnormalities, and neurological alterations in regions affected by the virus [68]. Similar concerns relate to the current SARS-CoV-2 pandemic, since maternal cytokine storm (mainly, IL-6 and IL-17) and intra-uterine inflammation might interfere with the fetal epigenetic machinery [69]. In fact, beside the vertical transmission, maternal infections may impact fetal neurodevelopment through the maternal immune activation (MIA). Several studies reported an increased risk of ASD in the offspring of mothers with active autoimmune diseases during pregnancy. Particularly, exposure to psoriasis, systemic lupus erythematosus, rheumatic arthritis, and autoimmune thyroid disease could significantly increase the risk of ASD [70–72]. In mothers with autoimmune diseases a pathogenetic effect is suggested for maternal autoantibodies and cytokines crossing placental barrier and the brain–blood barrier [73,74]. A meta-analysis showed that maternal autoimmune diseases were associated with a 34% increased risk of ASD in offspring, compared with the control groups [75]. Correlations between postnatally ASD-specific maternal autoantibodies and maternal metabolic conditions during gestation have been reported [76].

Neuroinflammation could damage fetal brain tissue and exert adverse influence on brain development [56]. Cytokines, activated T cells, autoantibodies, and microglia—the macrophages of the central nervous system—exert a pivotal role on antigen presence and cytokines production [56,77].

Maternal autoantibodies targeted against the Folate Receptor α (FRα) deserve to be mentioned in this section. Folate plays a key role in neural development during the embryo-fetal period and the early years of life [78]. Folate plays an essential role in cell-to-cell communication and in purine, methylation, and redox metabolic pathways. Since its concentration in the brain is several folds higher than in plasma, it relies on active import mechanisms, based on FRα, to cross both placental and brain barriers, but the transport is inhibited by anti-FRα autoantibodies (FRAAs) [79]. Animal models demonstrated a correlation between the exposition of pregnant dams to FRAAs and ASD-like features in the offspring [79]. This is consistent with the finding of more severe ASD symptoms in autistic children from mothers positive for FRAAs [78]. The relevance of this mechanism is confirmed further in life by the higher prevalence of FRAAs in children with ASD compared to controls, since FRAAs are detected in 58–76% of children with ASD [80] and blood titers of these autoantibodies correlate with folate levels in the cerebrospinal fluid [80,81]. This discovery of the impairment of folate metabolism has recently led to encouraging treatment opportunities [80].

1.5. Interplay between Epigenetics and Immune Response in Neurodevelopment

Currently, several studies are addressed to maternal immune activation (MIA) and compounding evidence supports a role for MIA at specific time frames in the pathogenesis of ASD. Several risk factors and pathogenetic pathways may converge and influence fetal brain development through the intra-uterine immune environment. It has been hypothesized that MIA is an effector arm of the epigenetic dysregulation, and a pivotal role of maternal immune response has been suggested for the downstream behavioral phenotypes observed in ASD and other neuropsychiatric disorders in offspring [82–84].

Animal studies show a link between MIA and ASD-like outcomes in offspring; correlation is shown with numerous environmental factors, including infections, toxin exposures, maternal stress, and maternal obesity, all of which impact maternal immune response [85]. Therefore, immune activation is a common pathogenetic pathway triggered by numerous infectious agents and environmental factors [86]. Changes in gestational immune environment are correlated with increased risk for neurodevelopmental disorders [87]. This is consistent with the increased risk for ASD and schizophrenia in the offspring of mothers with autoimmunity [88], allergy, asthma [89], maternal acute stress [90], depression [91], and exposure to environmental pollutants [92]—all conditions correlated with the activation of the maternal immune response [66,93].

Animal models made it possible to study the effects of MIA on fetal brain development [83,94–96]. DNA hypomethylation and hypermethylation have both been observed in these animal models and in their offspring. Animal models for MIA are obtained by in utero injection of a synthetic double-stranded mimetic of the RNA molecule (polyinosinic:polycytidylic acid-polyI:C), which triggers an immune response of both innate and adaptive immune regulatory mechanisms in the pregnant rodent female, through the activation of TLR3 and subsequent expression of interferon-1 [97]. The offspring of pregnant mice treated with Poly I:C display all the core deficits associated with ASD [98].

Tang et al. used the MIA mouse model and demonstrated significant epigenetic changes in response to polyI:C exposure in utero. Specifically, the study found that differential abnormalities in histone acetylation occurred in the cortex and hippocampus in response to polyI:C exposure; a majority of the observed abnormalities occurred in juvenile mice, prior to the onset of behavioral phenotypes; genes in the glutamate receptor signaling pathway were particularly associated with epigenetic changes in response to prenatal immune activation [94]. MIA was found to dysregulate key aspects of fetal brain gene expression that are highly relevant to the pathophysiology affecting ASD. For instance, transcriptional and translational programs, that are downstream targets of highly ASD-penetrant FMR1 and CHD8 genes, are heavily affected by MIA [83], as well as genes relevant for gamma-aminobutyric acidergic differentiation and signaling and Wnt signaling (that is, a group of signal transduction pathways that regulate crucial aspects of cell fate determination, cell migration, cell polarity, neural patterning, and organogenesis during embryonic development) [96]. Moreover, the changes were markedly influenced by the precise timing of prenatal immune activation, since the early and late gestational windows clearly differed in terms of the altered methylation pattern they induced. Particularly, late prenatal immune activation induced methylation changes in genes critical for GABAergic cell development and functions [96].

Non-coding RNAs, such as microRNAs, represent a further epigenetic mechanism. They resulted in being differentially expressed in brain tissue [40] and in the periphery (i.e., serum/plasma, saliva) [41] in ASD subjects compared to controls. Notably, most differences in ASD patients involved immune response and protein synthesis regulation [99].

Abnormalities in immune response in ASD brain are also reported [96]. Genome-wide transcriptomic studies demonstrate that ASD brains are enriched for "activated" M2 microglial genes and innate immune response-related genes [100]. Nardone et al. determined the presence of many dysregulated CpGs in two cortical regions in brain tissue from people with ASD: Brodmann area 10 (BA10) and Brodmann area 24 (BA24) [101]. Findings in BA10 showed very significant enrichment for genomic areas responsible for immune functions among the hypomethylated CpGs, whereas genes related to synaptic membrane were enriched among hypermethylated CpGs. An inverse correlation links gene expression and DNA methylation. It was reported that genes such as C1Q, C3, ITGB2 (C3R), and TNF-α, important molecules in immune response and implicated also in synaptic pruning and microglial cell specification, are among the hypomethylated (and overexpressed) genes in ASD [101].

Several studies have focused on the association between human leukocyte antigen (HLA) genes and the risk of ASD [102,103]. HLA is a complex genetic region with a pivotal role in some autoimmune diseases and in response towards infection, but also in fetal tolerization. Therefore, HLA impact in ASD may not be ascribed to a single specific HLA gene, but rather to a series of different genes which may intervene at different stages. HLA class I molecules were demonstrated to play a complex and significant role in brain development [104].

HLA class I and HLA-G interact with killer immunoglobulin like receptors (KIR) expressed by natural killer (NK) cells, the effectors of innate immunity. During pregnancy, NK are highly concentrated within the uterine mucosa, at the fetal/maternal interface. NK may be activated or inhibited through the interaction of specific activating and/or inhibitory KIR with HLA-C and non-classical HLA-G molecules on fetal trophoblast. KIR–HLA interaction has been largely demonstrated to play an important role in pregnancy complications. Notably, complications of pregnancy are, together with autoimmunity, very common in ASD mothers [88,105–109].

A skewing of the KIR-HLA complexes, in which activating molecules prevail, was shown in ASD children [110] and their mothers [103]. Moreover, an important role has been suggested for non-classical HLA-G polymorphisms in ASD mothers [111] as well as in women with recurrent spontaneous abortions [112,113]. The generation of a poorly tolerogenic fetal environment results in MIA and may be associated with pregnancy complications as well as with ASD development [111,114]. KIR genes may be regulated by switch on/switch off epigenetic signaling; DNA methylation plays a crucial role in shaping the KIR repertoire, supporting the importance of epigenetic mechanisms as regulatory switches in the immune system early in life [115].

The driving mediators of MIA-associated ASD pathology are most likely elevations in maternal cytokines and chemokines. Therefore, MIA can be considered as a 'priming condition' for neurodevelopmental disorders, a susceptibility background on which further risk factors can then be established [116], behaving as 'multiple hits' with synergistic effects. These can be infectious agents, any kind of immune stimulation and exposure to toxic substances (particularly, alcohol and drugs) [93]. In MIA murine model, a pro-inflammatory phenotype of T lymphocytes and myeloid cells are common findings [66,87]. Confirming the close relationship and interdependence between the nervous system and the immune system [117], reconstitution of MIA offspring with normal bone marrow improves repetitive behaviors and anxiety, suggesting that some MIA phenotypes are causally related to immune and nervous system imbalances [65].

Elevations of cytokines and chemokines in both maternal serum and amniotic fluid are associated with an increased risk of ASD [118]. Maternal cytokines that cross the placenta, such as IL-6 and IL-4, may alter fetal epigenetic machinery [82]. Particularly, IL-6 and IL-17 may favor inflammation either at the placenta or directly in the developing fetal brain [119]. IL-6 has been identified as a key intermediary of the pathways whereby MIA alters fetal brain development. Maternal IL-6 crossing the placenta can directly affect the development of the fetal brain [120], and animal models show that IL-6 is critical for mediating the behavioral and transcriptional changes in the offspring [121]. Recently, the importance of T helper 17 (Th17) lymphocytes and IL-17a effector cytokine in inducing autism-like phenotypes, acting on the developing fetal brain, has been demonstrated. It is likely that some environmental factors related to the onset of ASD follow this pathway. Structural similarities found between IL-17 family-cytokines and the neurotrophins (proteins regulating survival, development, and functions of neurons) suggest that the IL17Ra pathway has a physiological function in the fetal and adult brain [119].

Maternal cytokines and chemokines, in addition to their activity as immune mediators, are involved in migration of neuronal precursors, neuronal maintenance, synaptic pruning, and neuroplasticity [122]. Sotgiu et al. recently reviewed the numerous abnormalities in immune pathways involved in embryo-fetal neurodevelopment and linked to ASD. The authors confirmed MIA as a predisposing condition for a multiple-step frailty in brain growth, suggesting the importance of care addressed to women before and during pregnancy [123].

Discussion of immune response in pregnancy cannot leave out the microbiota. During pregnancy, one should consider both the placental microbiota and the maternal microbiota. As for the former, for a long time fetus and placenta have been considered to be sterile. Currently, mounting evidence suggests the occurrence of a fetal microbial colonization; moreover, placenta has been reported to harbor a specific microbiota [124]. Even though the 'sterile womb' paradigm is debated and results are conflicting, there is convincing evidence that the composition of the maternal microbiota may impact on fetal immune development prior to delivery. The maternal microbiota may exert an indirect effect on the fetus via maternal factors such as maternal immune responses, microbial metabolites that cross the placenta [125,126], or more indirectly via factors that may mediate epigenetic programming in the fetus, such as diet [127] or stress [128], which also affect the maternal microbiota. The gut and vaginal maternal microbiota changes with gestation [129,130]. It is plausible that these changes have an adaptive value. It has been suggested that they allow the fetus to derive energy from the mother's blood more efficiently [129] and promote immune tolerance in the mother [131]. Studies on animal models suggest that transient changes in maternal microbiota during pregnancy drive fetal immune programming [125].

At present, available knowledge about the fine and delicate tuning of placental immune response and the numerous immune mechanisms impacting fetal neurodevelopment, put the maternal immune response in the spotlight, as one of the most relevant issues to be addressed in the care of pregnant mothers.

1.6. Take Home Message from the Interplay between MIA and Epigenetics in Pregnancy

The striking amount of studies showing the impact of maternal immune response on neurodevelopment and the interplay between MIA and the epigenetic machinery requires best efforts to support maternal well-being during pregnancy, as a crucial determinant of lifelong physical and mental health of humans [132]. In fact, the complex molecular machinery described above represents an adaptive response to events occurring during pregnancy, constituting predictable and potentially preventable events.

Numerous risk and protective factors have been demonstrated and linked to the onset of ASD in the offspring, providing suggestions for clinical practice. Emberti Gialloreti et al. recently reviewed risk and protective factors related to the occurrence of ASD in offspring, highlighting the need of care for maternal diet, nutraceutical supplementation, prevention and treatment of metabolic abnormalities, prevention from toxicant exposure, and numerous other factors linked with an increased risk for ASD [133]. Therefore, nutritional state and proper nutraceutical supplementation during pregnancy should be warranted and carefully monitored (enough/not too much). In fact a 'U shaped' relationship is reported between maternal multivitamin supplementation frequency and ASD occurrence in offspring [134]. As far the evaluation of risk factors, it is underscored that most exposure models from epidemiological literature may suffer from oversimplification in case the effects of single factors are evaluated separately. In fact, findings in animal models suggest that the study of synergistic–rather than single-effects seems to be correct [135], a concept raising a relevant methodological issue, consistent with the complexity of biological systems. Many studies assessed the frequency of potential environmental risk factors in pregnancy related to ASD in offspring. Grossi et al. highlight explicit associational schemes between risk factors and ASD outcome through a multivariable modeling of data using Auto Contractive Map artificial neural network (ANN). The authors suggest that ANN might highlight hidden trends and associations among the variables, thus revealing the risk profiles related to ASD [136]. Notably, the graph of the study shows that cesarean section, absence of breastfeeding, and early antibiotic use are close to the autism node. All these risk factors are linked to changes in the neonatal bacterial substrate, confirming the importance of the appropriate composition of the early microbial communities for the neurodevelopment [136]. A recent meta-analysis confirms the cesarean delivery as a risk factor for ASD [137]. As a whole, these findings encourage best efforts in favoring vaginal delivery; in case of C-section, the early restoring of a microbial balance should be a priority in primary prevention. In addition to the review of pregnancy risk factors, the methodological question is the most notable feature of the study by Grossi et al. [136]. The study provides relevant suggestions for both research and clinical practice, in order to build an ever-increasing database, which might be continuously fed by clinical, laboratory, and instrumental records. A future personalized application of machine learning systems in neurodevelopmental disorders might be the development of predictive models to track different risk profiles in the lifelong neuropsychiatric trajectory.

1.7. Neuroinflammation and Gut-Brain Axis in People with ASD

Findings pointing to cerebral inflammation in autoptic brains of autistic people aroused considerable interest pertaining to the involvement of the immune response in ASD [138]. The study showed neuroinflammatory activity in the cerebral cortex, white substance and cerebellum of autistic subjects. Furthermore, marked activation of microglia and astroglia was demonstrated [138].

More recently, growing evidence supported a role for dysregulated neuroinflammation. In a recent review by Matta et al., numerous studies are reported concerning reactive microglia and astrocytes, altered glial structure and function, cytokine profiles, and gut immune dysfunction in ASD people and animal models. The authors conclude that a strong evidence for nervous system interaction with immune pathways in ASD is demonstrated [139].

The association between ASD and immunological imbalance concerns both innate immunity and the specific response of T lymphocytes, with a shift towards a Th1-type pattern and prevalence of pro-inflammatory cytokines; increase of B lymphocytes, NK cells, and dendritic cells; and different patterns in the expression of surface markers [102]. Findings in brain tissue from individuals with ASD do not allow to establish the period in which neuroinflammation started and the ways whereby it interfered with the formation of the neural networks. Another open question concerns the sequence of events. It is not clear to what extent neuroinflammation is a contributory effector mechanism of neurodevelopmental disorder or rather whether immunological abnormalities are secondary to a systemic and complex biochemical/metabolic imbalance. In other words, to what extent neuroinflammation in ASD is primary (causal) or secondary (reactive)? As the immune system is primarily involved in tissue repair and homeostatic processes, immune findings in ASD could represent compensatory responses to dysfunctional network activities and cellular stress. Therefore, studies addressing the temporal dynamics of brain dysfunction with age and whether they are linked to the ongoing and dynamic immune changes are important areas for future research.

Taken together, findings about immune abnormalities support evidence of an early and ongoing dysfunction in the peripheral immune system and the brain of individuals with ASD [140].

Severe immune alterations are demonstrated also in the non-ASD siblings of ASD patients [141]. In particular, in both autistic children and their siblings, increase in the production of IL-10 and a skewing toward earlier, less differentiated lymphocyte subpopulations were showed. Notably, IL-10 has strong anti-inflammatory properties: This finding could thus be interpreted as a way whereby the immune system tries to counterbalance the inflammation present both in autistic patients and in their unaffected siblings [141].

Neuroinflammation in ASD shows crucial links with the gut–brain axis, a bidirectional neurohumoral communication system [142] orchestrated by the microbiota [143].

Research on gut–brain interactions in the last decades has provided evidence about the close interactions between the gut-associated immune system, enteric nervous system, and gut endocrine system [144]. Animal models and studies in humans seem to support a relationship between the gut microbiota and brain development; moreover, functions and studies on microbiomes have triggered great interest from professionals and the National Institute of Mental Health. The simultaneous presence of oxidative stress, mitochondrial dysfunction, and inflammation has been often observed in the brain of ASD people, which were correlated also with ASD symptoms, thus suggesting an inter-relationship between these anomalies [145].

1.8. Microbiome in the Crosstalk between Immune System, Gut, and Brain

A rapidly increasing amount of evidence point to host–microbe interactions at virtually all levels of complexity, ranging from direct cell-to-cell communication to extensive systemic signaling, involving various organs and systems, and starting even before conception. The traditional idea of an auxiliary function of the friendly 'intestinal flora? has shifted in the recent years to the assignment of the role of orchestra conductor in the psycho-neuro-endocrine system. Consistently, a growing number of research projects have been launched worldwide concerning this topic. The human microbiota consists of the 10–100 trillion symbiotic microbial cells harbored by each person. The set of genes of the microbiota is collectively known as the microbiome [146], encoding for at least 100 times more genes than our genome [147] and suggesting the 'question 'who is harboring whom?'. As a whole, each individual should be considered an "holobiont harboring an hologenome'. The GI tract is the most heavily inhabited organ with micro-organisms, harboring a huge diversity with more than 500 bacterial species. [147].

Dysbiosis—the state of unbalanced microbial communities—and its impact on the early shaping of the immune system has been demonstrated in the pathogenesis of a wide range of diseases [148–150], including neurodevelopmental and psychiatric conditions [151,152].

Colonization of the infant's gut represents the de novo assembly of a microbial community [153]. The infant's gut microbiota is established after birth, within the first three years. After childbirth, the neonate and microbiota develop in an orchestrated way. There is a strong influence on infant microbiota of maternal gut microbiota during pregnancy. Maternal gut strains have been shown to be more persistent in the infant gut and ecologically better adapted compared to those from other sources [154].

The early establishment of gut microbiota is affected by several factors such as delivery mode (cesarean delivery vs. vaginal delivery), breast milk vs. formula feeding, antibiotic usage, timing of the introduction of solid foods, and cessation of milk feeding [155].

Early life perturbations of the developing gut microbiota can impact neurodevelopment and potentially lead to adverse mental health outcomes later in life. Borre et al. compare the parallel early development of the intestinal microbiota and the nervous system. The concept of parallel and interacting microbial-neural critical windows opens new avenues for developing novel microbiota-based preventive and therapeutic interventions in early life [156].

Animal studies suggest that the microbiota may regulate microglia maturation and function by activating immune signaling pathways, the release of cytokines, and other inflammatory molecules [102,140,157], including inflammasomes activation [158].

Other mechanisms are involved in the communication between gut microbiota and the brain and have been proposed to explain the possible role of microbiota in neurodevelopmental disorders: direct activation of the vagus nerve [151]; production or alteration of neurotransmitters, including serotonin [151]; production of toxins [159]; aberrations in fermentation processes or products [160,161]; and dysbiosis-induced breakdown in gut integrity [162,163]. Interacting molecules may be produced by the gut microbiota, such as short-chain fatty acids (SCFA), which may cause the increase of gut permeability and then act on a range of other systems. SCFA may also affect epigenetic modifications. In particular, butyrate is a histone deacetylase inhibitor, contributing to the attainment of a less relaxed chromatin conformation. This small molecule can cross the blood–brain barrier and impacts epigenetic machineries in the brain [164]. Butyrate exerts anti-inflammatory and neuroprotective effects [165] and attenuates social behavior deficits in autism models [166]. It supports mitochondrial function, stimulating oxidative phosphorylation and fatty acid oxidation [167]. Its concentration has been shown to be reduced in fecal samples from ASD children [168], and its supplementation had a positive effect in lymphoblastoid cell lines derived from children with ASD under physiological stress, and, in particular, in cell lines with underlying mitochondrial dysfunction [169], providing interesting insight into links between ASD, mitochondria, and gut microbial communities and the possible clinical application. Microbiota may also mediate the availability of S-methyl-Methionine (SAM), the donor of methyl groups for DNA methylation (reviewed by Kaur et al., [170]) by producing folate for generation of SAM. Folate is generally obtained by appropriate diet. Notably, a key enzyme for regulating the availability of folate for either DNA synthesis or DNA methylation is methylenetetrahydrofolate reductase (MTHFR). Remarkably, some MTHFR genetic polymorphisms have been associated with ASD risk [134,171]. This is another example of how inadequate diet or gut dysbiosis may mimic genetic defects promoting the onset of ASD.

In addition, stress, as signaled via the hypothalamic-pituitary-adrenal (HPA) axis, is one top-down mechanism that may affect gut microbiota [172]. As far as the composition of microbiota in ASD subjects, conflicting results are reported by numerous studies. A shift in the microbiota in autistic individuals compared with controls was reported and included elevated Clostridia spp., Bacteriodetes, and Desulfovibrio spp. in ASD [160,163,173,174]. The complexity of community relationships within the microbiota and the current challenges on microbiota data analysis—risk of false positive discovery—might explain the wide variability of findings [175].

In addition to dysbiosis, compared to controls, ASD patients show an increase in gut permeability (the so-called 'leaky gut'), a finding supported by numerous studies showing alterations in gut barrier in ASD [176]. Among factors concurring to the diagnosis of gut permeability, loss of zonulin is one of the most important. As a 'biological door to inflammation' [177], higher levels of plasmatic zonulin are reported in people with ASD than controls [178].

Fecal calprotectin might be a useful biomarker in the assessment of gut–brain axis involvement. It identifies people with gut inflammation [179] and correlation between calprotectin levels and main domains of the autism diagnostic interview-revised (ADI-R) has been shown [180].

In addition to theoretical issues and laboratory data, clinical findings also support the hypothesis of a pivotal role of the gut–brain axis, immune activation, and microbiota in ASD. A high rate of allergy and gastrointestinal (GI) symptoms are reported in people with ASD [2]. Diarrhea, constipation, vomiting, reflux, abdominal pain/discomfort, flatus, and unusually foul-smelling stools are more frequent than in healthy controls [181,182]. In a large sample of adult ASD patients, GI complaints are reported in 21% of patients [183]. A meta-analysis from 'Pediatrics' confirmed a higher prevalence of GI symptoms among children with ASD compared with control children [12].

Abnormalities in GI motility and intestinal permeability have been reported [175]. Studies report a wide range of variability of GI symptoms, from 9 to 70% [184]. Differences in studied populations and different assessment tools for symptoms might explain these differences. What is not in dispute is that GI disturbances represent a topical issue among health needs for people with ASD, with severe impacts on wellbeing and variably contributing to behavioral abnormalities [182,184]. Difficulties in the recognition of pain in people with intellectual disability make it easy to underdiagnose pain and discomfort. The risk of underestimation is even higher in ASD, due to difficulties in communication and abnormalities in the neural integration of somatosensory afferent inputs. For this reason, proper tools for GI symptoms and pain evaluation should be systematically included in clinical assessment and parallel monitoring of behavioral symptoms and of any other ailment should be provided [185]. In fact, inputs from the internal environment, as well the influence of external environmental factors, represent antecedent events preceding behaviors, and requiring evaluation according to the behavioral functional analysis methodology [186]. Therefore, a preliminary medical assessment for the identification and treatment of pathophysiological comorbidities of ASD is expected to achieve optimal outcomes according to a multidisciplinary approach [187,188].

Neuroinflammation in ASD might have links with epilepsy [189]. In a population-register study, a quarter of children with ASD had epilepsy, in contrast to 1.5% of population-based controls [190]. Berg et al. report a prevalence of 7% among children with no motor deficits or severe intellectual disability, compared to 42% in people with motor deficits and severe intellectual disability [191]. The above-mentioned evidence of immunologic abnormalities in ASD suggests a possible role of neuroinflammation in the pathogenesis of epilepsy [192]. Inflammatory mediators, such as IL-1β (imterleukin-1 β), TNF (tumor necrosis factor), HMGB1 (high mobility group box 1), TGF- β (transforming growth factor-β), and prostaglandins, can alter neuronal, glial, and blood–brain barrier functions by activating transcriptional and post-translational mechanisms in brain cells. Furthermore, a role by brain mast cells in neuroinflammation is reported, and the involvement of these cells is hypothesized in the pathogenesis of epilepsy in a group of ASD people [192]. The impact of immune abnormalities on the occurrence of epilepsy in ASD is of utmost interest and deserves further study.

In summary, clinical findings confirm the pivotal role of immune abnormalities and the gut–brain axis in ASD. Therefore, expertise in medical assessment for comorbidities should be warranted.

1.9. Mitochondria/Oxidative Stress . . . and the 'Bad Trio'

Increasing and converging evidence suggests a pivotal role for mitochondria in neurodevelopmental disorders [193]. Beside the generation of energy in the form of ATP, mitochondria encompass a wide array of functions, ranging from metabolite and redox signaling to the regulation of nuclear gene expression and epigenetics [194–196].

Notably, energy provided by mitochondria oils the epigenetic machinery, allowing selective access to specific DNA sequences by regulating the various levels of chromatin structure, from nucleosomes to chromatin fibers [197]. In neurodevelopment, mitochondria emerged as key regulators of neural stem cell fate decisions, impacting neurogenesis both in neurodevelopment and in adult mature brains [198].

Many studies have shown that mitochondrial dysfunction contributes to placental pathology underpinning gestational disorders [199]. Mitochondria are sensitive stress targets in the placental microenvironment. Placenta development and a successful pregnancy are under a precise oxygen-dependent control of trophoblast migration/invasion [200] and maternal immunity [201], since a regulatory loop might exist between trophoblasts and maternal immune cell subsets, promoting the harmonious maternal–fetal crosstalk [202]. Persistent low oxygen pressure, leading to failed trophoblast invasion, promotes inadequate spiral artery remodeling, a characteristic of preeclampsia [200].

Mitochondrial dysfunction and oxidative stress are two major and interconnected metabolic abnormalities associated with ASD, since oxidative stress causes mitochondrial dysfunction and dysfunctional mitochondria produce Reactive Oxygen Species (ROS) [203]. Thus, mitochondrial dysfunction can be at the same time the cause and/or the result of oxidative stress. In fact, excessive free radical production can lead to mitochondrial damage, and, in turn, the damaged mitochondria are prone to release increased amounts of ROS; this process is maximized in what has been termed 'Ros-induced ROS release' [204], but is also a common evidence in pathologies characterized by chronic oxidative stress. Under this perspective, the primary source of mitochondrial dysfunction may be oxidative stress itself, which in turn may originate from manifold ROS-generating processes, including chronic inflammation [205], metabolic dysfunctions [206,207], exposure to heavy metals [208], and other environmental issues. Indeed, several environmental factors, including toxicants, microbiome metabolites, and an oxidized microenvironment are shown to modulate mitochondrial function in ASD tissues [203,209]. Both intrinsic and extrinsic stressors can impact the interplay by increasing ROS and/or reducing mitochondrial function, thus prompting the establishment of a vicious circle [203,210]. Numerous genetic abnormalities are associated with mitochondrial dysfunction in ASD [210–212]. Furthermore, several environmental factors, including toxicants, microbiome metabolites, and an oxidized microenvironment are shown to modulate mitochondrial function in ASD tissues [203,209].

Traditional biomarkers commonly used to identify mitochondrial dysfunction include lactate, pyruvate, alanine, and creatine kinase. A meta-analysis by Rossignol and Frye demonstrated that ASD was associated with higher levels in lactate, pyruvate, lactate-to-pyruvate ratio, alanine, creatine kinase, ammonia, and aspartate aminotransferase (AST), and in decreased carnitine concentration [210,211]. Among mitochondrial dysfunctions, abnormal activity of the electron transport chain (ETC) enzyme complexes—the machinery fueling energy production—is reported in ASD children. Notably, these abnormalities are found in mucosal samples taken both from rectum and caecum and might explain gut dysmotility, higher sensitivity to oxidative stress, and abnormal functioning of enterocytes [213]. Oxidative stress results in damaged proteins and lipids in the cell, and consequently impacts enterocyte function. Therefore, dysbiosis (that is imbalance in microbial metabolites) and oxidative stress might explain abnormal mitochondrial function in the caecum [213]. Additionally, gut dysmotility caused by mitochondrial dysfunction would explain constipation observed in ASD and other GI symptoms [210,211]. Interestingly, GI problems similar to those of autistic children have also been noted in children affected by genetic syndromes in which mitochondrial dysfunctions play a central role in the etiopathogenesis and having ASD among clinical features, such as Down syndrome and Rett syndrome [210,211,214], again suggesting a link between mitochondrial dysfunction, GI problems, and microbiota in ASD people.

Numerous studies have reported biomarkers representing abnormalities in fatty acid metabolism in ASD [215]. ASD patients from Saudi Arabia were found to have elevations in saturated fatty acids and depressions in polyunsaturated fatty acids as compared to age-matched controls [216], consistently with previous results suggesting polyunsaturated fatty acids, carnitine, and lactate as biomarkers of brain energy in children with ASD [217].

Children with ASD show low levels of the reduced form of glutathione (GSH), the major intracellular antioxidant responsible for maintaining redox homeostasis and for reducing ROS in the cytosol and mitochondria [215]. In addition, more than 30% of ASD patients have elevations in acyl-carnitine, a cofactor carrying long-chain and very-long-chain fatty-acids into the mitochondria. Interestingly, this same pattern of GSH and acyl-carnitine abnormalities found in children with ASD [218] was also found in the rodent propionic acid (PPA) model of ASD [219]—PPA being one of the most important microbial metabolites believed to cause systematic mitochondrial dysfunction [218]—thus providing further evidence for the association among PPA, mitochondrial dysfunction, and ASD [220].

This is consistent with finding of higher levels of PPA in fecal microbiota and metabolome of children with ASD [161]. Balance in microbial metabolites (enough/not too much) significantly impacts mitochondrial functions and influences GI activity. For example, butyrate is converted into acetyl-CoA, which then is utilized in the citric cycle for NADH production. NADH, on the other hand, is utilized by the mitochondrial ETC complex I, the main site of entrance of reducing equivalents into the ETC, crucial for respiration and energy production, and the main site of ROS production when it is dysfunctional [213].

Therefore, at least part of the effects of dysbiosis on neurodevelopment and GI involvement in ASD seems to be mediated by mitochondrial impairment [210,211,221].

There are at least three possible connections between the GI tract and mitochondrial abnormalities in ASD [222]. First, mitochondrial dysfunction itself could result in GI dysfunction [223]. Secondly, there are common exposures to environmental stressors that are associated with ASD that can affect both the mitochondria and the GI tract: pesticides and heavy metals [224], exposure to drugs such as acetaminophen [225] or antibiotics, either during pregnancy [226] or early in life [227–229], and more likely the exposure to all these and other factors taken together [230]. Another plausible connection between gut and mitochondrial impairment is represented by cell wall agents (i.e., lipopolysaccharide, [231]) or metabolites from enteric bacteria [160,221] and their effect on mitochondrial functions.

Among bacterial metabolites, the aforesaid propionate (PPA) is seemingly the Short Chain Fatty Acid mostly produced by micro-organisms prevalent in the gut of ASD patients, including Clostridia spp., Bacteriodetes, and Desulfovibrio spp. in ASD [163,173,174,232]. Furthermore, propionate is universally used as a preservative in processed food due to its anti-fungal characteristics [233].

Maternal PPA exposure is one of the possible mechanisms interfering with neural wiring during early stages of embryonic neural development and leading to a shift of glial cells towards an inflammatory pattern [233]. Notably, the exposition of human fetal-derived neural stem cells to PPA resulted in downregulation of PTEN expression and a consequent differentiation shift to gliosis and neuroinflammation [233].

Another important point involving fatty acids is the organizational and functional integrity of the cellular membrane. The membrane phospholipids—the building blocks of membranes—are characterized by a balance in the diverse fatty acid residues (saturated, monounsaturated, and polyunsaturated), which varies from tissue to tissue in the same body [234], and is a condition-sine-qua-non for the normal health of the cells. An inadequate dietary intake, poor availability of specific enzymes, and oxidative stress alter the membrane lipids and the functionality of embedded proteins. Indeed, impairment in function of erythrocyte membrane proteins and lipids have been demonstrated as consequences of increased oxidative stress in ASD. A very significant reduction of Na+/K+-ATPase activity (-66%, $p < 0.0001$), a reduction of erythrocyte membrane fluidity, and alteration in erythrocyte fatty acid membrane profile (increase in monounsaturated fatty acids, decrease in EPA and DHA-ω3 with a consequent increase in ω6/ω3 ratio) were found in ASD children compared to controls [235]. Interestingly, some clinical features of children with ASD (in particular, hyperactivity and cognitive development) showed correlation with some parameters of the lipidomic profile (saturated fatty acids, arachidonic acid) and membrane fluidity, highlighting a pathogenetic key-point in ASD and a potential use of membrane lipidome profile as useful biomarker for personalized therapeutic supplementation [236]. The importance of a correct membrane concentration of DHA-ω3 was confirmed in a study of membrane lipidome, showing that the decrease of this fatty acid is not attributable to dietary differences between healthy and diseased children, as evaluated by food questionnaire indicating, for example, fish consumption. Moreover, statistical significance test of the ROC curve for DHA (p value = 0.0424) with a cut-off value at 4.08% gave a significant odds ratio corresponding to 6.23 (p value = 0.017; IC 95%: [1.3956–27.8412]), indicating that individuals with values of DHA < 4.08% (cut-off) have a probability of being autistic 6.23 times higher than those with DHA > 4.08%. [237]. A correlation between the reduced membrane fluidity and striking morphological abnormalities in the shape of red blood cells was also demonstrated [238], where most of the biological alterations resulted to be ascribed to oxidative stress [238]. As noticed by the authors, findings suggest a plausible dysfunction of erythrocytes in tissue oxygenation [238]. If so, a chronic state of hypoxia in tissues is expected to worsen the oxidative stress, contributing to a vicious loop and ongoing deterioration of health in ASD people.

A relevant increase in oxidative damage markers was further confirmed by protein glycation, oxidation, and nitration adducts and amino acid metabolome in plasma and urine of children with ASD [239]. Findings in people with ASD could be well described by the striking definition of 'pervasive oxidative stress'. Rossignol and Frye reviewed interplay between oxidative stress and immune activation [210,211]. The increase in the gene expression of IL6 and the stress protein HSP70i was demonstrated in ASD children [240]. Furthermore, the study of the protein expression of the antioxidant enzyme family of peroxiredoxins showed a significant increase in plasma of ASD children, supporting the link between oxidative stress and neuroinflammation in ASD [240]. The interplay between mitochondria and immune response represent a complex bidirectional system involving numerous mechanisms. Metabolic pathways such as tricarboxylic acid cycle, oxidative phosphorylation, and fatty acid oxidation impact macrophage polarization and T cell differentiation; mitochondrial ROS control immune cell transcription, metabolism, and NLRP3-mediated inflammation; mitochondrial DNA can be released from mitochondria into the cytosol and activate the NLRP3 inflammasome and production of IL-1β and IL-18 [241]. Findings are consistent with the aforesaid immune abnormalities in ASD [140], including higher inflammasome activation (in particular, NLRP3 activation) than in controls [158].

In summary, the literature findings reported above suggest in ASD the existence of a vicious circle between dysbiosis, immune response, and mitochondrial dysfunction/oxidative stress, a 'bad trio' which might start from the embryo-fetal period, impact neurodevelopment, and even might cause a progressive worsening of the neurological disorder. In fact, the same 'bad trio', if not stopped, might go on and contribute to the worsening of the systemic disorder through all life.

The interplay between the main effector pathways causing the ASD phenotype and acting during the embryo-fetal stage all through life is illustrated in Figure 1.

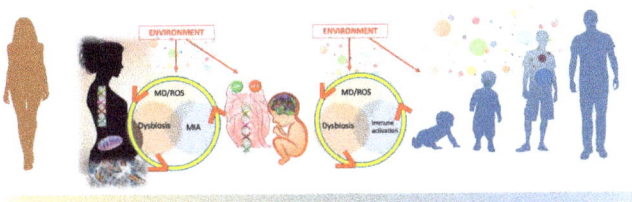

Figure 1. Interplay between the main determinants of Autism Spectrum Disorder. MD, Mitochondrial dysfunction; MIA, Maternal Immune Activation; ROS, Reactive Oxygen Species. In the new individual, matrilinear transfer of mitochondria and microbiota adds to the genetic information stored in the maternal and paternal germinal cells. Environmental factors as a whole may directly affect the epigenetic machinery, as it happens with heavy metals, or may influence the interconnected molecular pathways involved in the 'bad trio' (mitochondrial dysfunction (MT)/oxidative stress (ROS) plus maternal immune activation (MIA) plus dysbiosis). The 'omniscient placenta' [51] drives the metabolic and epigenetic regulation of fetal programming, hence influencing the ontogenesis and the crucial early stages of neurodevelopment. The epigenome— similarly to a software switching genes on and off [29]—is programmed in an adaptive and predictive sense by the intrauterine and cellular microenvironment, setting the limits of physiological adaptations to the postnatal environment and influencing the lifelong risk for diseases [43]. After birth, the same mechanisms involving environmental factors and the 'bad trio' are at play, and may continue to undermine human health lifelong. As for neurodevelopment, the maximum impact occurs in the first two years of life, which is the crucial time window for brain wiring.

1.10. Metabolomics: A Promising 'Meaningful Web' Describing a Biochemical Fingerprint

The evolving spectrum of clinical presentation and of laboratory findings in ASD offers the challenge to understand and respond to similarly evolving health needs of a growing number of people. Therefore, ASD is a paradigmatic situation urgently requiring a dynamic and personalized approach. The availability of suitable diagnostic tools capable of grasping the biological complexity seems to be the starting point.

Currently, sensitive, specific and early biomarkers are not available to detect ASD before the clinical onset of behavioral abnormalities; therefore, professionals have at their disposal only standardized clinical tools—interviews and behavioral scales—to make diagnosis. In the complex biological scenario beyond behavior in ASD, so distant from a linear model of 'a symptom, a biomarker', metabolomics opens new interesting avenues. In fact, it describes the individual molecular phenotype and allows monitoring of its changes over time.

The molecular phenotype closely reflects the result of interplay between genomics, transcriptomics, proteomics, environmental factors, and gut microbiota [242], and might thus be associated with the type and degree of the behavioral/cognitive impairment and with functional neuroimaging [243].

Metabolomic approach represents the phenotype by the detection and the representation of metabolites, low-molecular-weight end-products of cellular metabolic pathways, which in turn are influenced by genetic and nongenetic factors. Metabolomics allows the systematic identification and quantification of the global collection of all metabolites, namely the metabolome, recognizable either in biological fluids (e.g., urine) or in tissues [244]. Metabolites can be identified and characterized in their elemental composition, molecular charge and mass, stereochemical orientation, and order of atoms [245]. Metabolomics accurately identifies metabolites involved in the same pathway as well as the metabolic network shaped by nodes (metabolites) and their interactions (scale-free network models) [246]. In other words, metabolomics provides a personalized description through a 'meaningful web', representing the individual biochemical fingerprint.

Today, high throughput technologies like proton nuclear magnetic resonance (1H NMR) spectroscopy, liquid chromatography, and gas chromatography coupled with mass spectrometry (LCMS and GCMS, respectively) and further sophisticated analytical methods are outstanding tools that allow researchers to accurately explore the metabolome and its variations over time in various perinatal conditions involved in ASD etiology, for example perturbations of the gut–brain axis, due to gut dysbiosis, increased intestinal permeability, inflammation, oxidative stress/mitochondrial dysfunction, well representing the 'juniper bush' of ASD [242].

This means a great opportunity to search for new highly sensitive and specific biomarkers for early diagnosis of ASD, risk of regressive ASD [247], and further disorders in neurodevelopment and psychopathology, up to adulthood [248,249]. In a similar way to that of other neuropsychiatric disorders, ASD may be closely associated with several maternal, fetal, and perinatal epigenetic factors that influence brain development and maturation [250,251]. Metabolomics allows the discovery of biomarkers for an early diagnosis and the monitoring of fetal and perinatal programming [252]. The detection of biochemical patterns suggestive for the vicious circle within the 'bad trio'—involving maternal dysbiosis, immune activation, and oxidative stress—could allow early and personalized interventions during pregnancy, with the possibility to closely monitor the effects of treatment through changes in metabolomic profile. The urinary metabolome of ASD children has been extensively studied, and some studies have been devoted also to the analysis of the plasma metabolome. Mussap et al. reviewed most relevant metabolic pathways and key metabolites implicated in ASD. The most discriminant metabolites in ASD were involved in amino acid metabolism, antioxidant status, nicotinic acid metabolism, and mitochondrial function [253]. Most of the studies in ASD reported abnormalities in gut bacterial-derived compounds and in intermediary compounds of the Krebs cycle [254–256], confirming the aforesaid pivotal role of oxidative stress, microbiota, and abnormalities in mitochondrial function in ASD [203,210,211,221].

In summary, metabolomics approach opens very promising perspectives in diagnosis and follow-up in ASD, allowing an early understanding of the individual ASD patient, with evolving and unique needs.

2. New Methods for Renewed Diagnostic Tools: Machine Learning System in EEG

ASD is associated with abnormal neural connectivity [257–262], and some abnormalities in brain development might be already detectable at birth.

Currently, neural connectivity is a theoretical construct that is hard to be measured, but research in network science and time series analysis suggests that the neural network structure—a marker of neural activity—is measurable by EEG [263].

Hustler et al. described three types of cortical construction abnormalities in ASD (a) alterations to columnar structure that have significant implications for the organization of cortical circuits and connectivity; (b) alterations to synaptic spines on individual cortical units that may underlie specific types of connectional changes; and (c) alterations within the cortical sub-plate—a region that plays a role in proper cortical development and in regulating interregional communication in the mature brain [264]. The relevant involvement of the cerebral cortex in the substantial alteration of the cortical circuitry explains the unique pattern of deficits and strengths that characterize cognitive function. These findings make electroencephalography (EEG) a plausible useful tool to detect these abnormalities.

The EEG can measure neural activity and may provide a useful tool to early detect ASD in children, thus allowing the opportunity for early intervention. The potential usefulness of EEG in ASD has been reviewed almost ten years ago [259], in order to examine evidence for the utility of three methods of EEG signal analysis in the ASD diagnosis and subtype delineation. All studies identified significant differences between ASD and non-ASD subjects, confirming the presence of specific EEG abnormalities. However, due to the high heterogeneity in the results, findings could not be generalized and none of the methods, if taken alone, has been proposed as a new diagnostic tool [259].

Recent studies on this topic open new avenues and might represent a turning point for the early diagnosis of ASD based on the analysis of electroencephalographic tracing (EEG) supported by new adaptive artificial systems (ANNs). It was hypothesized that the atypical organization of the cerebral cortex in ASD might translate into an EEG signature detectable through powerful analytical systems such as ANNs [265–267].

Using particularly advanced machine learning systems, it has been possible to build a software able to distinguish almost perfectly the EEG from subjects with ASD from those of neurotypical controls or with different neuropsychiatric disorders.

The new system, called MS-ROM/I-FAST, belongs to the family of systems developed by the Semeion Research Centre. MS-ROM/I-FAST is a new and complex algorithm for the blind classification of the original EEG trace of each subject, through the recording and analysis of a few minutes of their EEG without any preliminary pre-processing [266]. A first pilot study assessed the discriminatory power of the methodology in distinguishing subjects with ASD from neurotypical controls. After the MS-ROM/I-FAST pre-processing, the overall predictive capacity of the different automatic learning systems in distinguishing autistic cases from the controls was constantly 100% [266]. Notably, these results were obtained at different times and in separate experiments performed on the same training and testing subsets. Furthermore, the similarities between the weight matrices of the neural networks measured with appropriate algorithms were not influenced by the age of the subjects, suggesting that the networks read invariant characteristics related to the disconnection signature in the brain [266]. The results of the pilot study have been recently confirmed. EEG data from ASD children were compared with EEG from controls affected by other neuropsychiatric disorders. With the training-testing protocol, the overall predictive capacity of the machine learning system used to distinguish between ASD and controls was constantly over 90% [267]. Along this research area, it would be of utmost interest to extend EEG tracks recording within the first year of life, with the purpose to use this technique as a specific, sensitive, non-invasive, non-expensive tool for early detection of the signature predictive for ASD. The potential usefulness of this methodology might be extended to find out possible different EEG signature in ASD subgroups with different onset (early/regressive autism) and different phenotypes. Furthermore, this tool could monitor the evolution of EEG abnormalities, find hidden links with clinical and laboratory biomarkers and monitor the effect of therapeutic interventions.

3. Discussion

Big data from basic research performed over the last ten years need to be translated into clinical practice. Knowledge about the increasing complexity in the etiopathogenetic pathways of diseases is the premise for the suitable adaptation of strategies for prevention, diagnosis, and treatment according to the evolving health needs of the population. In neurodevelopmental disorders—in particular in ASD—most current statistical methods do not seem suitable to study not linear, complex, and fuzzy interactions involving genome, epigenome, environmental factors, and nervous–immune-endocrine interplay, and to do so along a pathway that starts even before conception.

Most of available studies have been designed on the basis of methods developed in the first half of the past century, when the scenario was dominated by acute infectious diseases and linear models apparently succeeded in describing the phenomenon. In the last century, the epidemiological scenario has profoundly and dramatically changed, and traditional methods seem to be able to assess only a very small part of the phenomena, if compared to their intrinsic complexity. Consequently, the development of methods consistent with the complexity of the phenomena seems to be the premise for personalized medicine, able to avoid the narrow view of what is well known, leaving out the broader horizon of the unknown.

ASD is a paradigmatic condition within the epidemiological transition occurring in the last decades toward the prevalence of non-communicable disorders and diseases, which requires a plausible pathogenetic mechanism able to explain both epidemiological and clinical findings, that is the combination of the striking increase in prevalence with the multifaceted phenotype. The need for a scientific consensus on a comprehensive paradigm is much more than a theoretical issue. In fact, the coherent translation of the pathogenetic model into clinical practice is the premise for effective preventive strategies and comprehensive answers to the complex health needs of ASD people.

In order to do so, a dynamic and systemic perspective—starting with the care for women's health before pregnancy occurs—seems to be the most promising approach to face this major public health issue, both for current needs and in the future perspective.

Embryo-fetal brain development is profoundly influenced by numerous interacting environmental factors, named 'exposome' as a whole. Both in intrauterine and in post-natal life, environmental information converges on three major interacting/overlapping pathways: dysbiosis, mitochondrial impairment/oxidative stress, and immune activation (named MIA during pregnancy). As a whole, the three above-mentioned effector pathways—as a pathogenetic trio-impact epigenetic machinery. The matrilinear transmission of both microbiota and mitochondria [268,269] further enforces the need for effective women's health programs, which are even more important in the presence of known risk factors for ASD, such as of the occurrence of neurodevelopmental disorders in previous offspring.

Prenatal factors are expected to influence development more than all others, and are not limited to brain alone. The multifaceted phenotype and endophenotype found in ASD people are consistent with a multisystemic and evolving disorder. In fact, metabolomic data concerning the 'bad trio' are representative of a systemic and evolving inflammatory syndrome. Findings seem consistent with the high prevalence of obesity in ASD and obesity-related disorders (type 2 diabetes mellitus, hypertension, hyperlipidemia, and nonalcoholic fatty liver disease/nonalcoholic steatohepatitis) [270] and of metabolic syndrome in psychiatric disorders [271]. The issue is of the utmost importance and presents fundamental healthcare issues. Among the environmental factors, diet is in the spotlight as a fundamental tool for prevention and care in ASD. In particular, considering the frequent eating disorders [272] and use of edible reinforcers in educational intervention [273], the risk of nutritional imbalance seems to be high in people with ASD and could—at least in part—explain findings consistent with metabolic syndrome and oxidative stress [206,207,270]. Therefore, converging evidence suggests to include nutritional experts in the panel of professionals in the healthcare model addressed to people with ASD. In fact, besides the energy intake, diet impacts microbiota [274,275], immune function [276], and lipidic cell membrane profile [277]. In other words, diet impacts most of the fundamental pathogenetic mechanisms demonstrated in ASD. Consistently, an individualized and monitored dietetic plan may play a central role in preventive strategies and care in ASD.

The proposal of a personalized nutrition plan is only an example aimed at glimpsing the value of interdisciplinary models for clinical cooperation. Suitable diagnostic and monitoring tools are required to grasp the whole complexity of ASD and translate it into concise information, easy to be used by clinicians. Currently, metabolomics and machine learning systems seem to be respectively the 'materials and methods' of a foreseen tremendous impact both in research and clinical practice in the field of ASD.

The dynamic trajectory of individual brain connectome and the 'multiple-hits' frailty encourage best efforts to attain the early detection of any biological abnormality potentially impacting neurodevelopment, in order to restore the best balance as soon as possible, hopefully in the period of maximum neuroplasticity. Waiting for the availability of metabolomics in clinical practice in the next years, the question arises as to how to start transferring current biological knowledge into medical advice as soon as possible. The involvement and relevance of the gut–brain axis, dysbiosis, increase in intestinal permeability, and abnormal lipidic composition in cell membranes in ASD provide some useful suggestions for the adaptation of clinical assessment. Biomarkers such as fecal calprotectin, zonulin, erythrocyte fat profile, analysis of the microbiota, and of fecal microbial metabolites (mainly, lactate, propionic acid, and butyrate) characterize subgroups of people requiring specific diagnostic and therapeutic interventions addressed to expected and easily testable organic needs. The inclusion of such biomarkers in clinical trials is expected to contribute to the proper evaluation of the effectiveness of interventions on behavioral outcomes.

4. Conclusions

Current hardships experienced by autistic people and by their families, and the expected worsening of their troubles in the coming years are telling all of us that it is not time to rest on laurels.

Perhaps it is time to stop a while and take stock of the situation, in order to prevent the plethora of data by the literature that might take the scientific community away from people's needs instead of match them.

Therefore, 'joining the dots' seems to be the premise for a comprehensive and effective healthcare model addressed to ASD people. A multidisciplinary approach and interdisciplinary sharing of knowledge seem to be the only way to answer their complex, evolving, and unique needs. Figure 2 suggests an interdisciplinary healthcare model that is coherent with the contents of this review and comprehensive of their translation into clinical practice.

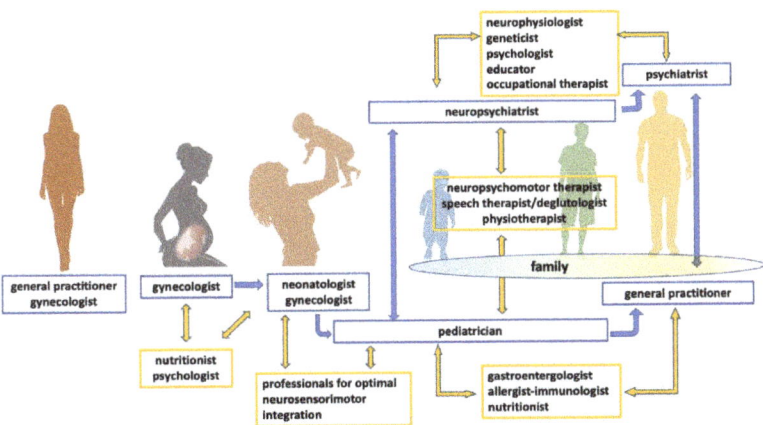

Figure 2. Mother's health is the premise for a successful intrauterine life. During pregnancy, the gynecologist ensures the best control of risk factors and the enhancement of protective factors, largely related to proper maternal nutrition and supplementation. After birth, the baby–mother dyad is supported by the neonatologist–gynecologist duo. The qualified support for the well-being of the mother is integrated by neonatal care, which includes the best conditions of neurosensory-motor integration aimed at the physiological postnatal neuronal wiring. With variable times and modalities—mostly depending on the outcome of the pregnancy and the characteristics of the newborn—the child's care is subsequently entrusted to the pediatrician, who provides suggestions for a positive physical and neuro-psychomotor development. In case of clinical abnormalities, the pediatrician prompts diagnostic pathways and early interdisciplinary interventions based on clinical and laboratory findings. In the event of motor and/or socio-communicative abnormalities, the pediatrician consults the neuropsychiatrist, who shall consider whether to include standardized diagnostic tools for ASD in the clinical assessment. The diagnosis of ASD is followed by further diagnostic evaluations (neurophysiologist, geneticist), functional assessment, and timely psychoeducational evidence-based interventions. The neuropsychiatrist orchestrates the cooperation of numerous professionals (psychologist, educator, occupational therapist), monitors the results, and tailors the supports according to the evolving skills and needs. In parallel with the neuropsychiatrist, the pediatrician prompts a clinical assessment according to the expected comorbidities in ASD, involving in particular gastroenterologist, allergist-immunologist, and nutritionist. A close collaboration with the neuropsychiatrist allows the best integration of physical and neuropsychiatric aspects, involving at the same time professionals linked both to the pediatric and the neuropsychiatric sides. The transition towards adulthood requires a handover on both levels of intervention, from the pediatrician to the general practitioner for the biological features, and from the neuropsychiatrist to the psychiatrist for the psychiatric sphere. The connection between the two levels (body and mind) is maintained even in adulthood. It should be noted that the above described structured model acquires worth and meaning if it places in the center the person with ASD and his/her family, as the main stakeholders of a flexible model, able to adapt to the evolving needs and favoring the highest level of feasible well-being.

The author panel proposing the review well represents the 'spectrum' of expertise required for advice in the evaluation of ASD patients. In other words, the heterogeneity of their expertise represents the implementation of the need for developing 'skills in communication and social interaction' that is the intriguing challenge that ASD is posing to all of us.

Author Contributions: Conceptualization, C.P. (Cristina Panisi), E.B., F.R.G., V.F., M.M. (Marina Marini); methodology, C.P. (Cristina Piras), F.R.G.; writing—original draft preparation, C.P. (Cristina Panisi), L.M (Lucia Migliore), F.R.G., M.M. (Marina Marini), V.F.; writing—review and editing, C.P. (Cristina Piras), M.M. (Marina Marini), A.S., F.R.G., P.M.A., F.B., P.M.B., A.B., M.B., E.B., A.C., M.C., L.C., C.F., V.F., N.G., A.G., E.G., R.K., A.M., L.M. (Lucio Moderato), L.M. (Lucia Migliore)., D.M., M.M. (Michele Mussap), V.P., M.P., A.P., C.P. (Cristina Piras), P.P., M.S., T.T., R.A.V., D.V., S.V., L.V.,A.P. All authors have read and agreed to the published version of the manuscript.

Funding: This research received no external funding.

Institutional Review Board Statement: Not applicable.

Informed Consent Statement: Not applicable.

Data Availability Statement: Not applicable.

Acknowledgments: We express our appreciation to all persons with ASD and to their families, who have taught us so much.

Conflicts of Interest: The authors declare no conflict of interest.

References

1. American Psychiatric Association. *Diagnostic and Statistical Manual of Mental Disorders (DSM-5)*, 5th ed.; American Psychiatric Association: Arlington, VA, USA, 2013.
2. Aldinger, K.A.; Lane, C.J.; Veenstra-VanderWeele, J.; Levitt, P. Patterns of Risk for Multiple Co-Occurring Medical Conditions Replicate Across Distinct Cohorts of Children with Autism Spectrum Disorder. *Autism. Res.* **2015**, *8*, 771–781. [CrossRef]
3. Maenner, M.J.; Shaw, K.A.; Baio, J.; Washington, A.; Patrick, M.; DiRienzo, M.; Christensen, D.L.; Wiggins, L.D.; Pettygrove, S.; Andrews, J.G.; et al. Prevalence of Autism Spectrum Disorder Among Children Aged 8 Years Autism and Developmental Disabilities Monitoring Network, 11 Sites, United States, 2016. *MMWR Surveill. Summ.* **2020**, *69*, 1–12. [CrossRef]
4. Cusick, S.E.; Georgieff, M.K. The Role of Nutrition in Brain Development: The Golden Opportunity of the "First 1000 Days". *J. Pediatr.* **2016**, *175*, 16–21. [CrossRef] [PubMed]
5. Fleming, T.P.; Velazquez, M.A.; Eckert, J.J. Embryos, DOHaD and David Barker. *J. Dev. Orig. Health Dis.* **2015**, *6*, 377–383. [CrossRef] [PubMed]
6. Barger, B.D.; Campbell, J.M.; McDonough, J.D. Prevalence and onset of regression within autism spectrum disorders: A meta-analytic review. *J. Autism Dev. Disord.* **2013**, *43*, 817–828. [CrossRef]
7. Bölte, S.; Mahdi, S.; de Vries, P.J.; Granlund, M.; Robison, J.E.; Shulman, C.; Swedo, S.; Tonge, B.; Wong, V.; Zwaigenbaum, L.; et al. The Gestalt of functioning in autism spectrum disorder: Results of the international conference to develop final consensus International Classification of Functioning, Disability and Health core sets. *Autism* **2019**, *23*, 449–467. [CrossRef] [PubMed]
8. Jonsson, U.; Alaie, I.; Löfgren Wilteus, A.; Zander, E.; Marschik, P.B.; Coghill, D.; Bölte, S. Annual Research Review: Quality of life and childhood mental and behavioural disorders a critical review of the research. *J. Child Psychol. Psychiatry* **2017**, *58*, 439–469. [CrossRef] [PubMed]
9. Holwerda, A.; van der Klink, J.J.; Groothoff, J.W.; Brouwer, S. Predictors for work participation in individuals with an Autism spectrum disorder: A systematic review. *J. Occup. Rehabil.* **2012**, *22*, 333–352. [CrossRef]
10. Hertz-Picciotto, I.; Delwiche, L. The rise in autism and the role of age at diagnosis. *Epidemiology* **2009**, *20*, 84–90. [CrossRef]
11. Mead, J.; Ashwood, P. Evidence supporting an altered immune response in ASD. *Immunol. Lett.* **2015**, *163*, 49–55. [CrossRef]
12. McElhanon, B.O.; McCracken, C.; Karpen, S.; Sharp, W.G. Gastrointestinal symptoms in autism spectrum disorder: A meta-analysis. *Pediatrics* **2014**, *133*, 872–883. [CrossRef] [PubMed]
13. Sandin, S.; Lichtenstein, P.; Kuja-Halkola, R.; Larsson, H.; Hultman, C.M.; Reichenberg, A. The familial risk of autism. *JAMA* **2014**, *311*, 1770–1777. [CrossRef] [PubMed]
14. Tick, B.; Bolton, P.; Happé, F.; Rutter, M.; Rijsdijk, F. Heritability of autism spectrum disorders: A meta-analysis of twin studies. *J. Child Psychol. Psychiatry* **2016**, *57*, 585–595. [CrossRef] [PubMed]
15. Bai, D.; Yip, B.H.K.; Windham, G.C.; Sourander, A.; Francis, R.; Yoffe, R.; Glasson, E.; Mahjani, B.; Suominen, A.; Leonard, H.; et al. Association of Genetic and Environmental Factors With Autism in a 5-Country Cohort. *JAMA Psychiatry* **2019**, *76*, 1035–1043. [CrossRef] [PubMed]

16. Grove, J.; Ripke, S.; Als, T.D.; Mattheisen, M.; Walters, R.K.; Won, H.; Pallesen, J.; Agerbo, E.; Andreassen, O.A.; Anney, R.; et al. Identification of common genetic risk variants for autism spectrum disorder. *Nat. Genet.* **2019**, *51*, 431–444. [CrossRef]
17. Di Gregorio, E.; Riberi, E.; Belligni, E.F.; Biamino, E.; Spielmann, M.; Ala, U.; Calcia, A.; Bagnasco, I.; Carli, D.; Gai, G.; et al. Copy number variants analysis in a cohort of isolated and syndromic developmental delay/intellectual disability reveals novel genomic disorders, position effects and candidate disease genes. *Clin. Genet.* **2017**, *92*, 415–422. [CrossRef]
18. Velinov, M. Genomic Copy Number Variations in the Autism Clinic-Work in Progress. *Front. Cell. Neurosci.* **2019**, *13*, 57. [CrossRef]
19. Zhou, J.; Park, C.Y.; Theesfeld, C.L.; Wong, A.K.; Yuan, Y.; Scheckel, C.; Fak, J.J.; Funk, J.; Yao, K.; Tajima, Y.; et al. Whole-genome deep-learning analysis identifies contribution of noncoding mutations to autism risk. *Nat. Genet.* **2019**, *51*, 973–980. [CrossRef]
20. Hu, V.W. From genes to environment: Using integrative genomics to build a "systems-level" understanding of autism spectrum disorders. *Child Dev.* **2013**, *84*, 89–103. [CrossRef]
21. Biamino, E.; Di Gregorio, E.; Belligni, E.F.; Keller, R.; Riberi, E.; Gandione, M.; Calcia, A.; Mancini, C.; Giorgio, E.; Cavalieri, S.; et al. A novel 3q29 deletion associated with autism, intellectual disability, psychiatric disorders, and obesity. *Am. J. Med. Genet B Neuropsychiatr. Genet.* **2016**, *171B*, 290–299. [CrossRef]
22. Cauda, F.; Nani, A.; Costa, T.; Palermo, S.; Tatu, K.; Manuello, J.; Duca, S.; Fox, P.T.; Keller, R. The morphometric co-atrophy networking of schizophrenia, autistic and obsessive spectrum disorders. *Hum Brain Mapp.* **2018**, *39*, 1898–1928. [CrossRef] [PubMed]
23. Mannion, A.; Leader, G. An investigation of comorbid psychological disorders, sleep problems, gastrointestinal symptoms and epilepsy in children and adolescents with autism spectrum disorder: A two year follow-up. *Res. Autism Spectr. Disord.* **2016**, *22*, 20–33. [CrossRef]
24. Hallmayer, J.; Cleveland, S.; Torres, A.; Phillips, J.; Cohen, B.; Torigoe, T.; Miller, J.; Fedele, A.; Collins, J.; Smith, K.; et al. Genetic heritability and shared environmental factors among twin pairs with autism. *Arch. Gen. Psychiatry* **2011**, *68*, 1095–1102. [CrossRef]
25. Vogel Ciernia, A.; LaSalle, J. The landscape of DNA methylation amid a perfect storm of autism aetiologies. *Nat. Rev. Neurosci.* **2016**, *17*, 411–423. [CrossRef]
26. Hannon, E.; Schendel, D.; Ladd-Acosta, C.; Grove, J.; iPSYCH-Broad ASD Group; Hansen, C.S.; Andrews, S.V.; Hougaard, D.M.; Bresnahan, M.; Mors, O.; et al. Elevated polygenic burden for autism is associated with differential DNA methylation at birth. *Genome Med.* **2018**, *10*, 19. [CrossRef] [PubMed]
27. Dupont, C.; Armant, D.R.; Brenner, C.A. Epigenetics: Definition, mechanisms and clinical perspective. *Semin. Reprod. Med.* **2009**, *27*, 351–357. [CrossRef] [PubMed]
28. Strohman, R.C. Linear genetics, non-linear epigenetics: Complementary approaches to understanding complex diseases. *Integr. Physiol. Behav. Sci.* **1995**, *30*, 273–282. [CrossRef]
29. Goldberg, A.D.; Allis, C.D.; Bernstein, E. Epigenetics: A landscape takes shape. *Cell* **2007**, *128*, 635–638. [CrossRef] [PubMed]
30. Kiefer, J.C. Epigenetics in development. *Dev. Dyn.* **2007**, *236*, 1144–1156. [CrossRef]
31. Spiers, H.; Hannon, E.; Schalkwyk, L.C.; Smith, R.; Wong, C.C.; O'Donovan, M.C.; Bray, N.J.; Mill, J. Methylomic trajectories across human fetal brain development. *Genome Res.* **2015**, *25*, 338–352. [CrossRef] [PubMed]
32. Linnér, A.; Almgren, M. Epigenetic programming-The important first 1000 days. *Acta Paediatr.* **2020**, *109*, 443–452. [CrossRef] [PubMed]
33. De Rubeis, S.; He, X.; Goldberg, A.P.; Poultney, C.S.; Samocha, K.; Cicek, A.E.; Kou, Y.; Liu, L.; Fromer, M.; Walker, S.; et al. Synaptic, transcriptional and chromatin genes disrupted in autism. *Nature* **2014**, *515*, 209–215. [CrossRef]
34. Lasalle, J.M. Autism genes keep turning up chromatin. *OA Autism* **2013**, *1*, 14. [CrossRef] [PubMed]
35. Amir, R.E.; Van den Veyver, I.B.; Wan, M.; Tran, C.Q.; Francke, U.; Zoghbi, H.Y. Rett syndrome is caused by mutations in X-linked MECP2, encoding methyl-CpG-binding protein 2. *Nat. Genet.* **1999**, *23*, 185–188. [CrossRef]
36. Chahrour, M.; Jung, S.Y.; Shaw, C.; Zhou, X.; Wong, S.T.; Qin, J.; Zoghbi, H.Y. MeCP2, a key contributor to neurological disease, activates and represses transcription. *Science* **2008**, *320*, 1224–1229. [CrossRef] [PubMed]
37. Jiang, Y.H.; Bressler, J.; Beaudet, A.L. Epigenetics and human disease. *Annu. Rev. Genom. Hum. Genet.* **2004**, *5*, 479–510. [CrossRef]
38. Zhao, X.; Pak, C.; Smrt, R.D.; Jin, P. Epigenetics and Neural developmental disorders: Washington DC, September 18 and 19, 2006. *Epigenetics* **2007**, *2*, 126–134. [CrossRef]
39. Dall'Aglio, L.; Muka, T.; Cecil, C.A.M.; Bramer, W.M.; Verbiest, M.M.P.J.; Nano, J.; Hidalgo, A.C.; Franco, O.H.; Tiemeier, H. The role of epigenetic modifications in neurodevelopmental disorders: A systematic review. *Neurosci. Biobehav. Rev.* **2018**, *94*, 17–30. [CrossRef]
40. Stamova, B.; Ander, B.P.; Barger, N.; Sharp, F.R.; Schumann, C.M. Specific Regional and Age-Related Small Noncoding RNA Expression Patterns Within Superior Temporal Gyrus of Typical Human Brains Are Less Distinct in Autism Brains. *J. Child Neurol.* **2015**, *30*, 1930–1946. [CrossRef]
41. Mundalil Vasu, M.; Anitha, A.; Thanseem, I.; Suzuki, K.; Yamada, K.; Takahashi, T.; Wakuda, T.; Iwata, K.; Tsuji, M.; Sugiyama, T.; et al. Serum microRNA profiles in children with autism. *Mol. Autism* **2014**, *5*, 40. [CrossRef] [PubMed]
42. Hicks, S.D.; Rajan, A.T.; Wagner, K.E.; Barns, S.; Carpenter, R.L.; Middleton, F.A. Validation of a Salivary RNA Test for Childhood Autism Spectrum Disorder. *Front. Genet.* **2018**, *9*, 534. [CrossRef] [PubMed]
43. Gluckman, P.D.; Hanson, M.A. Living with the past: Evolution, development, and patterns of disease. *Science* **2004**, *305*, 1733–1736. [CrossRef] [PubMed]
44. Gluckman, P.D.; Hanson, M.A.; Low, F.M. The role of developmental plasticity and epigenetics in human health. *Birth Defects Res. C Embryo Today* **2011**, *93*, 12–18. [CrossRef] [PubMed]

45. Burgio, E. Environment and Fetal Programming: The origins of some current "pandemics". *J. Pediatr. Neonat. Individual. Med.* **2015**, *4*, 2.
46. Vineis, P.; Stringhini, S.; Porta, M. The environmental roots of non-communicable diseases (NCDs) and the epigenetic impacts of globalization. *Environ. Res.* **2014**, *133*, 424–430. [CrossRef]
47. Godfrey, K.M.; Costello, P.M.; Lillycrop, K.A. The developmental environment, epigenetic biomarkers and long-term health. *J. Dev. Orig. Health Dis.* **2015**, *6*, 399–406. [CrossRef]
48. Barker, D.J.; Eriksson, J.G.; Forsén, T.; Osmond, C. Fetal origins of adult disease: Strength of effects and biological basis. *Int. J. Epidemiol.* **2002**, *31*, 1235–1239. [CrossRef]
49. Shapiro, J.A. A 21st century view of evolution: Genome system architecture, repetitive DNA, and natural genetic engineering. *Gene* **2005**, *345*, 91–100. [CrossRef]
50. Nugent, B.M.; Bale, T.L. The omniscient placenta: Metabolic and epigenetic regulation of fetal programming. *Front. Neuroendocrinol.* **2015**, *39*, 28–37. [CrossRef]
51. Coan, P.M.; Burton, G.J.; Ferguson-Smith, A.C. Imprinted genes in the placenta–A review. *Placenta* **2005**, *26*, S10–S20. [CrossRef]
52. Hochberg, Z.; Feil, R.; Constancia, M.; Fraga, M.; Junien, C.; Carel, J.C.; Boileau, P.; Le Bouc, Y.; Deal, C.L.; Lillycrop, K.; et al. Child health, developmental plasticity, and epigenetic programming. *Endocr. Rev.* **2011**, *32*, 159–224. [CrossRef] [PubMed]
53. LaSalle, J.M. A genomic point-of-view on environmental factors influencing the human brain methylome. *Epigenetics* **2011**, *6*, 862–869. [CrossRef] [PubMed]
54. Day, J.J.; Childs, D.; Guzman-Karlsson, M.C.; Kibe, M.; Moulden, J.; Song, E.; Tahir, A.; Sweatt, J.D. DNA methylation regulates associative reward learning. *Nat. Neurosci.* **2013**, *16*, 1445–1452. [CrossRef] [PubMed]
55. Podobinska, M.; Szablowska-Gadomska, I.; Augustyniak, J.; Sandvig, I.; Sandvig, A.; Buzanska, L. Epigenetic Modulation of Stem Cells in Neurodevelopment: The Role of Methylation and Acetylation. *Front. Cell. Neurosci.* **2017**, *11*, 23. [CrossRef] [PubMed]
56. Gesundheit, B.; Rosenzweig, J.P.; Naor, D.; Lerer, B.; Zachor, D.A.; Procházka, V.; Melamed, M.; Kristt, D.A.; Steinberg, A.; Shulman, C.; et al. Immunological and autoimmune considerations of Autism Spectrum Disorders. *J. Autoimmun.* **2013**, *44*, 1–7. [CrossRef] [PubMed]
57. Filiano, A.J.; Gadani, S.P.; Kipnis, J. Interactions of innate and adaptive immunity in brain development and function. *Brain Res.* **2015**, *1617*, 18–27. [CrossRef] [PubMed]
58. Deverman, B.E.; Patterson, P.H. Cytokines and CNS development. *Neuron* **2009**, *64*, 61–78. [CrossRef] [PubMed]
59. Bilbo, S.D.; Schwarz, J.M. The immune system and developmental programming of brain and behavior. *Front. Neuroendocrinol.* **2012**, *33*, 267–286. [CrossRef]
60. Schwarz, J.M.; Bilbo, S.D. Sex, glia, and development: Interactions in health and disease. *Horm. Behav.* **2012**, *62*, 243–253. [CrossRef]
61. Kipnis, J. Immune system: The "seventh sense". *J. Exp. Med.* **2018**, *215*, 397–398. [CrossRef]
62. Chess, S. Autism in children with congenital rubella. *J. Autism Child Schizophr.* **1971**, *1*, 33–47. [CrossRef] [PubMed]
63. Chess, S. Follow-up report on autism in congenital rubella. *J. Autism Child Schizophr.* **1977**, *7*, 69–81. [CrossRef] [PubMed]
64. Patterson, P.H. Immune involvement in schizophrenia and autism: Etiology, pathology and animal models. *Behav. Brain Res.* **2009**, *204*, 313–321. [CrossRef]
65. Reisinger, S.; Khan, D.; Kong, E.; Berger, A.; Pollak, A.; Pollak, D.D. The poly(I:C)-induced maternal immune activation model in preclinical neuropsychiatric drug discovery. *Pharmacol. Ther.* **2015**, *149*, 213–226. [CrossRef] [PubMed]
66. Knuesel, I.; Chicha, L.; Britschgi, M.; Schobel, S.A.; Bodmer, M.; Hellings, J.A.; Toovey, S.; Prinssen, E.P. Maternal immune activation and abnormal brain development across CNS disorders. *Nat. Rev. Neurol.* **2014**, *10*, 643–660. [CrossRef] [PubMed]
67. Lee, B.K.; Magnusson, C.; Gardner, R.M.; Blomström, Å.; Newschaffer, C.J.; Burstyn, I.; Karlsson, H.; Dalman, C. Maternal hospitalization with infection during pregnancy and risk of autism spectrum disorders. *Brain Behav. Immun.* **2015**, *44*, 100–105. [CrossRef]
68. Vianna, P.; Gomes, J.D.A.; Boquett, J.A.; Fraga, L.R.; Schuch, J.B.; Vianna, F.S.L.; Schuler-Faccini, L. Zika Virus as a Possible Risk Factor for Autism Spectrum Disorder: Neuroimmunological Aspects. *Neuroimmunomodulation* **2018**, *25*, 320–327. [CrossRef]
69. Forestieri, S.; Marcialis, M.A.; Migliore, L.; Panisi, C.; Fanos, V. Relationship between pregnancy and coronavirus: What we know. *J. Matern. Fetal Neonatal Med.* **2020**, 1–12. [CrossRef]
70. Keil, A.; Daniels, J.L.; Forssen, U.; Hultman, C.; Cnattingius, S.; Söderberg, K.C.; Feychting, M.; Sparen, P. Parental autoimmune diseases associated with autism spectrum disorders in offspring. *Epidemiology* **2010**, *21*, 805–808. [CrossRef]
71. Lyall, K.; Pauls, D.L.; Spiegelman, D.; Ascherio, A.; Santangelo, S.L. Pregnancy complications and obstetric suboptimality in association with autism spectrum disorders in children of the Nurses' Health Study II. *Autism Res.* **2012**, *5*, 21–30. [CrossRef]
72. Brown, A.S.; Surcel, H.M.; Hinkka-Yli-Salomäki, S.; Cheslack-Postava, K.; Bao, Y.; Sourander, A. Maternal thyroid autoantibody and elevated risk of autism in a national birth cohort. *Prog. Neuropsychopharmacol. Biol. Psychiatry* **2015**, *57*, 86–92. [CrossRef] [PubMed]
73. Singer, H.S.; Morris, C.; Gause, C.; Pollard, M.; Zimmerman, A.W.; Pletnikov, M. Prenatal exposure to antibodies from mothers of children with autism produces neurobehavioral alterations: A pregnant dam mouse model. *J. Neuroimmunol.* **2009**, *211*, 39–48. [CrossRef]
74. Braunschweig, D.; Van de Water, J. Maternal autoantibodies in autism. *Arch. Neurol.* **2012**, *69*, 693–699. [CrossRef] [PubMed]
75. Chen, S.W.; Zhong, X.S.; Jiang, L.N.; Zheng, X.Y.; Xiong, Y.Q.; Ma, S.J.; Qiu, M.; Huo, S.T.; Ge, J.; Chen, Q. Maternal autoimmune diseases and the risk of autism spectrum disorders in offspring: A systematic review and meta-analysis. *Behav. Brain Res.* **2016**, *296*, 61–69. [CrossRef]

76. Krakowiak, P.; Walker, C.K.; Tancredi, D.; Hertz-Picciotto, I.; Van de Water, J. Autism-specific maternal anti-fetal brain autoantibodies are associated with metabolic conditions. *J. Autism Res.* **2017**, *10*, 89–98. [CrossRef] [PubMed]
77. Croen, L.A.; Braunschweig, D.; Haapanen, L.; Yoshida, C.K.; Fireman, B.; Grether, J.K.; Kharhfr, M.; Hansen, R.L.; Ashwood, P.; Van de Water, J. Maternal mid-pregnancy autoantibodies to fetal brain protein: The early markers for autism study. *Biol. Psychiatry* **2008**, *64*, 583–588. [CrossRef] [PubMed]
78. Ramaekers, V.T.; Sequeira, J.M.; DiDuca, M.; Vrancken, G.; Thomas, A.; Philippe, C.; Peters, M.; Jadot, A.; Quadros, E.V. Improving Outcome in Infantile Autism with Folate Receptor Autoimmunity and Nutritional Derangements: A Self-Controlled Trial. *Autism. Res. Treat.* **2019**, *2019*, 7486431. [CrossRef] [PubMed]
79. Sequeira, J.M.; Desai, A.; Berrocal-Zaragoza, M.I.; Murphy, M.M.; Fernandez-Ballart, J.D.; Quadros, E.V. Exposure to Folate Receptor Alpha Antibodies during Gestation and Weaning Leads to Severe Behavioral Deficits in Rats: A Pilot Study. *PLoS ONE* **2016**, *11*, e0152249. [CrossRef]
80. Frye, R.E.; Rossignol, D.A.; Scahill, L.; McDougle, C.J.; Huberman, H.; Quadros, E.V. Treatment of folate metabolism abnormalities in Autism Spectrum Disorder. *Semin. Pediatr. Neurol.* **2020**, *35*, 100835. [CrossRef]
81. Frye, R.E.; Sequeira, J.M.; Quadros, E.V.; James, S.J.; Rossignol, D.A. Cerebral folate receptor autoantibodies in autism spectrum disorder. *Mol. Psychiatry* **2013**, *18*, 369–381. [CrossRef]
82. Nardone, S.; Elliott, E. The Interaction between the Immune System and Epigenetics in the Etiology of Autism Spectrum Disorders. *Front. Neurosci.* **2016**, *10*, 329. [CrossRef] [PubMed]
83. Lombardo, M.V.; Moon, H.M.; Su, J.; Palmer, T.D.; Courchesne, E.; Pramparo, T. Maternal immune activation dysregulation of the fetal brain transcriptome and relevance to the pathophysiology of autism spectrum disorder. *Mol. Psychiatry* **2018**, *23*, 1001–1013. [CrossRef] [PubMed]
84. Conway, F.; Brown, A.S. Maternal Immune Activation and Related Factors in the Risk of Offspring Psychiatric Disorders. *Front. Psychiatry* **2019**, *10*, 430. [CrossRef] [PubMed]
85. Phillips, N.L.H.; Roth, T.L. Animal Models and Their Contribution to Our Understanding of the Relationship Between Environments, Epigenetic Modifications, and Behavior. *Genes* **2019**, *10*, 47. [CrossRef]
86. Parker-Athill, E.C.; Tan, J. Maternal immune activation and autism spectrum disorder: Interleukin-6 signaling as a key mechanistic pathway. *Neurosignals* **2010**, *18*, 113–128. [CrossRef]
87. Estes, M.L.; McAllister, A.K. Immune mediators in the brain and peripheral tissues in autism spectrum disorder. *Nat. Rev. Neurosci.* **2015**, *16*, 469–486. [CrossRef]
88. Sweeten, T.L.; Bowyer, S.L.; Posey, D.J.; Halberstadt, G.M.; McDougle, C.J. Increased prevalence of familial autoimmunity in probands with pervasive developmental disorders. *Pediatrics* **2003**, *112*, e420. [CrossRef]
89. Patel, S.; Masi, A.; Dale, R.C.; Whitehouse, A.J.O.; Pokorski, I.; Alvares, G.A.; Hickie, I.B.; Breen, E.; Guastella, A.J. Social impairments in autism spectrum disorder are related to maternal immune history profile. *Mol. Psychiatry* **2018**, *23*, 1794–1797. [CrossRef]
90. Hompes, T.; Izzi, B.; Gellens, E.; Morreels, M.; Fieuws, S.; Pexsters, A.; Schops, G.; Dom, M.; Van Bree, R.; Freson, K.; et al. Investigating the influence of maternal cortisol and emotional state during pregnancy on the DNA methylation status of the glucocorticoid receptor gene (NR3C1) promoter region in cord blood. *J. Psychiatr. Res.* **2013**, *47*, 880–891. [CrossRef]
91. Liu, Y.; Murphy, S.K.; Murtha, A.P.; Fuemmeler, B.F.; Schildkraut, J.; Huang, Z.; Overcash, F.; Kurtzberg, J.; Jirtle, R.; Iversen, E.S.; et al. Depression in pregnancy, infant birth weight and DNA methylation of imprint regulatory elements. *Epigenetics* **2012**, *7*, 735–746. [CrossRef]
92. Carter, C.J.; Blizard, R.A. Autism genes are selectively targeted by environmental pollutants including pesticides, heavy metals, bisphenol A, phthalates and many others in food, cosmetics or household products. *Neurochem. Int.* **2016**, *S0197-0186*, 30197–30198. [CrossRef] [PubMed]
93. Estes, M.L.; McAllister, A.K. Maternal immune activation: Implications for neuropsychiatric disorders. *Science* **2016**, *353*, 772–777. [CrossRef] [PubMed]
94. Tang, B.; Jia, H.; Kast, R.J.; Thomas, E.A. Epigenetic changes at gene promoters in response to immune activation in utero. *Brain Behav. Immun.* **2013**, *30*, 168–175. [CrossRef] [PubMed]
95. Reisinger, S.N.; Kong, E.; Khan, D.; Schulz, S.; Ronovsky, M.; Berger, S.; Horvath, O.; Cabatic, M.; Berger, A.; Pollak, D.D. Maternal immune activation epigenetically regulates hippocampal serotonin transporter levels. *Neurobiol. Stress* **2016**, *4*, 34–43. [CrossRef]
96. Richetto, J.; Massart, R.; Weber-Stadlbauer, U.; Szyf, M.; Riva, M.A.; Meyer, U. Genome-wide DNA Methylation Changes in a Mouse Model of Infection-Mediated Neurodevelopmental Disorders. *Biol. Psychiatry* **2017**, *81*, 265–276. [CrossRef]
97. Alexopoulou, L.; Holt, A.C.; Medzhitov, R.; Flavell, R.A. Recognition of double-stranded RNA and activation of NF-kappaB by Toll-like receptor 3. *Nature* **2001**, *413*, 732–738. [CrossRef] [PubMed]
98. Malkova, N.V.; Yu, C.Z.; Hsiao, E.Y.; Moore, M.J.; Patterson, P.H. Maternal immune activation yields offspring displaying mouse versions of the three core symptoms of autism. *Brain Behav. Immun.* **2012**, *26*, 607–616. [CrossRef]
99. Da SilvaVaccaro, T.; Sorrentino, J.M.; Salvador, S.; Veit, T.; Souza, D.O.; de Almeida, R.F. Alterations in the MicroRNA of the Blood of Autism Spectrum Disorder Patients: Effects on Epigenetic Regulation and Potential Biomarkers. *Behav. Sci.* **2018**, *8*, 75. [CrossRef]

100. Gupta, S.; Ellis, S.E.; Ashar, F.N.; Moes, A.; Bader, J.S.; Zhan, J.; West, A.B.; Arking, D.E. Transcriptome analysis reveals dysregulation of innate immune response genes and neuronal activity-dependent genes in autism. *Nat. Commun.* **2014**, *5*, 5748. [CrossRef]
101. Nardone, S.; Sams, D.S.; Reuveni, E.; Getselter, D.; Oron, O.; Karpuj, M.; Elliott, E. DNA methylation analysis of the autistic brain reveals multiple dysregulated biological pathways. *Transl. Psychiatry* **2014**, *4*, e433. [CrossRef]
102. Ashwood, P.; Krakowiak, P.; Hertz-Picciotto, I.; Hansen, R.; Pessah, I.; Van de Water, J. Elevated plasma cytokines in autism spectrum disorders provide evidence of immune dysfunction and are associated with impaired behavioral outcome. *Brain Behav. Immun.* **2011**, *25*, 40–45. [CrossRef]
103. Guerini, F.R.; Bolognesi, E.; Chiappedi, M.; Manca, S.; Ghezzo, A.; Agliardi, C.; Zanette, M.; Littera, R.; Carcassi, C.; Sotgiu, S.; et al. Activating KIR molecules and their cognate ligands prevail in children with a diagnosis of ASD and in their mothers. *Brain Behav. Immun.* **2014**, *36*, 54–60. [CrossRef] [PubMed]
104. Boulanger, L.M.; Shatz, C.J. Immune signalling in neural development, synaptic plasticity and disease. *Nat. Rev. Neurosci.* **2004**, *5*, 521–531. [CrossRef]
105. Comi, A.M.; Zimmerman, A.W.; Frye, V.H.; Law, P.A.; Peeden, J.N. Familial clustering of autoimmune disorders and evaluation of medical risk factors in autism. *J. Child Neurol.* **1999**, *14*, 388–394. [CrossRef]
106. Croen, L.A.; Grether, J.K.; Yoshida, C.K.; Odouli, R.; Van de Water, J. Maternal autoimmune diseases, asthma and allergies, and childhood autism spectrum disorders: A case-control study. *Arch. Pediatr. Adolesc. Med.* **2005**, *159*, 151–157. [CrossRef] [PubMed]
107. Atladóttir, H.O.; Thorsen, P.; Østergaard, L.; Schendel, D.E.; Lemcke, S.; Abdallah, M.; Partner, E.T. Maternal infection requiring hospitalization during pregnancy and autism spectrum disorders. *J. Autism Dev. Disord.* **2010**, *40*, 1423–1430. [CrossRef]
108. Altevogt, B.M.; Hanson, S.L.; Leshner, A.I. Autism and the environment: Challenges and opportunities for research. *Pediatrics* **2008**, *121*, 1225–1229. [CrossRef] [PubMed]
109. Colucci, F. The role of KIR and HLA interactions in pregnancy complications. *Immunogenetics* **2017**, *69*, 557–565. [CrossRef]
110. Torres, A.R.; Westover, J.B.; Gibbons, C.; Johnson, R.C.; Ward, D.C. Activating killer-cell immunoglobulin-like receptors (KIR) and their cognate HLA ligands are significantly increased in autism. *Brain Behav. Immun.* **2012**, *26*, 1122–1127. [CrossRef]
111. Guerini, F.R.; Bolognesi, E.; Chiappedi, M.; Ghezzo, A.; Canevini, M.P.; Mensi, M.M.; Vignoli, A.; Agliardi, C.; Zanette, M.; Clerici, M. An HLA-G(*)14bp insertion/deletion polymorphism associates with the development of autistic spectrum disorders. *Brain Behav. Immun.* **2015**, *44*, 207–212. [CrossRef]
112. Christiansen, O.B.; Kolte, A.M.; Dahl, M.; Larsen, E.C.; Steffensen, R.; Nielsen, H.S.; Hviid, T.V. Maternal homozygosity for a 14 base pair insertion in exon 8 of the HLA-G gene and carriage of HLA class II alleles restricting HY immunity predispose to unexplained secondary recurrent miscarriage and low birth weight in children born to these patients. *Hum. Immunol.* **2012**, *73*, 699–705. [CrossRef] [PubMed]
113. Hylenius, S.; Andersen, A.M.; Melbye, M.; Hviid, T.V. Association between HLA-G genotype and risk of pre-eclampsia: A case-control study using family triads. *Mol. Hum. Reprod.* **2004**, *10*, 237–246. [CrossRef]
114. Guerini, F.R.; Bolognesi, E.; Chiappedi, M.; Ghezzo, A.; Manca, S.; Zanette, M.; Sotgiu, S.; Mensi, M.M.; Zanzottera, M.; Agliardi, C.; et al. HLA-G*14bp Insertion and the KIR2DS1-HLAC2 Complex Impact on Behavioral Impairment in Children with Autism Spectrum Disorders. *Neuroscience* **2018**, *370*, 163–169. [CrossRef] [PubMed]
115. Uhrberg, M. Shaping the human NK cell repertoire: An epigenetic glance at KIR gene regulation. *Mol. Immunol.* **2005**, *42*, 471–475. [CrossRef] [PubMed]
116. Blomström, Å.; Karlsson, H.; Gardner, R.; Jörgensen, L.; Magnusson, C.; Dalman, C. Associations Between Maternal Infection During Pregnancy, Childhood Infections, and the Risk of Subsequent Psychotic Disorder–A Swedish Cohort Study of Nearly 2 Million Individuals. *Schizophr. Bull.* **2016**, *42*, 125–133. [CrossRef] [PubMed]
117. Kipnis, J. Multifaceted interactions between adaptive immunity and the central nervous system. *Science* **2016**, *353*, 766–771. [CrossRef] [PubMed]
118. Jones, K.L.; Croen, L.A.; Yoshida, C.K.; Heuer, L.; Hansen, R.; Zerbo, O.; DeLorenze, G.N.; Kharrazi, M.; Yolken, R.; Ashwood, P.; et al. Autism with intellectual disability is associated with increased levels of maternal cytokines and chemokines during gestation. *Mol. Psychiatry* **2017**, *22*, 273–279. [CrossRef] [PubMed]
119. Choi, G.B.; Yim, Y.S.; Wong, H.; Kim, S.; Kim, H.; Kim, S.V.; Hoeffer, C.A.; Littman, D.R.; Huh, J.R. The maternal interleukin-17a pathway in mice promotes autism-like phenotypes in offspring. *Science* **2016**, *351*, 933–939. [CrossRef]
120. Zaretsky, M.V.; Alexander, J.M.; Byrd, W.; Bawdon, R.E. Transfer of inflammatory cytokines across the placenta. *Obstet. Gynecol.* **2004**, *103*, 546–550. [CrossRef]
121. Smith, S.E.; Li, J.; Garbett, K.; Mirnics, K.; Patterson, P.H. Maternal immune activation alters fetal brain development through interleukin-6. *J. Neurosci.* **2007**, *27*, 10695–10702. [CrossRef]
122. Boulanger, L.M. Immune proteins in brain development and synaptic plasticity. *Neuron* **2009**, *64*, 93–109. [CrossRef]
123. Sotgiu, S.; Manca, S.; Gagliano, A.; Minutolo, A.; Melis, M.A.; Pisuttu, G.; Scoppola, C.; Bolognesi, E.; Clerici, M.; Guerini, F.R.; et al. Immune regulation of neurodevelopment at the mother-foetus interface: The case of autism. *Clin. Transl. Immunol.* **2020**, e1211. [CrossRef]
124. Aagaard, K.; Ma, J.; Antony, K.M.; Ganu, R.; Petrosino, J.; Versalovic, J. The placenta harbors a unique microbiome. *Sci. Transl. Med.* **2014**, *6*, 237ra65. [CrossRef] [PubMed]

125. Gomez de Agüero, M.; Ganal-Vonarburg, S.C.; Fuhrer, T.; Rupp, S.; Uchimura, Y.; Li, H.; Steinert, A.; Heikenwalder, M.; Hapfelmeier, S.; Sauer, U.; et al. The maternal microbiota drives early postnatal innate immune development. *Science* **2016**, *351*, 1296–1302. [CrossRef] [PubMed]
126. Romano-Keeler, J.; Weitkamp, J.H. Maternal influences on fetal microbial colonization and immune development. *Pediatr. Res.* **2015**, *77*, 189–195. [CrossRef] [PubMed]
127. Hoffman, D.J.; Reynolds, R.M.; Hardy, D.B. Developmental origins of health and disease: Current knowledge and potential mechanisms. *Nutr. Rev.* **2017**, *75*, 951–970. [CrossRef] [PubMed]
128. Weaver, I.C.; Korgan, A.C.; Lee, K.; Wheeler, R.V.; Hundert, A.S.; Goguen, D. Stress and the Emerging Roles of Chromatin Remodeling in Signal Integration and Stable Transmission of Reversible Phenotypes. *Front. Behav. Neurosci.* **2017**, *11*, 41. [CrossRef] [PubMed]
129. Koren, O.; Goodrich, J.K.; Cullender, T.C.; Spor, A.; Laitinen, K.; Bäckhed, H.K.; Gonzalez, A.; Werner, J.J.; Angenent, L.T.; Knight, R.; et al. Host remodeling of the gut microbiome and metabolic changes during pregnancy. *Cell* **2012**, *150*, 470–480. [CrossRef] [PubMed]
130. Aagaard, K.; Riehle, K.; Ma, J.; Segata, N.; Mistretta, T.A.; Coarfa, C.; Raza, S.; Rosenbaum, S.; Van den Veyver, I.; Milosavljevic, A.; et al. A metagenomic approach to characterization of the vaginal microbiome signature in pregnancy. *PLoS ONE* **2012**, *7*, e36466. [CrossRef] [PubMed]
131. Blaser, M.J.; Dominguez-Bello, M.G. The Human Microbiome before Birth. *Cell Host. Microbe.* **2016**, *20*, 558–560. [CrossRef]
132. Hackman, D.A.; Farah, M.J.; Meaney, M.J. Socioeconomic status and the brain: Mechanistic insights from human and animal research. *Nat. Rev. Neurosci.* **2010**, *11*, 651–659. [CrossRef] [PubMed]
133. Emberti Gialloreti, L.; Mazzone, L.; Benvenuto, A.; Fasano, A.; Alcon, A.G.; Kraneveld, A.; Moavero, R.; Raz, R.; Riccio, M.P.; Siracusano, M.; et al. Risk and Protective Environmental Factors Associated with Autism Spectrum Disorder: Evidence-Based Principles and Recommendations. *J. Clin. Med.* **2019**, *8*, 217. [CrossRef] [PubMed]
134. Raghavan, R.; Riley, A.W.; Volk, H.; Caruso, D.; Hironaka, L.; Sices, L.; Hong, X.; Wang, G.; Ji, Y.; Brucato, M.; et al. Maternal Multivitamin Intake, Plasma Folate and Vitamin B12 Levels and Autism Spectrum Disorder Risk in Offspring. *Paediatr. Perinat. Epidemiol.* **2018**, *32*, 100–111. [CrossRef] [PubMed]
135. Bilbo, S.D.; Block, C.L.; Bolton, J.L.; Hanamsagar, R.; Tran, P.K. Beyond infection Maternal immune activation by environmental factors, microglial development, and relevance for autism spectrum disorders. *Exp. Neurol.* **2018**, *299*, 241–251. [CrossRef]
136. Grossi, E.; Migliore, L.; Muratori, F. Pregnancy risk factors related to autism: An Italian case-control study in mothers of children with autism spectrum disorders (ASD), their siblings and of typically developing children. *J. Dev. Orig. Health Dis.* **2018**, *9*, 442–449. [CrossRef] [PubMed]
137. Zhang, T.; Sidorchuk, A.; Sevilla-Cermeno, L.; Vilaplana-Perez, A.; Chang, Z.; Larsson, H.; Mataix-Cols, D.; Fernandez de la Cruz, L. Association of cesarean delivery with risk of neurodevelopmental and psychiatric disorders in the offspring: A systematic review and meta-analysis. *JAMA Netw. Open* **2019**, *2*, e1910236. [CrossRef] [PubMed]
138. Vargas, D.L.; Nascimbene, C.; Krishnan, C.; Zimmerman, A.W.; Pardo, C.A. Neuroglial activation and neuroinflammation in the brain of patients with autism. *Ann. Neurol.* **2005**, *57*, 67–81. [CrossRef] [PubMed]
139. Matta, S.M.; Hill-Yardin, E.L.; Crack, P.J. The influence of neuroinflammation in Autism Spectrum Disorder. *Brain Behav. Immun.* **2019**, *79*, 75–90. [CrossRef]
140. Onore, C.; Careaga, M.; Ashwood, P. The role of immune dysfunction in the pathophysiology of autism. *Brain Behav. Immun.* **2012**, *26*, 383–392. [CrossRef]
141. Saresella, M.; Marventano, I.; Guerini, F.R.; Mancuso, R.; Ceresa, L.; Zanzottera, M.; Rusconi, B.; Maggioni, E.; Tinelli, C.; Clerici, M. An autistic endophenotype results in complex immune dysfunction in healthy siblings of autistic children. *Biol. Psychiatry* **2009**, *66*, 978–984. [CrossRef]
142. Li, Q.; Zhou, J.M. The microbiota-gut-brain axis and its potential therapeutic role in autism spectrum disorder. *Neuroscience* **2016**, *324*, 131–139. [CrossRef] [PubMed]
143. El Aidy, S.; Dinan, T.G.; Cryan, J.F. Gut Microbiota: The Conductor in the Orchestra of Immune-Neuroendocrine Communication. *Clin. Ther.* **2015**, *37*, 954–967. [CrossRef] [PubMed]
144. Mayer, E.A. Gut feelings: The emerging biology of gut-brain communication. *Nat. Rev. Neurosci.* **2011**, *12*, 453–466. [CrossRef] [PubMed]
145. Rossignol, D.A.; Frye, R.E. Evidence linking oxidative stress, mitochondrial dysfunction, and inflammation in the brain of individuals with autism. *Front. Physiol.* **2014**, *5*, 150. [CrossRef]
146. Turnbaugh, P.J.; Ley, R.E.; Hamady, M.; Fraser-Liggett, C.M.; Knight, R.; Gordon, J.I. The human microbiome project. *Nature* **2007**, *449*, 804–810. [CrossRef]
147. Qin, J.; Li, R.; Raes, J.; Arumugam, M.; Burgdorf, K.S.; Manichanh, C.; Nielsen, T.; Pons, N.; Levenez, F.; Yamada, T.; et al. A human gut microbial gene catalogue established by metagenomic sequencing. *Nature* **2010**, *464*, 59–65. [CrossRef]
148. Littman, D.R.; Pamer, E.G. Role of the commensal microbiota in normal and pathogenic host immune responses. *Cell Host Microbe* **2011**, *10*, 311–323. [CrossRef] [PubMed]
149. Blumberg, R.; Powrie, F. Microbiota, disease, and back to health: A metastable journey. *Sci. Transl. Med.* **2012**, *4*, 137rv7. [CrossRef]
150. Hooper, L.V.; Littman, D.R.; Macpherson, A.J. Interactions between the microbiota and the immune system. *Science* **2012**, *336*, 1268–1273. [CrossRef]

151. Ho, P.; Ross, D.A. More Than a Gut Feeling: The Implications of the Gut Microbiota in Psychiatry. *Biol. Psychiatry* **2017**, *81*, e35–e37. [CrossRef]
152. Vuong, H.E.; Hsiao, E.Y. Emerging Roles for the Gut Microbiome in Autism Spectrum Disorder. *Biol. Psychiatry* **2017**, *81*, 411–423. [CrossRef] [PubMed]
153. Costello, E.K.; Stagaman, K.; Dethlefsen, L.; Bohannan, B.J.; Relman, D.A. The application of ecological theory toward an understanding of the human microbiome. *Science* **2012**, *336*, 1255–1262. [CrossRef] [PubMed]
154. Ferretti, P.; Pasolli, E.; Tett, A.; Asnicar, F.; Gorfer, V.; Fedi, S.; Armanini, F.; Truong, D.T.; Manara, S.; Zolfo, M.; et al. Mother-to-Infant Microbial Transmission from Different Body Sites Shapes the Developing Infant Gut Microbiome. *Cell Host Microbe* **2018**, *24*, 133–145.e5. [CrossRef] [PubMed]
155. Francino, M.P. Early development of the gut microbiota and immune health. *Pathogens* **2014**, *3*, 769–790. [CrossRef] [PubMed]
156. Borre, Y.E.; O'Keeffe, G.W.; Clarke, G.; Stanton, C.; Dinan, T.G.; Cryan, J.F. Microbiota and neurodevelopmental windows: Implications for brain disorders. *Trends Mol. Med.* **2014**, *20*, 509–518. [CrossRef]
157. Erny, D.; Hrabě Macfabe, D.F.; Short-chain, A.L.; Jaitin, D.; Wieghofer, P.; Staszewski, O.; David, E.; Keren-Shaul, H.; Mahlakoiv, T.; Jakobshagen, K.; et al. Host microbiota constantly control maturation and function of microglia in the CNS. *Nat. Neurosci.* **2015**, *18*, 965–977. [CrossRef]
158. Saresella, M.; Piancone, F.; Marventano, I.; Zoppis, M.; Hernis, A.; Zanette, M.; Trabattoni, D.; Chiappedi, M.; Ghezzo, A.; Canevini, M.P.; et al. Multiple inflammasome complexes are activated in autistic spectrum disorders. *Brain Behav. Immun.* **2016**, *57*, 125–133. [CrossRef]
159. Finegold, S.M.; Molitoris, D.; Song, Y.; Liu, C.; Vaisanen, M.L.; Bolte, E.; McTeague, M.; Sandler, R.; Wexler, H.; Marlowe, E.M.; et al. Gastrointestinal microflora studies in late-onset autism. *Clin. Infect. Dis.* **2002**, *35*, S6–S16. [CrossRef]
160. Macfabe, D.F. Short-chain fatty acid fermentation products of the gut microbiome: Implications in autism spectrum disorders. *Microb. Ecol. Health Dis.* **2012**, *23*. [CrossRef]
161. De Angelis, M.; Piccolo, M.; Vannini, L.; Siragusa, S.; De Giacomo, A.; Serrazzanetti, D.I.; Cristofori, F.; Guerzoni, M.E.; Gobbetti, M.; Francavilla, R. Fecal microbiota and metabolome of children with autism and pervasive developmental disorder not otherwise specified. *PLoS ONE* **2013**, *8*, e76993. [CrossRef]
162. Fasano, A. Leaky gut and autoimmune diseases. *Clin. Rev. Allergy Immunol.* **2012**, *42*, 71–78. [CrossRef] [PubMed]
163. Hsiao, E.Y.; McBride, S.W.; Hsien, S.; Sharon, G.; Hyde, E.R.; McCue, T.; Codelli, J.A.; Chow, J.; Reisman, S.E.; Petrosino, J.F.; et al. Microbiota modulate behavioral and physiological abnormalities associated with neurodevelopmental disorders. *Cell* **2013**, *155*, 1451–1463. [CrossRef] [PubMed]
164. Carey, N.; La Thangue, N.B. Histone deacetylase inhibitors: Gathering pace. *Curr. Opin. Pharmacol.* **2006**, *6*, 369–375. [CrossRef] [PubMed]
165. Lanza, M.; Campolo, M.; Casili, G.; Filippone, A.; Paterniti, I.; Cuzzocrea, S.; Esposito, E. Sodium butyrate exerts neuroprotective effects in spinal cord injury. *Mol. Neurobiol.* **2019**, *56*, 3937–3947. [CrossRef]
166. Kratsman, N.; Getselter, D.; Elliott, E. Sodium butyrate attenuates social behavior deficits and modifies the transcription of inhibitory/excitatory genes in the frontal cortex of an autism model. *Neuropharmacology* **2016**, *102*, 136–145. [CrossRef]
167. Hong, J.; Jia, Y.; Pan, S.; Jia, L.; Li, H.; Han, Z.; Cai, D.; Zhao, R. Butyrate alleviates high fat diet-induced obesity through activation of adiponectin-mediated pathway and stimulation of mitochon- drial function in the skeletal muscle of mice. *Oncotarget* **2016**, *7*, 56071–56082. [CrossRef]
168. Liu, S.; Li, E.; Sun, Z.; Fu, D.; Duan, G.; Jiang, M.; Yu, Y.; Mei, L.; Yang, P.; Tang, Y.; et al. Altered gut microbiota and short chain fatty acids in Chinese children with autism spectrum disorder. *Sci. Rep.* **2019**, *9*, 287. [CrossRef]
169. Rose, S.; Bennuri, S.C.; Davis, J.E.; Wynne, R.; Slattery, J.C.; Tippett, M.; Delhey, L.; Melnyk, S.; Kahler, S.G.; MacFabe, D.F.; et al. Butyrate enhances mitochondrial function during oxidative stress in cell lines from boys with autism. *Transl. Psychiatry* **2018**, *8*, 42. [CrossRef]
170. Kaur, H.; Singh, Y.; Singh, S.; Singh, R.B. Gut microbiome mediated epigenetic regulation of brain disorder and application of machine learning for multi-omics data analysis. *Genome* **2020**. [CrossRef]
171. Sadeghiyeh, T.; Dastgheib, S.A.; Mirzaee-Khoramabadi, K.; Morovati-Sharifabad, M.; Akbarian-Bafghi, M.J.; Poursharif, Z.; Mirjalili, S.R.; Neamatzadeh, H. Association of MTHFR 677C>T and 1298A>C polymorphisms with susceptibility to autism: A systematic review and meta-analysis. *Asian J. Psychiatr.* **2019**, *46*, 54–61. [CrossRef]
172. Cryan, J.F.; Dinan, T.G. Mind-altering microorganisms: The impact of the gut microbiota on brain and behaviour. *Nat. Rev. Neurosci.* **2012**, *13*, 701–712. [CrossRef] [PubMed]
173. MacFabe, D.F.; Cain, N.E.; Boon, F.; Ossenkopp, K.P.; Cain, D.P. Effects of the enteric bacterial metabolic product propionic acid on object-directed behavior, social behavior, cognition, and neuroinflammation in adolescent rats: Relevance to autism spectrum disorder. *Behav. Brain Res.* **2011**, *217*, 47–54. [CrossRef] [PubMed]
174. Strati, F.; Cavalieri, D.; Albanese, D.; De Felice, C.; Donati, C.; Hayek, J.; Jousson, O.; Leoncini, S.; Renzi, D.; Calabrò, A.; et al. New evidences on the altered gut microbiota in autism spectrum disorders. *Microbiome* **2017**, *5*, 24. [CrossRef] [PubMed]
175. Ding, H.T.; Taur, Y.; Walkup, J.T. Gut Microbiota and Autism: Key Concepts and Findings. *J. Autism Dev. Disord.* **2017**, *47*, 480–489. [CrossRef]
176. de Magistris, L.; Familiari, V.; Pascotto, A.; Sapone, A.; Frolli, A.; Iardino, P.; Carteni, M.; De Rosa, M.; Francavilla, R.; Riegler, G.; et al. Alterations of the intestinal barrier in patients with autism spectrum disorders and in their first-degree relatives. *J. Pediatr. Gastroenterol. Nutr.* **2010**, *51*, 418–424. [CrossRef]

177. Fasano, A. Zonulin and its regulation of intestinal barrier function: The biological door to inflammation, autoimmunity, and cancer. *Physiol. Rev.* **2011**, *91*, 151–175. [CrossRef]
178. Fasano, A.; Hill, I. Serum Zonulin, Gut Permeability, and the Pathogenesis of Autism Spectrum Disorders: Cause, Effect, or an Epiphenomenon? *J. Pediatr.* **2017**, *188*, 15–17. [CrossRef]
179. Kushak, R.I.; Buie, T.M.; Murray, K.F.; Newburg, D.S.; Chen, C.; Nestoridi, E.; Winter, H.S. Evaluation of Intestinal Function in Children with Autism and Gastrointestinal Symptoms. *J. Pediatr. Gastroenterol. Nutr.* **2016**, *62*, 687–691. [CrossRef]
180. Babinská, K.; Tomova, A.; Celušáková, H.; Babková, J.; Repiská, G.; Kubranská, A.; Filčíková, D.; Siklenková, L.; Ostatníková, D. Fecal calprotectin levels correlate with main domains of the autism diagnostic interview-revised (ADI-R) in a sample of individuals with autism spectrum disorders from Slovakia. *Physiol. Res.* **2017**, *66*, S517–S522. [CrossRef]
181. Nikolov, R.N.; Bearss, K.E.; Lettinga, J.; Erickson, C.; Rodowski, M.; Aman, M.G.; McCracken, J.T.; McDougle, C.J.; Tierney, E.; Vitiello, B.; et al. Gastrointestinal symptoms in a sample of children with pervasive developmental disorders. *J. Autism Dev. Disord.* **2009**, *39*, 405–413. [CrossRef]
182. Buie, T.; Campbell, D.B.; Fuchs, G.J., 3rd; Furuta, G.T.; Levy, J.; Vandewater, J.; Whitaker, A.H.; Atkins, D.; Bauman, M.L.; Beaudet, A.L.; et al. Evaluation, diagnosis, and treatment of gastrointestinal disorders in individuals with ASDs: A consensus report. *Pediatrics* **2010**, *125*, S1–S18. [CrossRef] [PubMed]
183. Keller, R.; Chieregato, S.; Bari, S.; Castaldo, R.; Rutto, F.; Chiocchetti, A.; Dianzani, U. Autism in Adulthood: Clinical and Demographic Characteristics of a Cohort of Five Hundred Persons with Autism Analyzed by a Novel Multistep Network Model. *Brain Sci.* **2020**, *10*, 416. [CrossRef]
184. Adams, J.B.; Johansen, L.J.; Powell, L.D.; Quig, D.; Rubin, R.A. Gastrointestinal flora and gastrointestinal status in children with autism–comparisons to typical children and correlation with autism severity. *BMC Gastroenterol.* **2011**, *11*, 22. [CrossRef] [PubMed]
185. Whitney, D.G.; Shapiro, D.N. National Prevalence of Pain among Children and Adolescents with Autism Spectrum Disorders. *JAMA Pediatr.* **2019**, *173*, 1203–1205. [CrossRef] [PubMed]
186. Iwata, B.A.; Deleon, I.G.; Roscoe, E.M. Reliability and validity of the functional analysis screening tool. *J. Appl. Behav. Anal.* **2013**, *46*, 271–284. [CrossRef] [PubMed]
187. Frye, R.E.; Rossignol, D.A. Identification and Treatment of Pathophysiological Comorbidities of Autism Spectrum Disorder to Achieve Optimal Outcomes. *Clin. Med. Insights Pediatr.* **2016**, *10*, 43–56. [CrossRef] [PubMed]
188. Guinchat, V.; Cravero, C.; Lefèvre-Utile, J.; Cohen, D. Multidisciplinary treatment plan for challenging behaviors in neurodevelopmental disorders. *Handb. Clin. Neurol.* **2020**, *174*, 301–321. [CrossRef]
189. Keller, R.; Basta, R.; Salerno, L.; Elia, M. Autism, epilepsy, and synaptopathies: A not rare association. *Neurol. Sci.* **2017**, *38*, 1353–1361. [CrossRef]
190. Mouridsen, S.E.; Rich, B.; Isager, T. A longitudinal study of epilepsy and other central nervous system diseases in individuals with and without a history of infantile autism. *Brain Dev.* **2011**, *33*, 361–366. [CrossRef]
191. Berg, A.T.; Plioplys, S. Epilepsy and autism: Is there a special relationship? *Epilepsy Behav.* **2012**, *23*, 193–198. [CrossRef]
192. Theoharides, T.C.; Zhang, B. Neuro-inflammation, blood-brain barrier, seizures and autism. *J. Neuroinflamm.* **2011**, *8*, 168. [CrossRef] [PubMed]
193. Valenti, D.; Lidia de Bari, L.; Bianca De Filippis, B.; Alexandra Henrion-Caude, A.; Vacca, R.A. Mitochondrial dysfunction as a central actor in intellectual disability-related diseases: An overview of Down syndrome, autism, Fragile X and Rett syndrome. *Neurosci. Biobehav. Rev.* **2014**, *46*, 202–217. [CrossRef] [PubMed]
194. Chandel, N.S. Mitochondria as signaling organelles. *BMC Biol.* **2014**, *12*, 34. [CrossRef] [PubMed]
195. Khacho, M.; Slack, R.S. Mitochondrial and Reactive Oxygen Species Signaling Coordinate Stem Cell Fate Decisions and Life Long Maintenance. *Antioxid. Redox Signal.* **2018**, *28*, 1090–1101. [CrossRef]
196. Bahat, A.; Gross, A. Mitochondrial plasticity in cell fate regulation. *J. Biol. Chem.* **2019**, *294*, 13852–13863. [CrossRef] [PubMed]
197. Wright, R.H.; Fernandez-Fuentes, N.; Oliva, B.; Beato, M. Insight into the machinery that oils chromatin dynamics. *Nucleus* **2016**, *7*, 532–539. [CrossRef]
198. Khacho, M.; Harris, R.; Slack, R.S. Mitochondria as central regulators of neural stem cell fate and cognitive function. *Nat. Rev. Neurosci.* **2019**, *20*, 34–48. [CrossRef]
199. Mandò, C.; Anelli, G.M.; Novielli, C.; Panina-Bordignon, P.; Massari, M.; Mazzocco, M.I.; Cetin, I. Impact of Obesity and Hyperglycemia on Placental Mitochondria. *Oxid. Med. Cell. Longev.* **2018**, *2018*, 2378189. [CrossRef] [PubMed]
200. Farrell, A.; Alahari, S.; Ermini, L.; Tagliaferro, A.; Litvack, M.; Post, M.; Caniggia, I. Faulty oxygen sensing disrupts angiomotin function in trophoblast cell migration and predisposes to preeclampsia. *JCI Insight* **2019**, *4*, e127009. [CrossRef] [PubMed]
201. Figueiredo, A.S.; Schumacher, A. The T helper type 17/regulatory T cell paradigm in pregnancy. *Immunology* **2016**, *148*, 13–21. [CrossRef] [PubMed]
202. Wang, S.; Qian, J.; Sun, F.; Li, M.; Ye, J.; Li, M.; Du, M.; Li, D. Bidirectional regulation between 1st trimester HTR8/SVneo trophoblast cells and in vitro differentiated Th17/Treg cells suggest a fetal-maternal regulatory loop in human pregnancy. *Am. J. Reprod. Immunol.* **2019**, *81*, e13106. [CrossRef] [PubMed]
203. Rose, S.; Niyazov, D.M.; Rossignol, D.A.; Goldenthal, M.; Kahler, S.G.; Frye, R.E. Clinical and Molecular Characteristics of Mitochondrial Dysfunction in Autism Spectrum Disorder. *Mol. Diagn. Ther.* **2018**, *22*, 571–593. [CrossRef] [PubMed]

204. Zorov, D.B.; Filburn, C.R.; Klotz, L.O.; Zweier, J.L.; Sollott, S.J. Reactive oxygen species (ROS)-induced ROS release: A new phenomenon accompanying induction of the mitochondrial permeability transition in cardiac myocytes. *J. Exp. Med.* **2000**, *192*, 1001–1014. [CrossRef] [PubMed]
205. Tschopp, J.; Schroder, K. NLRP3 inflammasome activation: The convergence of multiple signalling pathways on ROS production? *Nat. Rev. Immunol.* **2010**, *10*, 210–215. [CrossRef]
206. Engin, A. Endothelial Dysfunction in Obesity. *Adv. Exp. Med. Biol.* **2017**, *960*, 345–379. [CrossRef]
207. Newsholme, P.; Cruzat, V.F.; Keane, K.N.; Carlessi, R.; Homem de Bittencourt, P.I., Jr. Molecular mechanisms of ROS production and oxidative stress in diabetes. *Biochem. J.* **2016**, *473*, 4527–4550. [CrossRef]
208. Jomova, K.; Jenisova, Z.; Feszterova, M.; Baros, S.; Liska, J.; Hudecova, D.; Rhodes, C.J.; Valko, M. Arsenic: Toxicity, oxidative stress and human disease. *J. Appl. Toxicol.* **2011**, *31*, 95–107. [CrossRef]
209. Meyer, U. Developmental neuroinflammation and schizophrenia. *Prog. Neuropsychopharmacol. Biol. Psychiatry* **2013**, *42*, 20–34. [CrossRef] [PubMed]
210. Rossignol, D.A.; Frye, R.E. A review of research trends in physiological abnormalities in autism spectrum disorders: Immune dysregulation, inflammation, oxidative stress, mitochondrial dysfunction and environmental toxicant exposures. *Mol. Psychiatry* **2012**, *17*, 389–401. [CrossRef]
211. Rossignol, D.A.; Frye, R.E. Mitochondrial dysfunction in autism spectrum disorders: A systematic review and meta-analysis. *Mol. Psychiatry* **2012**, *17*, 290–314. [CrossRef]
212. Walker, S.J.; Langefeld, C.D.; Zimmerman, K.; Schwartz, M.Z.; Krigsman, A. A molecular biomarker for prediction of clinical outcome in children with ASD, constipation, and intestinal inflammation. *Sci. Rep.* **2019**, *9*, 5987. [CrossRef]
213. Rose, S.; Bennuri, S.C.; Murray, K.F.; Buie, T.; Winter, H.; Frye, R.E. Mitochondrial dysfunction in the gastrointestinal mucosa of children with autism: A blinded case-control study. *PLoS ONE* **2017**, *12*, e0186377. [CrossRef]
214. Vacca, R.A.; Bawari, S.; Valenti, D.; Tewari, D.; Nabavi, S.F.; Shirooie, S.; Sah, A.N.; Volpicella, M.; Braidy, N.; Nabavi, S.M. Down syndrome: Neurobiological alterations and therapeutic targets. *Neurosci. Biobehav. Rev.* **2019**, *98*, 234–255. [CrossRef] [PubMed]
215. Frye, R.E. Biomarker of abnormal energy metabolism in children with autism spectrum disorder. *N. Am. J. Med. Sci.* **2012**, *5*, 141–147. [CrossRef]
216. El-Ansary, A.K.; Bacha, A.G.; Al-Ayahdi, L.Y. Plasma fatty acids as diagnostic markers in autistic patients from Saudi Arabia. *Lipids Health Dis.* **2011**, *10*, 62. [CrossRef] [PubMed]
217. Mostafa, G.A.; El-Gamal, H.A.; El-Wakkad, A.S.E.; El-Shorbagy, O.E.; Hamza, M.M. Polyunsaturated fatty acids, carnitine and lactate as biological markers of brain energy in autistic children. *Int. J. Child Neuropsychiatry* **2005**, *2*, 179–188.
218. Frye, R.E.; Melnyk, S.; Macfabe, D.F. Unique acyl-carnitine profiles are potential biomarkers for acquired mitochondrial disease in autism spectrum disorder. *Transl. Psychiatry* **2013**, *3*, e220. [CrossRef] [PubMed]
219. MacFabe, D.F.; Cain, D.P.; Rodriguez-Capote, K.; Franklin, A.E.; Hoffman, J.E.; Boon, F.; Taylor, A.R.; Kavaliers, M.; Ossenkopp, K.P. Neurobiological effects of intraventricular propionic acid in rats: Possible role of short chain fatty acids on the pathogenesis and characteristics of autism spectrum disorders. *Behav. Brain Res.* **2007**, *176*, 149–169. [CrossRef]
220. Foley, K.A.; MacFabe, D.F.; Kavaliers, M.; Ossenkopp, K.P. Sexually dimorphic effects of prenatal exposure to lipopolysaccharide, and prenatal and postnatal exposure to propionic acid, on acoustic startle response and prepulse inhibition in adolescent rats: Relevance to autism spectrum disorders. *Behav. Brain Res.* **2015**, *278*, 244–256. [CrossRef] [PubMed]
221. Frye, R.E.; Delatorre, R.; Taylor, H.; Slattery, J.; Melnyk, S.; Chowdhury, N.; James, S.J. Redox metabolism abnormalities in autistic children associated with mitochondrial disease. *Transl. Psychiatry* **2013**, *3*, e273. [CrossRef]
222. Frye, R.E.; Rose, S.; Slattery, J.; MacFabe, D.F. Gastrointestinal dysfunction in autism spectrum disorder: The role of the mitochondria and the enteric microbiome. *Microb. Ecol. Health Dis.* **2015**, *26*, 27458. [CrossRef] [PubMed]
223. Amiot, A.; Tchikviladzé, M.; Joly, F.; Slama, A.; Hatem, D.C.; Jardel, C.; Messing, B.; Lombès, A. Frequency of mitochondrial defects in patients with chronic intestinal pseudo-obstruction. *Gastroenterology* **2009**, *137*, 101–109. [CrossRef] [PubMed]
224. Rossignol, D.A.; Genuis, S.J.; Frye, R.E. Environmental toxicants and autism spectrum disorders: A systematic review. *Transl. Psychiatry* **2014**, *4*, e360. [CrossRef] [PubMed]
225. Parker, W.; Hornik, C.D.; Bilbo, S.; Holzknecht, Z.E.; Gentry, L.; Rao, R.; Lin, S.S.; Herbert, M.R.; Nevison, C.D. The role of oxidative stress, inflammation and acetaminophen exposure from birth to early childhood in the induction of autism. *J. Int. Med. Res.* **2017**, *45*, 407–438. [CrossRef]
226. Atladóttir, H.Ó.; Henriksen, T.B.; Schendel, D.E.; Partner, E.T. Autism after infection, febrile episodes, and antibiotic use during pregnancy: An exploratory study. *Pediatrics* **2012**, *130*, e1447–e1454. [CrossRef]
227. Fallon, J. Could one of the most widely prescribed antibiotics amoxicillin/clavulanate "augmentin" be a risk factor for autism? *Med. Hypotheses* **2005**, *64*, 312–315. [CrossRef]
228. Kalghatgi, S.; Spina, C.S.; Costello, J.C.; Liesa, M.; Morones-Ramirez, J.R.; Slomovic, S.; Molina, A.; Shirihai, O.S.; Collins, J.J. Bactericidal antibiotics induce mitochondrial dysfunction and oxidative damage in Mammalian cells. *Sci. Transl. Med.* **2013**, *5*, 192ra85. [CrossRef]
229. Mezzelani, A.; Landini, M.; Facchiano, F.; Raggi, M.E.; Villa, L.; Molteni, M.; De Santis, B.; Brera, C.; Caroli, A.M.; Milanesi, L.; et al. Environment, dysbiosis, immunity and sex-specific susceptibility: A translational hypothesis for regressive autism pathogenesis. *Nutr. Neurosci.* **2015**, *18*, 145–161. [CrossRef]

230. Good, P. Evidence the U.S. autism epidemic initiated by acetaminophen (Tylenol) is aggravated by oral antibiotic amoxicillin/clavulanate (Augmentin) and now exponentially by herbicide glyphosate (Roundup). *Clin. Nutr. Espen* **2018**, *23*, 171–183. [CrossRef]
231. Bullón, P.; Román-Malo, L.; Marín-Aguilar, F.; Alvarez-Suarez, J.M.; Giampieri, F.; Battino, M.; Cordero, M.D. Lipophilic antioxidants prevent lipopolysaccharide-induced mitochondrial dysfunction through mitochondrial biogenesis improvement. *Pharmacol. Res.* **2015**, *91*, 1–8. [CrossRef]
232. Hsiao, E.Y. Gastrointestinal issues in autism spectrum disorder. *Harv. Rev. Psychiatry* **2014**, *22*, 104–111. [CrossRef]
233. Abdelli, L.S.; Samsam, A.; Naser, S.A. Propionic Acid Induces Gliosis and Neuro-inflammation through Modulation of PTEN/AKT Pathway in Autism Spectrum Disorder. *Sci. Rep.* **2019**, *9*, 8824. [CrossRef] [PubMed]
234. Harayama, T.; Riezman, H. Understanding the diversity of membrane lipid composition. *Nat. Rev. Mol. Cell Biol.* **2018**, *19*, 281–296. [CrossRef] [PubMed]
235. Ghezzo, A.; Visconti, P.; Abruzzo, P.M.; Bolotta, A.; Ferreri, C.; Gobbi, G.; Malisardi, G.; Manfredini, S.; Marini, M.; Nanetti, L.; et al. Oxidative Stress and Erythrocyte Membrane Alterations in Children with Autism: Correlation with Clinical Features. *PLoS ONE* **2013**, *8*, e66418. [CrossRef]
236. Ferreri, C.; Masi, A.; Sansone, A.; Giacometti, G.; Larocca, A.V.; Menounou, G.; Scanferlato, R.; Tortorella, S.; Rota, D.; Conti, M.; et al. Fatty Acids in Membranes as Homeostatic, Metabolic and Nutritional Biomarkers: Recent Advancements in Analytics and Diagnostics. *Diagnostics* **2017**, *7*, 1. [CrossRef] [PubMed]
237. Giacometti, G.; Ferreri, C.; Sansone, A.; Chatgilialoglu, C.; Marzetti, C.; Spyratou, E.; Georgakilas, G.A.; Marini, M.; Abruzzo, P.M.; Bolotta, A.; et al. High predictive values of RBC membrane-based diagnostics by biophotonics in an integrated approach for Autism Spectrum Disorders. *Sci. Rep.* **2017**, *7*, 9854. [CrossRef] [PubMed]
238. Bolotta, A.; Battistelli, M.; Falcieri, E.; Ghezzo, A.; Manara, M.C.; Manfredini, S.; Marini, M.; Posar, A.; Visconti, P.; Abruzzo, P.M. Oxidative Stress in Autistic Children Alters Erythrocyte Shape in the Absence of Quantitative Protein Alterations and of Loss of Membrane Phospholipid Asymmetry. *Oxid. Med. Cell Longev.* **2018**, *2018*, 6430601. [CrossRef]
239. Anwar, A.; Abruzzo, P.M.; Pasha, S.; Rajpoot, K.; Bolotta, A.; Ghezzo, A.; Marini, M.; Posar, A.; Visconti, P.; Thornalley, P.J.; et al. Advanced glycation endproducts, dityrosine and arginine transporter dysfunction in autism a source of biomarkers for clinical diagnosis. *Mol. Autism* **2018**, *9*, 3. [CrossRef]
240. Abruzzo, P.M.; Matté, A.; Bolotta, A.; Federti, E.; Ghezzo, A.; Guarnieri, T.; Marini, M.; Posar, A.; Siciliano, A.; De Franceschi, L.; et al. Plasma peroxiredoxin changes and inflammatory cytokines support the involvement of neuro-inflammation and oxidative stress in Autism Spectrum Disorder. *J. Transl. Med.* **2019**, *17*, 332. [CrossRef]
241. Angajala, A.; Lim, S.; Phillips, J.B.; Kim, J.H.; Yates, C.; You, Z.; Tan, M. Diverse Roles of Mitochondria in Immune Responses: Novel Insights Into Immuno-Metabolism. *Front. Immunol.* **2018**, *9*, 1605. [CrossRef]
242. Fanos, V.; Noto, A.; Mussap, M. The juniper bush of autism spectrum disorder (ASD): Metabolomics, microbiomics, acetaminophen. What else? *J. Pediatr. Neonat. Individual. Med.* **2018**, *7*, e070205. [CrossRef]
243. Hazlett, H.C.; Gu, H.; Munsell, B.C.; Kim, S.H.; Styner, M.; Wolff, J.J.; Elison, J.T.; Swanson, M.R.; Zhu, H.; Botteron, K.N.; et al. Early brain development in infants at high risk for autism spectrum disorder. *Nature* **2017**, *542*, 348–351. [CrossRef] [PubMed]
244. Zamboni, N.; Saghatelian, A.; Patti, G.J. Defining the metabolome: Size, flux, and regulation. *Mol. Cell.* **2015**, *58*, 699–706. [CrossRef] [PubMed]
245. Zampieri, M.; Sekar, K.; Zamboni, N.; Sauer, U. Frontiers of high-throughput metabolomics. *Curr. Opin. Chem. Biol.* **2017**, *36*, 15–23. [CrossRef]
246. Rajula, H.S.R.; Mauri, M.; Fanos, V. Scale-free networks in metabolomics. *Bioinformation* **2018**, *14*, 140–144. [CrossRef]
247. Elsabbagh, M.; Johnson, M.H. Getting answers from babies about autism. *Trends Cogn. Sci.* **2010**, *14*, 81–87. [CrossRef]
248. Estes, M.L.; McAllister, A.K. IMMUNOLOGY. Maternal TH17 cells take a toll on baby's brain. *Science* **2016**, *351*, 919–920. [CrossRef]
249. Manchia, M.; Fanos, V. Targeting aggression in severe mental illness: The predictive role of genetic, epigenetic, and metabolomic markers. *Prog. Neuropsychopharmacol. Biol. Psychiatry* **2017**, *77*, 32–41. [CrossRef]
250. Faa, G.; Manchia, M.; Pintus, R.; Gerosa, C.; Marcialis, M.A.; Fanos, V. Fetal programming of neuropsychiatric disorders. *Birth Defects Res. C Embryo Today.* **2016**, *108*, 207–223. [CrossRef]
251. Fanni, D.; Gerosa, C.; Rais, M.; Ravarino, A.; Van Eyken, P.; Fanos, V.; Faa, G. The role of neuropathological markers in the interpretation of neuropsychiatric disorders: Focus on fetal and perinatal programming. *Neurosci. Lett.* **2018**, *669*, 75–82. [CrossRef]
252. Hagenbeek, F.A.; Kluft, C.; Hankemeier, T.; Bartels, M.; Draisma, H.H.; Middeldorp, C.M.; Berger, R.; Noto, A.; Lussu, M.; Pool, R.; et al. Discovery of biochemical biomarkers for aggression: A role for metabolomics in psychiatry. *Am. J. Med. Genet. B Neuropsychiatr. Genet.* **2016**, *171*, 719–732. [CrossRef] [PubMed]
253. Mussap, M.; Noto, A.; Fanos, V. Metabolomics of autism spectrum disorders: Early insights regarding mammalian-microbial cometabolites. *Expert Rev. Mol. Diagn.* **2016**, *16*, 869–881. [CrossRef] [PubMed]
254. Bitar, T.; Mavel, S.; Emond, P.; Nadal-Desbarats, L.; Lefèvre, A.; Mattar, H.; Soufia, M.; Blasco, H.; Vourc'h, P.; Hleihel, W.; et al. Identification of metabolic pathway disturbances using multimodal metabolomics in autistic disorders in a Middle Eastern population. *J. Pharm. Biomed. Anal.* **2018**, *152*, 57–65. [CrossRef]

255. Noto, A.; Fanos, V.; Barberini, L.; Grapov, D.; Fattuoni, C.; Zaffanello, M.; Casanova, A.; Fenu, G.; De Giacomo, A.; De Angelis, M.; et al. The urinary metabolomics profile of an Italian autistic children population and their unaffected siblings. *J. Matern. Fetal Neonatal Med.* **2014**, *27*, 46–52. [CrossRef] [PubMed]
256. Lussu, M.; Noto, A.; Masili, A.; Rinaldi, A.C.; Dessì, A.; De Angelis, M.; De Giacomo, A.; Fanos, V.; Atzori, L.; Francavilla, R. The urinary 1 H-NMR metabolomics profile of an italian autistic children population and their unaffected siblings. *Autism Res.* **2017**, *10*, 1058–1066. [CrossRef]
257. Wang, J.; Barstein, J.; Ethridge, L.E.; Mosconi, M.W.; Takarae, Y.; Sweeney, J.A. Resting state EEG abnormalities in autism spectrum disorders. *J. Neurodev. Disord.* **2013**, *5*, 1–14. [CrossRef]
258. Belmonte, M.K.; Allen, G.; Beckel-Mitchener, A.; Boulanger, L.M.; Carper, R.A.; Webb, S.J. Autism and abnormal development of brain connectivity. *J. Neurosci.* **2004**, *24*, 9228–9231. [CrossRef]
259. Assaf, M.; Jagannathan, K.; Calhoun, V.D.; Miller, L.; Stevens, M.C.; Sahl, R.; O'Boyle, J.G.; Schultz, R.T.; Pearlson, G.D. Abnormal functional connectivity of default mode sub-networks in autism spectrum disorder patients. *Neuroimage* **2010**, *53*, 247–256. [CrossRef]
260. Minshew, N.J.; Keller, T.A. The nature of brain dysfunction in autism: Functional brain imaging studies. *Curr. Opin. Neurol.* **2010**, *23*, 124–130. [CrossRef]
261. Sato, J.R.; Calebe Vidal, M.; de Siqueira Santos, S.; Brauer Massirer, K.; Fujita, A. Complex Network Measures in Autism Spectrum Disorders. *IEEE/ACM Trans. Comput. Biol. Bioinform.* **2018**, *15*, 581–587. [CrossRef]
262. Nelson, C.A., 3rd. Introduction to special issue on The Role of Connectivity in Developmental Disorders: Genetic and Neural Network Approaches. *Dev. Sci.* **2016**, *19*, 523. [CrossRef] [PubMed]
263. Bosl, W.; Tierney, A.; Tager-Flusberg, H.; Nelson, C. EEG complexity as a biomarker for autism spectrum disorder risk. *BMC Med.* **2011**, *9*, 18. [CrossRef] [PubMed]
264. Hutsler, J.J.; Casanova, M.F. Review: Cortical construction in autism spectrum disorder: Columns; connectivity and the subplate. *Neuropathol. Appl. Neurobiol.* **2016**, *42*, 115–134. [CrossRef] [PubMed]
265. Buscema, M.; Vernieri, F.; Massini, G.; Scrascia, F.; Breda, M.; Rossini, P.M.; Grossi, E. An improved I-FAST system for the diagnosis of Alzheimer's disease from unprocessed electroencephalograms by using robust invariant features. *Artif. Intell. Med.* **2015**, *64*, 59–74. [CrossRef]
266. Grossi, E.; Olivieri, C.; Buscema, M. Diagnosis of autism through EEG processed by advanced computational algorithms: A pilot study. *Comput. Methods Programs Biomed.* **2017**, *142*, 73–79. [CrossRef]
267. Grossi, E.; Buscema, M.; Della Torre, F.; Swatzyna, R.J. The "MS-ROM/IFAST" Model, a Novel Parallel Nonlinear EEG Analysis Technique, Distinguishes ASD Subjects from Children Affected With Other Neuropsychiatric Disorders with High Degree of Accuracy. *Clin. EEG Neurosci.* **2019**, *50*, 319–331. [CrossRef]
268. Wahlqvist, M.L. Ecosystem Dependence of Healthy Localities, Food and People. *Ann. Nutr. Metab.* **2016**, *69*, 75–78. [CrossRef]
269. Godoy-Vitorino, F. Human microbial ecology and the rising new medicine. *Ann. Transl. Med.* **2019**, *7*, 342. [CrossRef]
270. Shedlock, K.; Susi, A.; Gorman, G.H.; Hisle-Gorman, E.; Erdie-Lalena, C.R.; Nylund, C.M. Autism Spectrum Disorders and Metabolic Complications of Obesity. *J. Pediatr.* **2016**, *178*, 183–187.e1. [CrossRef]
271. Penninx, B.W.J.H.; Lange, S.M.M. Metabolic syndrome in psychiatric patients: Overview, mechanisms, and implications. *Dialogues Clin. Neurosci.* **2018**, *20*, 63–73. [CrossRef]
272. Huke, V.; Turk, J.; Saeidi, S.; Kent, A.; Morgan, J.F. Autism spectrum disorders in eating disorder populations: A systematic review. *Eur. Eat. Disord. Rev.* **2013**, *21*, 345–351. [CrossRef] [PubMed]
273. Fahmie, T.A.; Iwata, B.A.; Jann, K.E. Comparison of edible and leisure reinforcers. *J. Appl. Behav. Anal.* **2015**, *48*, 331–343. [CrossRef] [PubMed]
274. Conlon, M.A.; Bird, A.R. The impact of diet and lifestyle on gut microbiota and human health. *Nutrients* **2014**, *7*, 17–44. [CrossRef] [PubMed]
275. Berding, K.; Donovan, S.M. Diet can impact microbiota composition in children with autism spectrum disorder. *Front. Neurosci.* **2018**, *12*, 515. [CrossRef] [PubMed]
276. Goldsmith, J.R.; Sartor, R.B. The role of diet on intestinal microbiota metabolism: Downstream impacts on host immune function and health, and therapeutic implications. *J. Gastroenterol.* **2014**, *49*, 785–798. [CrossRef] [PubMed]
277. Murphy, K.J.; Meyer, B.J.; Mori, T.A.; Burke, V.; Mansour, J.; Patch, C.S.; Tapsell, L.C.; Noakes, M.; Clifton, P.A.; Barden, A.; et al. Impact of foods enriched with n-3 long-chain polyunsaturated fatty acids on erythrocyte n-3 levels and cardiovascular risk factors. *Br. J. Nutr.* **2007**, *97*, 749–757. [CrossRef]

MDPI
St. Alban-Anlage 66
4052 Basel
Switzerland
Tel. +41 61 683 77 34
Fax +41 61 302 89 18
www.mdpi.com

Journal of Personalized Medicine Editorial Office
E-mail: jpm@mdpi.com
www.mdpi.com/journal/jpm

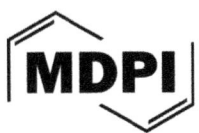

www.ingramcontent.com/pod-product-compliance
Lightning Source LLC
LaVergne TN
LVHW070656100526
838202LV00013B/977